PHASE II

ORTHODONTIC OCCLUSAL FINISHING
(RESEARCH PROJECT)

AREAS OF SKELETAL ANCHORAGE TOOTH MOVEMENT AREAS

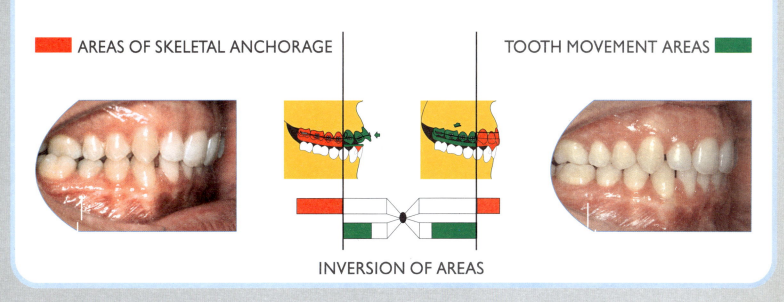

INVERSION OF AREAS

DENTAL ANCHORAGE TOOTH REQUIRING MOVING

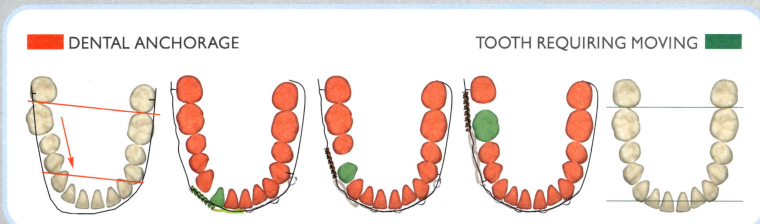

ANCHORAGE WITH MINI-SCREW IMPLANTS
Completing the anchorage stability options

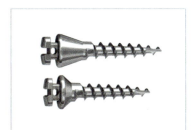 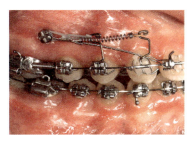 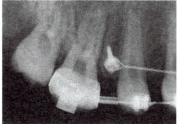

N.B. various anchorage types eliminate the need to rely on patients' compliance.

TREATING THE TRIAD:
TEETH, MUSCLES, TMJs

Giuseppe Cozzani

TREATING THE TRIAD

TEETH, MUSCLES, TMJs

Milan, Berlin, Chicago, Tokyo, Barcelona,
Istanbul, London, Moscow, New Delhi, Paris,
Peking, Prague, São Paulo, Seoul, Warsaw

Dr. Giuseppe Cozzani
MD, Specialist in Orthodontics
Authorized Private Clinic
Via Vailunga, 37- 19125 La Spezia, Italy
telephone: Studio: +39 0187 511088
             Courses +39 0187 510597
             Fax: +39 0187 515100
e-mail: segreteria@giuseppecozzani.it
http: www.giuseppecozzani.it

With the extraordinary assistance of:
Prof. Anthony A. Gianelly
   Chairman of the Department of Orthodontics – Henry M. Goldman
   School of Graduate Dentistry – Boston University
Dr. Fabio Ciuffolo
   D.D.S. – Ph.D – Specialist in Ortognathodontics,
   Private Practice in Pescara, Italy
Dr. Fabio Ferretti
   M.D. – Specialist in Odontostomatology & in Diagnostic Radiology –
   Advanced Studies in Orthodontics and Maxillo-facial Radiology
   – Private Practice in Livorno (Leghorn), Italy
   Operates at Leghorn Hospital Radiology Department
With the help of our staff:
Alberta Bombarda
Dr. Emanuele Crudo
Dr. Pietro Petroni
   Specialist in Orthognathodontics – Private Practice in Certaldo,
   Florence, Italy
Dr. Francesca Pastorelli
Andrea Bertelli (laboratory technician)
Rina Guidugli (for the outlines)
Barbara Rosellini (administration)
With the participation of:
Prof. Franco Mongini
   Director, Headache & Facial Pain Section, Department of
   Clinical Physiopathology, University of Turin, Italy
Prof. Piergiorgio Strata
   Scientific Director
   European Brain Research Institute
   Rita Levi Montalcini Foundation – Rome, Italy
Dr. Lorenzo Vanini
   Private Practice – San Fedele – Intelvi, Como, Italy
   Contract Professor of Reconstructive Dentistry –
   La Sapienza University – Rome, Italy

Dr. Franco Carlino
   Specialist in maxillo-facial surgery –
   Maxillo-facial Surgery Department II –
   Galeazzi Research Hospital (IRCCS) – Milan, Italy
Dr. Pier Francesco Carrara (Catania, Italy)
Dr.ssa Beatrice Caruso (Cagliari, Italy)
Dr. Giancarlo Coari (Orthopedic Specialist – La Spezia, Italy)
Prof. Felice Festa
   Chair of Orthognathodontics –
   Director of Orthognathodontics Specialization School –
   G. D'Annunzio University – Chieti, Italy
Prof. Gian Franco Franchi
   Professor, Advanced Technologies Postgraduate Courses –
   Universities of Florence & Pisa, Italy
Dr. Riccardo Giorgi (La Spezia, Italy)
Dr. Maria Paola Guarneri
   Research fellow – University of Ferrara, Italy
Dr. B. Giuliano Maino
   Contract Professor – University of Ferrara, Italy
Prof. Claudio Maioli
   Professor of Human Physiopathology – University of Brescia, Italy
Dr. Marialuisa Mandalà
   Director of Imagining Diagnostics Department
   – Main Hospital – Cannizzaro, Catania, Italy
Dr. Filippo Petroni
   (Specialist in Sports Medicine – Certaldo, Florence, Italy)
Dr. Paolo Ronchi
   Director of Maxillo-facial Surgery Department –
   S. Anna Main Hospital – Como, Italy
Prof. Giuseppe Siciliani
   Director of Orthognathodontics Specialization School –
   University of Ferrara
Prof. Maurizio Tonetti
   Director, European Research Group on Periodontology

Drawings & graphics: Maria Grazia Innocenti
Cover: Fabio Varini
3D images: Structura SAS, Ancona, Italy
             Radiology Centers: City Hospital, Leghorn, Italy
             (for MRI)
             DICRA – Massa Carrara, Italy (for CT scans)
             Fortis S.r.l. – Forte dei Marmi, Lucca, Italy

© 2011 Quintessenza Edizioni
Via Ciro Menotti, 65 - 20017 Rho, Milano (Italy)
www.quintessenzaedizioni.it

I dedicate this book to:

- *My mentor and friend Tony Gianelly*

- *My grandchildren, Michele, Filippo, and Jacopo*

- *The many instructors and pupils who for 40 years have given me the pleasure of listening and stimulating my mind with their many questions*

- *All young orthodontists, in the hope that they will not be distracted by technical simplification but instead reflect deeply on the individual characteristics of each patient during both diagnosis and treatment*

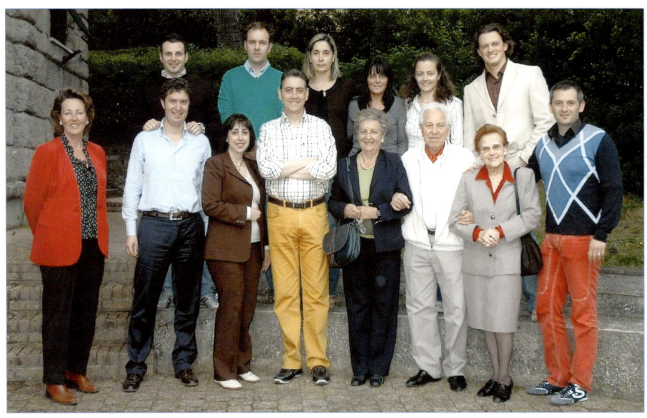

Our Staff

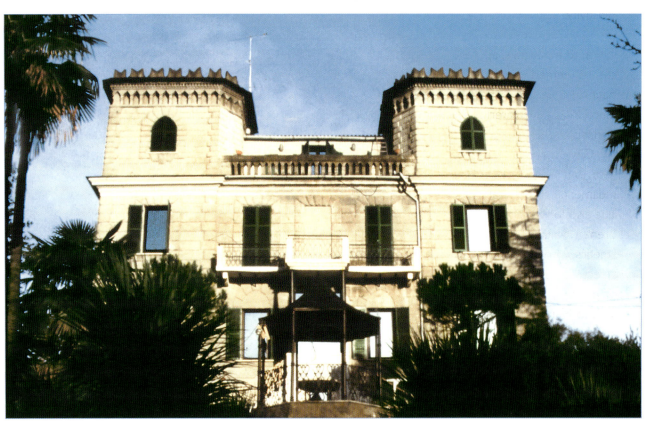

Villa Andreino

ACKNOWLEDGEMENTS

I wish to express my deepest gratitude to those who have walked alongside me at all stages of my long career:

- Tony Gianelly, for his incredible knowledge of the subject–a master at showing the way towards learning, a treasured friend who always found time to help me in whatever I asked, and a guide who would bring me back to the straight and narrow. I shall miss him;
- Fabio Ciuffolo, for his organization of the references, profound observations throughout the text, and assistance with the area of muscle pathology;
- Fabio Ferretti, for his never-failing help and profound knowledge of magnetic resonance, which have brought patient records to a level of rational objectivity.

In addition to my thanks, appreciation is owed to many for the esteemed level of their research on an international scale. These include:

- Franco Mongini, a forerunner and constant guide in diagnosis and therapy of musculoarticular disorders;
- Pier Giorgio Strata, whose research at the most prestigious levels of neuroscience has set forth fundamental theoretical and practical guidelines of value also for our specialty;
- Lorenzo Vanini, a champion of facial and smile esthetics, who never fails to support our search for a correct functional relationship between occlusion and posture;
- Giuliano Maino, who has integrated and fine-tuned orthodontic treatment with his "spider screw", of whose application he is a master;
- Maurizio Tonetti, whose love for periodontology is equalled only by his brilliance in teaching it. Our two specialties complement each other so well with many patients;
- Mario Martignoni, for his major contribution in integrating gnathology with the fundamental concepts of occlusal dynamics;
- Those great masters of dentistry and orthodontics who lectured on our courses in La Spezia: V. Alexander, A. Biaggi, J. Canut, N. Cetlin, C. Cugino, C. De Chiesa, Sir John Eccles (1963 Nobel Laureate in Medicine), T. Graeber, L. Johnston, R. Little, G. May, E. Muzi, M. Rosa, P. Stockli, P.K. Thomas, F. Toffenetti, F. Van der Linden, L. Wieslander, B. Zachrisson, Roth-Williams, among others.

Further thanks go to:

- Grazia Innocenti, for her unfailing interpretation of my ideas and creating the artwork illustrating them;
- Rina and Tosca, for a lifetime's generous unquestioning work;
- Pietro Petroni and Emanuele Crudo, who lend extraordinary care and impressive ability to the treatment of patients according to the new procedures of our Research Project;
- Alberta, for her uncommon efficiency and humanity;
- Andrea Bertelli, for his impeccable skill in the laboratory;
- Barbara, our good-natured and energetic secretary;
- Horst-Wolfgang Haase, extraordinary head of the Quintessence International Organization whose network has made it possible for me to publish my works in more languages than ever before;
- His team, especially Johannes Wolters and Juliane Richter, for their care with every detail.

THE BOOK

This book is dedicated to all those who take an interest in teeth, muscles, and temporomandibular joints and therefore all dentists who come into contact with other medical specialities, particularly in dealing with facial pain and postural problems.

BOOK SUMMARY

Contributions from:	25	prestigious contributors
Illustrations of:	50	patients with partial or complete documentation
New proposals:	23	pages dedicated entirely to color illustrations describing the underlying theories and related practical applications **(with a Graphic Summary on pages 92-93)**
	19	Considerations on specific subjects
Includes:	142	imaging diagnostics (CT-OPT-Tomograms-Cephalography)
	78	Magnetic Resonance Images
	101	3D mandibular translations (pre- and posttreatment)
	11	pages on diagnostic-therapeutic manipulation techniques
Presents:	272	drawings with color outlines
	12	3D virtual images predicting in detail Phase I musculoarticular rehabilitation,
Phase II		orthodontic occlusal finishing, and description of various splint types
	20	pages on splint fabrication laboratory techniques
	710	color photographs documenting treatment
Totals:	407	pages
	90	references cited

Innovative therapeutic proposals:
- In orthodontics: Research Project
- Anterior Repositioning Splint (ARS): adaptation "A"
  adaptation "B"

• Studies into:
- changes in condylar position following treatment
- the Invisalign method with dysfunctional patients
- dental and skeletal movements shown by cephalometry

FOREWORD

PRESENTATION of Prof. Anthony A. GIANELLY

This book is outstanding for a number of reasons. One is that it is an intelligent discussion of normal and abnormal temporomandibular joint (TMJ) function with superb diagrams, illustrations, and use of diagnostic criteria. A second is the large number of complete case reports of step-by-step procedures used to treat patients suffering from symptoms of pathology of teeth, muscles, and the TMJ.

A valuable inclusion is the descriptions of the various splints used in treatment, with clear indications of their use. In addition, the clinical management of the various splints, particularly the Anterior Repositioning Splint (ARS), is described and illustrated clearly and precisely.

The splints are also important components of the orthodontic treatment when finalization of occlusion is done by means of orthodontic treatment, both to stabilize mandibular position and control orthodontic movements.

The orthodontic treatment procedures are inventive and clearly illustrated and the results of the splint and orthodontic treatments are excellent both in terms of relief of symptomatology and final occlusal result.

Although the emphasis is on orthodontic treatment of temporomandibular disorder (TMD), surgical, prosthetic, and occlusal equilibration methods of treatment of patients with TMD are also included.

This book can be of benefit to all orthodontists and should be necessary reading for all orthodontists who treat TMD.

Prof. Anthony A. Gianelly, DMD, MD, PhD
Chairman of the Department of Orthodontics
Henry M. Goldman School of Graduate Dentistry,
Boston University

A PROFESSIONAL PROGRESSION:
From TEETH to MUSCLES to TMJ

Giuseppe Cozzani

When I started in my profession, I was fascinated by the world of orthodontics even though in those days it was based mainly on alignment of the TEETH.

It was not long before I realized that the MUSCLES also contributed. If we maintained normal muscle tone successful long-term results were obtained with the treatment; with muscle stress, pathology resulted.

Once treatment was completed it was often believed that the teeth had harmonized with the muscles, and no form of retention was applied.

To investigate the issue further, in 1968, my mentors, Prof Carnelutti and Prof Blasi, and I decided to conduct a study on 30 postorthodontic–treatment patients by fitting them with a stabilization splint to assess whether a dual bite persisted, ie, one with normal muscle tone, and therefore physiologic, and the other a maximum-intercuspation bite with muscle tension and therefore pathologic. The outcome, disappointingly, was that half the patients were in an unacceptable state. This was a significant experience in the development of our therapeutic postulations.

Towards the late 1970s, it became imperative to include consideration of the TMJs in order to complete an assessment of the stomatognathic apparatus and all its key components: TEETH, MUSCLES, and the TMJ. The literature was, and is, full of considerable discussion on diagnosis but relatively little on therapeutic proposals.

When William B. Farrar's inspirational ideas started to take hold in the early 1980s, it was clear that TMJ pathology needed to be addressed once and for all, by using an Anterior Repositioning Splint (ARS) based on Farrar's orthotic.

Magnetic resonance has recently added a further contribution by assisting with diagnosis and assessment of treatment outcome, by focusing less on centering the condyle within the fossa, but rather aiming for a dynamic concept of effective FUNCTION.

The ARS inspired by Farrar is essential to maintain correct musculoarticular position as established from the onset of treatment with PHASE I as a first procedure to relieve musculoarticular damage. The subsequent stage of orthodontic occlusal finishing, PHASE II, is proposed as a RESEARCH PROJECT based on differing types of anchorage (dental, skeletal, and temporary intraosseous mini-screws). These are potentially beneficial in all kinds of orthodontic treatment.

This book presents carefully weighed diagnostic approaches and related functional–recovery therapeutic procedures. While these may meet disagreement and criticism, it is hoped that they provide food for thought and discussion, without which no progress is ever made.

The illustrations and considerable clinical documentation occupy a large portion of the book in an attempt to assist in understanding the theoretic and practical solutions proposed.

William B. Farrar: ARS pioneer and his concepts

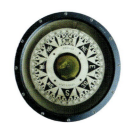

Treatment with the ARS, as pioneered by Dr Farrar, remains to this day the basis for recovery procedures. Time has been unable to alter his extraordinary insight and only has succeeded in helping it progress.

It seems a logical duty to pay tribute to the genius whose splint remains the best indicated therapeutic device to treat alterations to the musculoarticular structures.

Since the 1970s and 1980s, largely thanks to the many publications on the subject stemming from Dr Farrar[1-3], TMJ specialists became aware of a splint that advanced the mandible in order to treat TMJ dysfunction connected with:

- forms of condylodiscal dislocation;
- alterations to articular osseous extremities (internal derangement).

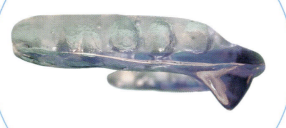

Disk repositioning

An anteriorly dislocated disk may be repositioned in approximately 30% of internal derangement cases, and the younger the patient and the lesser degree of initial reciprocal clicking, the higher the probability is of success. Repositioning with an ARS causes mandibular advance varying between 1.0 and 2.5 mm.

Unlocking

If the patient has TMJ lock due to total anterior discal dislocation, repositioning will take place following the appropriate unlocking maneuver and will be greater between 3.0 and 4.5 mm. Some weeks later the repositioning wedge/inclined plane is reduced by 1.5 to 2.0 mm from its original position, following the walk back procedure.

If discal dislocation is extreme

Farrar's principle was not to attempt recapture but instead to use a superior splint, which is a flat passive bite plane with incisal and canine rise. This splint could be used in order to treat dental occlusion while leaving the condylar position with its displaced disk, since the latter has shifted too far to be recaptured.

Occlusal finishing

After splint usage, Farrar goes on with extreme care to provide occlusal finishing, in order to establish a new intercuspation position in acceptable conditions of articular functionality.

THE TWO SCHOOLS OF THOUGHT

The ways in which the ARS is used differ considerably according to the authors concerned.

REVERSIBLE forms of treatment (WITHOUT FINISHING)	IRREVERSIBLE forms of treatment (WITH FINISHING)

REVERSIBLE forms of treatment (WITHOUT FINISHING)

Some authors do not endorse finishing and do not agree with the concept that ARS use must necessarily conclude as an irreversible form of treatment.

Those who do not secure the anteriorized position obtained with the ARS prefer to return the mandible to a position closer to or coinciding with the patient's original occlusion, by following a partial or total **walk-back procedure**.

ARS use is inconsistent. It may be worn **in terms of time** at night only or full-time, **and for periods lasting** from a few weeks to a few months. It is also variable in terms of space, going from a more anterior position in early treatment to a position closer to the patient's initial occlusion, which it reaches at the end of treatment.

Among these authors are:
- Williamson[4];
- Okeson[5];
- Solberg[6];
as well as many others, with whom they form the majority.

IRREVERSIBLE forms of treatment (WITH FINISHING)

Other authors apply a first phase of articular therapy and a second phase of occlusal finishing to adapt the occlusion to the new articular position obtained as a result of **assiduous ARS wear**, with the splint used night and day over a **longer period of time** (as much as 24-36 months).

The specialist responsible, must also aim to obtain anatomical and functional remodeling of the condyles, which will remain stable long-term precisely because they are supported by correct occlusion in harmony with the articular position.

Among the authors are:
- Eiji Tanaka[7].

The therapeutic protocols dealt with in the text with both PHASE I (musculoarticular recovery) and PHASE II (orthodontic occlusal finishing) are in line with the principle of IRREVERSIBLE ARTICULAR AND OCCLUSAL TREATMENT.

CONSIDERATIONS ON CHOOSING A SCHOOL OF THOUGHT: REVERSIBLE VERSUS IRREVERSIBLE

No matter the type of treatment planned, a clinician must always aim to achieve the best possible outcome. In the field of temporomandibular disorders (TMDs) there are many factors that may detract from an optimal solution, including the objective difficulty of the case, the patient's preference for a simpler and less expensive option, less-developed professional skill on the part of some operators, and others.

Conversely, it may occur that patient and clinician do not agree, with the clinician forced to refuse procedures which would damage the patient's ultimate wellbeing.

With these differing opinions, there is one major query: can severely damaged joints be treated with an acceptable lasting outcome?

The answer is unquestionably yes, provided that certain conditions of efficiency are met (see pages 160-161):

- Keep the condyle stable while away from the fossa, to permit rearrangement of the altered structures.
- Utilize long recovery times, unlike other joints of the body which are completely immobilized for only a matter of weeks. Immobilization is obviously impossible with TMD patients who need to be able to speak, eat, clean their teeth, and maintain a degree of social interaction.

It is therefore necessary to:

- Extend treatment for a greater number of months
- Continue to wear the ARS constantly for at least 20 to 22 hours per day in order to maintain the therapeutic position established at the start of treatment, both during the musculoarticular therapy and also during the subsequent orthodontic occlusal finishing (irreversible articular and occlusal treatments).

Having acknowledged these conditions as correct, the walk back procedure is no longer acceptable as it would involve abandoning the initial therapeutic position with a return – more or less – to the initial pathologic conditions.

It should be pointed out that an ARS (integrated as appropriate with other treatment such as medication, physiotherapy, counseling, etc) has wide-ranging effects and can provide the best possible rehabilitation of damaged musculoarticular structures.

Specifically it:

- relaxes the muscles, consequently relieving pain;
- places the condyle in the best therapeutic (not anatomical) functional position in relation to the fossa. In this context it is important to remember that condylar advance is not the only therapeutic direction since mandibular depression is also essential in correcting the relationships with a therapeutic position hardly ever in the center of the fossa but instead inferiorly and anteriorly (see clinical investigation on page 96 et seqq);
- helps restore axial alignment between condyle, disc/pseudodisc, and fossa;
- favors condylar head remodeling, thus also contributing to the best possible anatomical and functional compromise.

Although requiring commitment on the part of both doctor and patient, these choices can produce interesting results. When combined with necessary additional treatment such as surgery or prosthodontics, they allow the patient to recover a valid masticatory function.

PRELIMINARY OVERVIEW OF THE UNDERLYING PRINCIPLES AND CONSEQUENT CLINICAL IMPLICATIONS

PATHOLOGY

MUSCULOARTICULAR THERAPY
(to be applied as first-stage therapy,
with rare exceptions – see page 220)

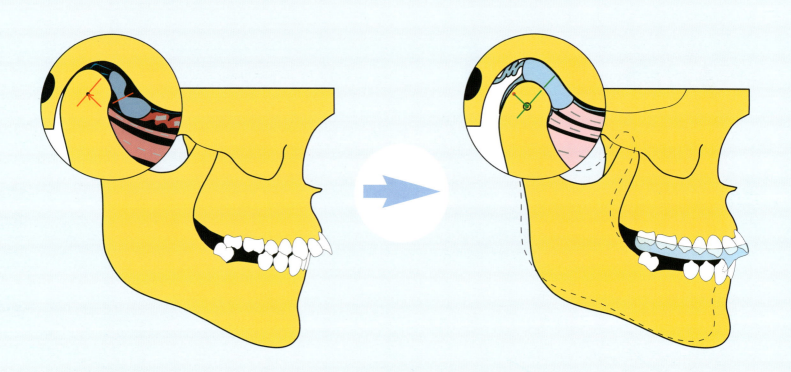

Normally, disk anteriorized and condyle posteriorized, with axial alignment lost: muscle tension and pain.

Recapture of disk/formation of pseudo disk as best as possible with ARS worn always; axial alignment restored with improvement in muscle tension hence relief of pain.

PHASE I: pages 85 through 202

PHASE II

ORTHODONTIC OCCLUSAL FINISHING:
RESEARCH PROJECT (to be applied, with rare
exceptions, as second-stage procedure)

OUTCOME:
EQUILIBRIUM

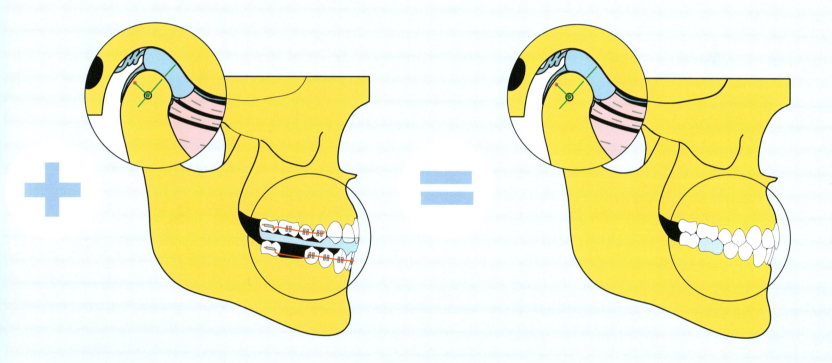

Dental rearrangement with orthodontics while
maintaining the splint.

FUNCTIONAL EFFICIENCY
between teeth, muscles and TMJ

PHASE II: pages 203 through 366

LIST OF CONSIDERATIONS

INDEX

CLINICAL APPROACH: LIST OF PATIENTS

We have listed all the patients illustrated in order to confirm the clinical approach of this book.

GENERAL TABLE OF CONTENTS   **page**

CHAPTER 1.   BASIC CONCEPTS

CHAPTER 2.   DIAGNOSIS: PATIENT RECORDS

CHAPTER 3.   Phase I: MUSCULOARTICULAR THERAPY

CHAPTER 4.   Phase II: ORTHODONTIC OCCLUSAL FINISHING

CHAPTER 5. CHILDREN AND TEMPOROMANDIBULAR DISORDERS

CHAPTER 6. INNOVATIVE ORTHODONTIC TREATMENT OF TEETH, MUSCLES AND TEMPOROMANDIBULAR DISORDERS

OVERVIEW

Edited by Prof Franco Mongini[8-10]

The etiologic factors and pathogenic mechanisms of headache, facial pain, and temporomandibular joint (TMJ) disorders and disorders affecting the craniocervicofacial musculature are subject to much controversy.

The reasons for lack of consensus are to be found in four main areas, which can be summarized as:

1. Differing etiologic factors may be found in the same patient.
2. When combined with differing pathogenic mechanisms, the same etiologic factors may involve joints and/or muscles thereby causing different and variable symptomatic profiles.
3. Problems originating from craniofacial structures may be complicated by superimposition of systemic factors.
4. Although the latter may be prevalent, they may be camouflaged as localized causes.

A further reason for perplexity lies in the still-common tendency to consider these pathologies as a single illness and consequently to lump them together under an umbrella term. The most frequently used is "craniomandibular disorders" while others currently found include "temporomandibular disorders", "TMJ pain dysfunction syndrome", "myofascial pain syndrome", etc.

As mentioned, a distinction may be made between local versus systemic etiologic factors.
The most important etiologic factors are:

1. Alterations to the jaw structures with mandibular dislocation when in maximum intercuspation
2. Neuromuscular alterations (parafunctions)
3. Altered posture of the head, neck and shoulders

The general or systemic factors which may complicate the situation are:

1. Hormone imbalance
2. Vascular alterations
3. Alterations to the central and/or peripheral nervous system
4. Psychologic disorders

It follows that patients with TMJ and/or muscle disorders may present one or more local factors, just as these factors may have greater or lesser relevance. Additionally, it must be ascertained what role, if any, is played by aggravating disorders, especially of a psychologic nature.

PRINCIPLES FOR DIAGNOSIS AND THERAPY

In order to avoid diagnostic errors it is essential that all relevant data be systematically collected and that no diagnosis should be made until the data is complete. Only an integrated, thoughtful analysis of findings from physical examination correlated as appropriate with test results can enable a correct profile of a patient suffering from headache or another form of dysfunction of the cranio–cervico–facial complex. Secondly, one must avoid the only-too-common trap of basing a diagnosis blindly on data from complex equipment such as electromyographs or electronic movement recorders, especially if the data is incorrectly or insufficiently interpreted through theories that have not been sufficiently confirmed from a scientific point of view.

The same is true for so-called "kinesiologic" tests, upon which decisions are sometimes made as to the suitability of an occlusal pattern for the patient and the relevance of this in identifying whether a pain syndrome actually originates in the head or elsewhere. It is easy to demonstrate that these tests almost always fail a blind study in which the operator has no prior knowledge of the situation being tested.

The testing protocol includes a clinical examination (inspection, palpation and auscultation of joint noise) with any recommended tests such as TMJ radiography and intraoral registration. However, if the clinical examination suggests myogenous pain where there is no sign of joint problems, there are reasonable grounds for omitting TMJ radiography. Intraoral registration is taken when a structural etiologic factor is suspected, with mandibular displacement in maximum intercuspation, and it is consequently likely that an orthopedic plate will be used for treatment.

Indicatively speaking, when formulating a diagnosis a fundamental distinction must be made between patients:
- Who present an essentially structural etiologic factor.
- Whose main etiologic factor is neuromuscular.
- In whom both factors are present.
- Who have etiologic factors of another type (segmental neurologic factors or systemic factors).
- In whom the latter factors are the only ones present or in any case are definitely prevailing.

While rather schematic, this distinction is of major importance for practical purposes. The responsibility of dental specialists is in fact to:
1. Ascertain the category to which the patient belongs;
2. Provide suitable treatment for the patients of the first three categories;
3. Coordinate treatment for patients from the fourth category with other specialists;
4. Send patients from the fifth category to other specialists, and refrain from any action which would alter the occlusion, at least for the time being.

PRINCIPLES FOR TREATMENT

Where there is discal dislocation without reduction, the dislocation must firstly be reduced. The patient will then be fitted with a retainer, physiotherapy, and/or exercises that will accelerate healing of the TMJ. If an intense parafunction is present, it will be useful to associate a cycle of biofeedback, relaxation exercises and if necessary a bland form of medication.

If the patient has a structural etiologic factor which has provoked discal dislocation with reduction, a plate will be applied in the therapeutic position established during the physical examination and perhaps confirmed with a bite registration.

Individuals whose sole or main problem is neuromuscular will be treated with local physiotherapy, biofeedback and appropriate medication if the disorder stems from clinical anxiety or depression. It should be remembered that in certain cases there may be a combination of two etiologic factors, both structural and neuromuscular, which together give rise to the pathology in question.

It is therefore important to assess whether the two factors have contributed in relatively equal measures to causing the patient's complaint, or whether one prevails over the other. For example, if a discal dislocation without reduction leads back to an evident structural factor, even though there may also be a neuromuscular component it will be necessary to proceed with reduction and fit an orthopedic plate to ensure that normal condylodiscal relationships are maintained, while simultaneously attempting to eliminate the neuromuscular factors.

Conversely, if the neuromuscular factor is more significant than the structural causes, and the articular lesion is not serious, priority should be given to removing the key causes of the disorder. Furthermore, a full-time plate should be avoided due to its excessive invasiveness and the consequent risk of aggravating the neuromuscular problem.

It is relatively common to find that local and systemic factors coexist, with the latter often in the form of a significant psychologic factor. The importance of detecting a psychologic component lies in the fact that treatment must be integrated with suitable means (pharmaceutical and other), which are not normally managed by a dental specialist.

A first screening of these patients can be done when recording patient history, according to the replies to a number of questions designed to detect disorders caused by anxiety, whether overt or somatised, or typical of depressive disorders. Where a high percentage of affirmative answers is noted in a patient also exhibiting local etiologic factors, treatment should be multifactorial from the start. Generally speaking, these patients should not be compelled to wear endoral plates, or wear them full-time, at least to begin with.

Where an orthopedic-acting plate is indicated on the grounds of a local structural factor, a flexible approach is recommended with the patient told to feel free to remove the plate whenever it were to accentuate his or her sense of discomfort or anxiety.

REFERENCES

1. Farrar WB. Differentiation of temporomandibular joint dysfunction to simplify treatment. J Prosthet Dent 1972;28:629–636.
2. Farrar WB. Disk derangement and dental occlusion: Changing concepts. Int J Periodontics Restorative Dent 1985;5:34–47
3. Farrar WB, McCarty WL Jr. A Clinical Outline of Temporomandibular Joint – Diagnosis and Treatment, Normandie Study Group for TMJ Dysfunction, 1983.
4. Williamson EH, Rosenzweig BJ. The treatment of temporomandibular disorders through repositioning splint therapy: A follow-up study. Cranio 1998;16:222–225.
5. Okeson JP. Il trattamento delle disfunzioni dell'occlusione e dei disordini temporomandibolari. 3^ ed. Bologna. Martina: 1993.
6. Solberg WK. Patologie Temporomandibolari, Ed. Scienza e Tecnica, 1991.
7. Tanaka E, Kikuchi K, Sasaki A, Tanne K. An adult case of TMJ osteoarthrosis treated with splint therapy and the subsequent orthodontic occlusal reconstruction: Adaptive change of the condyle during the treatment. Am J Orthod Dentofacial Orthop 2000;118:566–571.
8. Mongini F, Schmid W. Ortopedia Cranio Mandibolare e dell'ATM. Scienza e tecnica dentistica, Ed internaz. S.r.l. Milano, 1990.
9. Mongini F. ATM e muscolatura Cranio-cervico-facciale. Fisiopatologia e terapia. UTET, Torino, 1996.
10. Mongini F. Cefalee e Dolore Facciale. UTET, Torino, 1998.

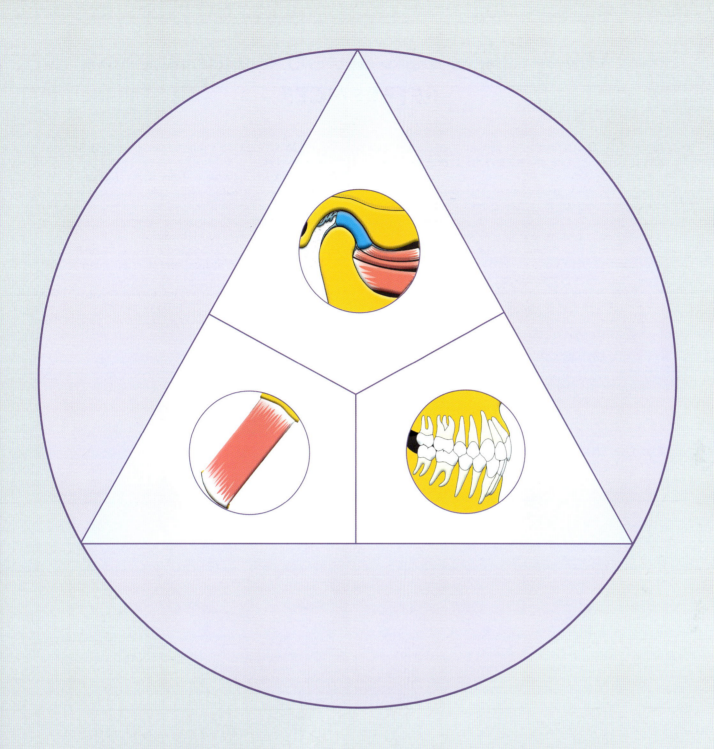

BASIC CONCEPTS

This chapter introduces the anatomy and physiopathology of the stomatognathic apparatus to aid readers' understanding of the philosophy behind the treatment of patients with temporomandibular disorders (TMDs). The chief components of the stomatognathic apparatus—teeth, muscles, and joints—are a set of functional subunits interacting as a whole under the control of the central nervous system. Proper individual diagnosis is essential to establishing an equally individual treatment plan, especially where irreversible procedures such as prosthodontics, surgery, and major orthodontic rehabilitation are contemplated—all of which will permanently affect the architecture of the stomatognathic apparatus.

FUNDAMENTALS

The guiding arch differs between traditional orthodontics (the mandible) and tooth, muscle, and joint disorders (the maxilla). Until recently, the mandible was—and often still is—considered the guiding arch except in patients suffering from dysfunctional problems. Today's orthodontists must move past the traditional guidelines when diagnosing and treating the stomatognathic apparatus. Precedence must be given the maxilla as the guiding arch where there is evidence of dual bite or, worse, signs of more serious musculoarticular pathology since the maxilla engages the anterior repositioning splint (ARS), which is commonly used as a key treatment aid (see page 145). Muscle-led closure must be systematically chosen at all stages of treatment. The therapeutic choice between dental closure (maximum intercuspation) and muscle-led closure (giving maximum function) must be made and maintained not only when starting treatment but also during every subsequent stage. Treatment causes changes that produce a series of new dual bites requiring correction. Maintaining muscle-led closure will cause the difference between closures to diminish further and further until it has disappeared altogether. At that point, the treatment goal is to adapt the teeth to the requirements of the muscles and joints (a fundamental aim of every dental specialty, including orthodontics), after which treatment may be concluded. (See page 46 onward.)

YESTERDAY...

FROM GNATHOLOGY:
THE SEARCH FOR CONDYLAR GEOMETRIC CENTERING
IN THE MANDIBULAR FOSSA

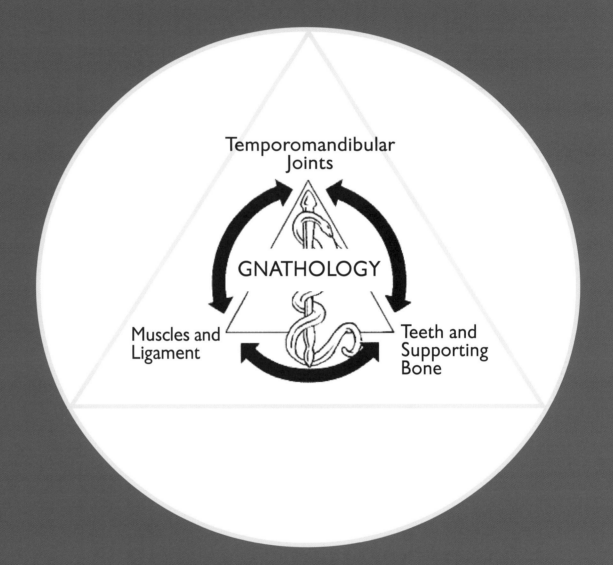

...TODAY

THE SEARCH FOR AXIAL ALIGNMENT BETWEEN CONDYLE, DISC, AND ARTICULAR SURFACE (FUNCTIONAL EFFICIENCY)

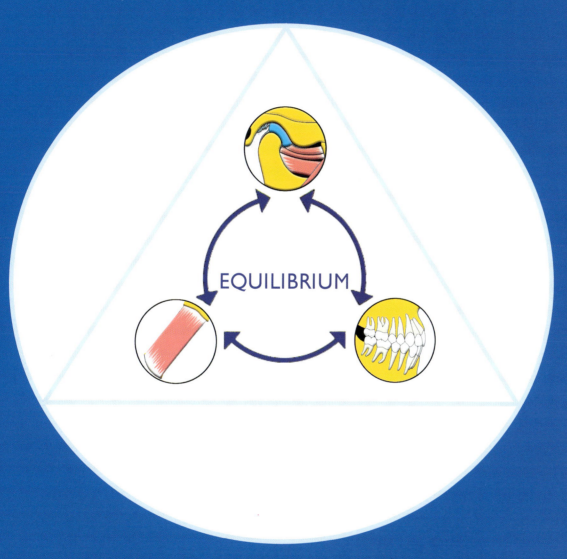

EQUILIBRIUM

THE INSEPARABLE TRIAD:
TEETH, MUSCLES, AND JOINTS

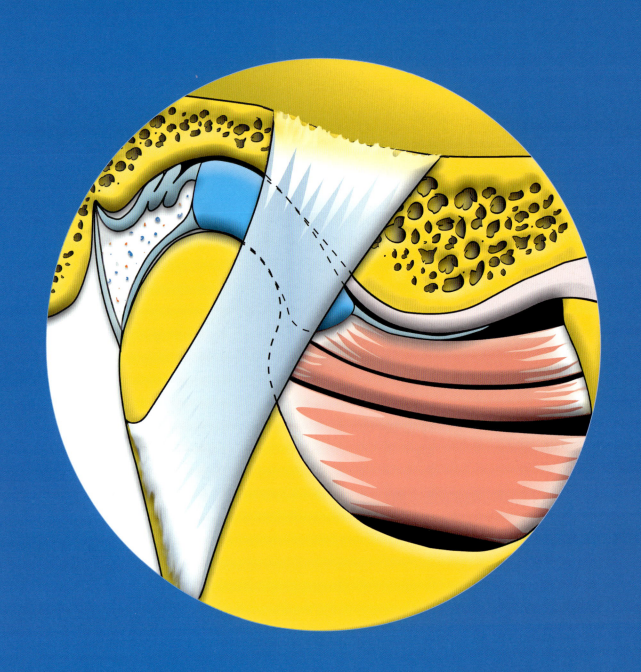

TEMPOROMANDIBULAR JOINTS

Section edited by Dr Fabio Ferretti

It is advisable to study the temporomandibular joint (TMJ) in depth[1,2] not only to understand its function and pathology but also to comprehend why this joint is of interest in primary imaging techniques such as computerized axial tomography and magnetic resonance imaging. The twin TMJs each consist of two anatomical compartments that are functionally interdependent with one another, with other oral and dental structures, and indeed, with almost the entire locomotor apparatus. Their role in opening and closing the jaw with a hinge movement in the sagittal plane places them in the category of ginglymus joints. Since the TMJs also permit sliding and translation movements, they also belong in the arthrodial class of joint, making them ginglymoarthrodial joints.

The TMJ is made up of two articulating structures: the mandibular condylar head and the mandibular fossa of the temporal bone. These two structures are connected by an interposed disc.

The **MANDIBULAR CONDYLE** is a bony apophysis of the mandibular ramus. It has a slim neck and an ellipsoid-shaped head with a mediolateral width greater than the anteroposterior length.

The **MANDIBULAR FOSSA** belongs to the squamous portion of the temporal bone. It is a semi-ellipsoid–shaped depression limited anteriorly by the anterior articular eminence and posteriorly by the postarticular crest (in close relationship with the internal auditory meatus). The extremely thin concavity of the depression, called the roof, relates with the cranial fossa. Only the anterior portion of the mandibular fossa, which extends from the roof to the anterior eminence, is the **true articulating surface**, often referred to simply as the **articulating surface** (see page 10).

The **ARTICULAR DISC** is a small fibrocartilaginous meniscus that supports dynamic loading and cushions

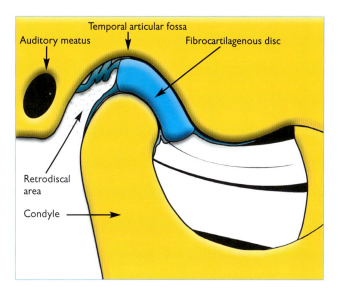

TMJ sagittal cross-section.

the joint's osseous articulating surfaces against pressure. It consists of dense connective tissue, having a high percentage of collagen fibers and few cells. The articular disc may be divided into three functional segments:

- **Anterior:** the relatively thick part leading into the tendinous bundles of the external pterygoid muscle.
- **Intermediate:** the slim avascular portion providing protection as the condyle glides against the anterior slope during opening movements. In normal conditions, it lies between the condyle and the anterior eminence when the jaws are open.
- **Posterior:** the thick band acting as a cushion between the condyle and the mandibular fossa roof when the jaws are closed. Posteriorly, it interacts with the retrodiscal area.

Closed mouth TMJ sagittal cross-section.

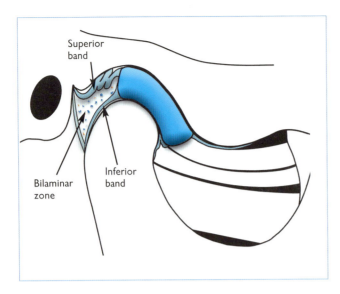

Open mouth TMJ sagittal cross-section.

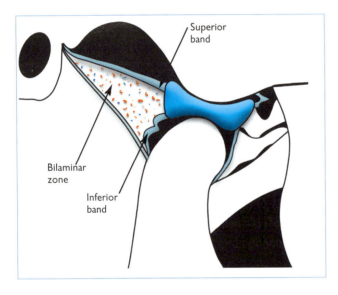

TMJ coronal cross-section.

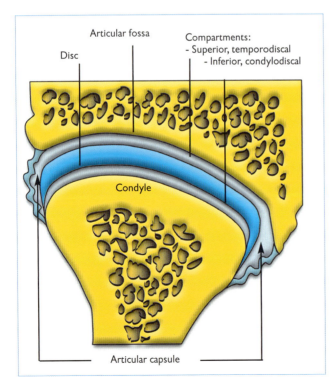

The **RETRODISCAL AREA** of the TMJ is the thick posterior band of the articular disc that continues backward into two fibrous bands. The elastic upper band originates from the postarticular crest whereas the lower band attaches to the posterior edge of the mandibular condyle. The area between these two bands is the bilaminar zone, or posterior ligament, a cushion of loose connective tissue enclosing a highly vascularized venous plexus. When the jaws are closed, the elastic upper band folds like an accordion, and there is little blood flow into the venous plexus. Conversely, when the jaws are opened, the upper band stretches, permitting the anterior condyle to glide under the pull of the contracting external pterygoid muscle, and the venous plexus dilates as blood flows in. The opposite occurs as the jaws close, and the venous plexus is squeezed as the condyle returns toward the fossa roof.

The **ARTICULAR CAPSULE** is a sleeve-shaped circular ligament. It is wide at its insertion base on the temporal bone and narrows around the neck of the mandibular condyle. The posterior segment consists of robust connective fibers that run vertically while the anterior fibers continue into the muscle fibers of the external pterygoid. The lateral portion is reinforced by bundles of the temporomandibular ligament, which explains how the mandible is able to perform ample anteroposterior movements while its lateral movements are far more limited.

Internally, the capsule is lined with synovial membrane and is divided into two distinct compartments, the temporodiscal and the condylodiscal. These compartments are separated by the disc, but both are lubricated by synovial fluid released by the synovial epithelium. The capsule also teems with nerve receptors responsible for proprioceptive sensoriality. These receptors transmit information along the auriculotemporal, masseteric, and posterior deep temporal nerves—mandibular divisions of the trigeminal nerve.

A number of **LIGAMENTOUS** structures border the articular capsule, the most important being the temporomandibular, stylomandibular, and sphenomandibular ligaments, which limit articular movements from surpassing their farthest extent.

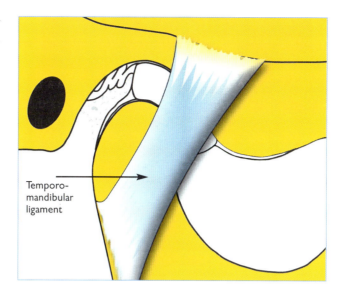

Temporo-
mandibular
ligament

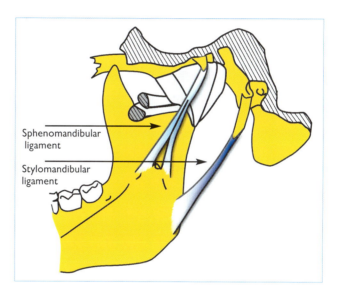

Sphenomandibular
ligament

Stylomandibular
ligament

TRUE ARTICULATING SURFACE

The TMJ fossa may be defined as the joint's true articulating surface, for it is within this space that the condyle-disc unit engages in a range of positions during mandibular excursions. The TMJ fossa is composed of the inclined anterior wall, which slopes downward and forward, and the anterior articular eminence, against which the condyle-disc unit glides during mouth opening and closure. The thickness of the cartilage increases in proportion to the forward movement, which protects against an increase in pressure on the articulating surface as the degree of condylar anterior translation increases.[3]

In contrast, neither the roof nor the posterior surface wall (near the auditory meatus) of the mandibular fossa takes an active part in articulating movements. Thus the morphology of the mandibular fossa roof, a thin bony lamella that lacks a cartilage lining, is totally unlike that of the true articulating surface.

In normal physiologic conditions when the mouth is closed, the condyle is held in place by pterygoid muscle tone and exerts pressure on the anterior wall. The pressure is partly absorbed by the interposed fibrocartilaginous disc. During the initial stage of opening, the condyle remains almost in the same position while purely rotating. Next, in the translation stage, increased muscle tone exerts even more pressure on the condyle and the true articulating surface until the jaws are fully open.

TMJ pathology is commonly caused by the long-term repetition of altered occlusal patterns resulting from an abnormal range of movements. In pathologic conditions, the condyle frequently experiences pressure from excessive nonaxial forces. *This is precisely the risk encountered with iatrogenous influences such as Class III elastics and Delaire face masks.* These forces slide the condyle against the posterior wall, which cannot tolerate pressure of any kind. Abnormal loading leads to tissue alteration in both condyle and fossa, and if the pressure persists, it eventually destroys live tissue.

True articulating surface

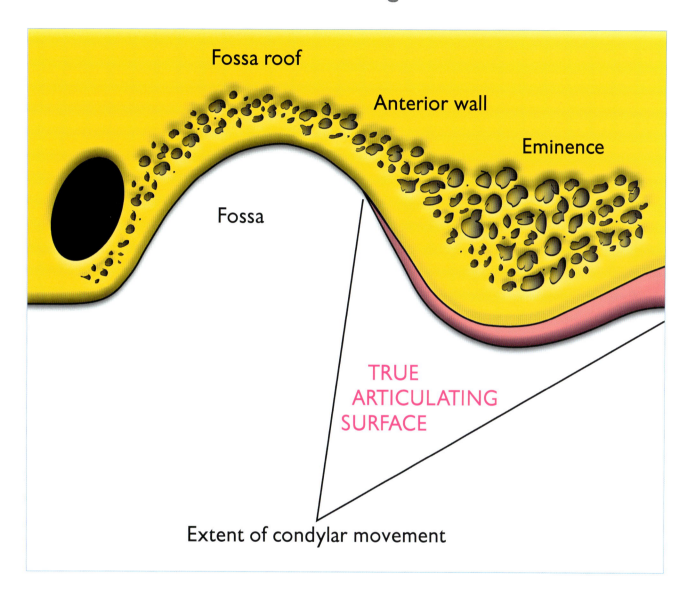

SKELETAL MUSCLE APPARATUS

Section edited by Prof Piergiorgio Strata

Under physiologic conditions, skeletal muscle fibers contract as a result of stimulation by α-motor neurons, each of which innervates from 10 to 1,600 muscle fibers. A motor unit consists of a complex of a single motor neuron and all the muscle fibers synapsed by it. Motor units containing a high number of muscle fibers belong to the muscles that sustain posture, such as the gastrocnemic muscle. Motor units containing a lower number of fibers belong to the muscles that control refined motions, such as those of the eyes. The muscles of the orofacial sphere consist of relatively small motor units. Movements within the masticatory sphere require high precision in order to perform functions such as controlling food in the mouth without biting the cheeks and tongue.

The motor neurons receive commands (1) from the periphery to control reflexes and posture and (2) from the upper centers to control voluntary movement and modulate the postural reflexes that maintain a suitable position of the body in space. Impulses from the upper centers can affect α-motor neurons. These impulses are also sent to the α-motor neurons to modulate sensitivity of the neuromuscular spindle and, consequently, regulate the myotatic reflexes that are the basis of normal postural tone. In addition, by modulating neuromuscular spindle sensitivity, the α-motor neurons make it possible for the spindle to provide a suitable response to the varying initial lengths of the muscle.

Muscle tone can be measured as resistance to passive distension of the muscle. Increased tone is referred to as muscle spasticity or rigidity. Spasticity is caused by increased activity of the α-motor neurons; rigidity is caused by an increase of descending motor input into the α-motor neurons. In pathologic conditions, muscle fibers may contract independently from the control of motor neurons. Similar conditions provoked by various local factors are also referred to as contractions, as in the case of caffeine-induced contraction.

There are essentially two types of muscle fibers, identified as slow-twitch (or red) and fast-twitch (or white):

- Slow-twitch muscle fibers have a high level of enzymes capable of transforming glucose into water and carbon dioxide (oxidative phosphorylation), which are rapidly excreted by the muscle. They are also dense with blood capillaries and contain myoglobin, which accounts for their red color. The fibers are capable of great stamina, and as such, they serve to maintain posture or carry a marathon runner over long distances.
- Fast-twitch (white) fibers have a low level of oxidative enzymes. They produce great force for short bursts of activity, as in weightlifting, but they also produce lactic acid, which causes tiring and becomes painful.

Each muscle has a different distribution of muscle fibers that depends on the tasks required of it. For example, slow-twitch fibers predominate in the masseter and external pterygoid muscles.

Muscle activity is monitored through electromyography, which records electrical activity within the muscle.

RELATIONSHIP BETWEEN INITIAL MUSCLE LENGTH AND FORCE OF CONTRACTION

The intensity of the contraction force of a muscle fiber is correlated with the fiber's initial length. There is an optimal length at which a muscle fiber generates its maximum contraction power. At this length, all actin-myosin crossbridges are functioning. At nonoptimal lengths, the number of functioning crossbridges is decreased. As a result, the force of contraction is diminished if the initial length is greater or less than the optimum.

In isolation, a muscle can no longer contract when the initial muscle length is reduced to 60% of the optimum, and this same incapacity exists when the initial length is increased to 175% of the optimum. However, these extremes do not occur in physiologic conditions. When a muscle is inserted into its connecting bones, initial muscle length may vary from the optimal length up to 30% in either direction. At the physiologic extremes, force of contraction is reduced by approximately half.

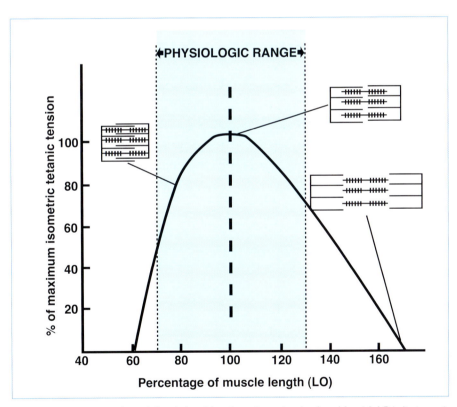

Relationship between initial muscle length (x axis) and muscle tension developed (y axis). LO indicates optimal length, considered 100%. This is the length at which a maximum contraction force of 100% is obtained. All greater and lesser lengths cause a reduction in the tension obtained.
The blue area indicates variations in length that the muscle is subjected to in physiologic conditions as a result of joint movement. Initial muscle lengths lying outside the blue area can be obtained only if the muscle is removed from its natural bone insertions, hence an isolated muscle. The inserts illustrate the sarcomeres with the molecules of myosin with their heads (center) and actin.

BASIC MUSCLE ANATOMY

MANDIBULAR ELEVATORS

PTERYGOID MUSCLE:

- External or lateral pterygoid:

  - Upper head

  - Lower head

- Internal or medial pterygoid

- MASSETER:

  - Deep layer

  - Superficial layer

- TEMPORALIS:

  - Anterior bundle

  - Medial bundle

  - Deep belly

DEPRESSORS MANDIBULAR

- Digastric

- Mylohyoid

- Stylohyoid

NECK MUSCLES

- Sternocleidomastoid

- Trapezius

MUSCLES OF MASTICATION: ELEVATOR MUSCLES

PTERYGOID MUSCLE

Of the various masticatory muscles (masseter, temporalis, internal and external pterygoid), the external (or lateral) pterygoid is the closest and most directly involved in dysfunctional pathology.

EXTERNAL PTERYGOID MUSCLE

The external pterygoid is the most important periarticular muscle affecting the TMJ. Its *superior head* inserts partly onto the articular capsule and disc in the anteromedial area and partly onto the mandibular condylar neck, then rises to enter the great wing of the sphenoid. The superior head stabilizes the mandible by holding the condyle-disc complex steady on the articular eminence.

The *inferior head* originates from the external surface of the lateral pterygoid plate. It is directed backward and laterally, inserting at the height of the neck of the condyle (pterygoid fovea). The inferior head is responsible for translation of the mandible, enabling it to follow the inclined plane of the articular eminence.

INTERNAL PTERYGOID MUSCLE

The internal (or medial) pterygoid arises from the medial face of the internal pterygoid plate, the maxillary tuberosity, and the pyramidal process of the palatine bone. Its fibers pass downward, laterally and posteriorly, and insert into the internal surface of the mandibular angle. Its action is similar to that of the masseter, with which it runs parallel.

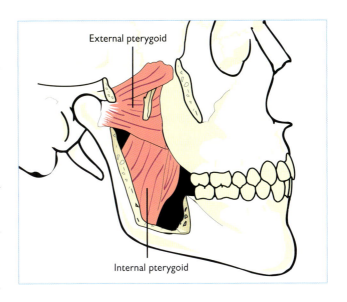

External pterygoid

Internal pterygoid

NORMAL

EXTERNAL PTERYGOID WITH NORMAL TENSION

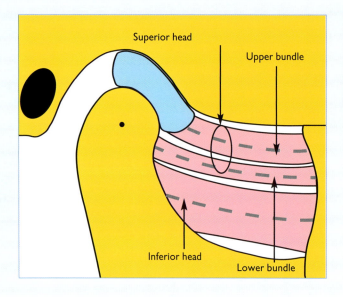
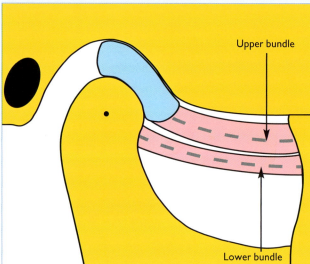

PATHOLOGY

EXTERNAL PTERYGOID: ALTERED DISTANCE BETWEEN BONE EXTREMITIES (MUSCLE STRESS)

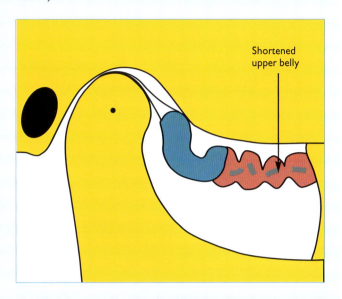

In pathologic conditions, the upper belly of the superior head of the external pterygoid shortens as the disc comes forward, and the lower belly stretches as the condyle moves backward.

CLINICAL IMPACT:

Very often, the external pterygoid is the first muscle to show painful symptoms and the last to regain normal tone.

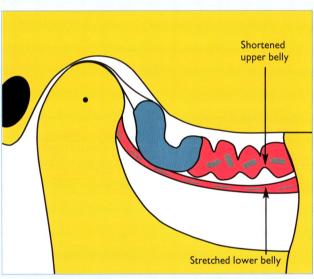

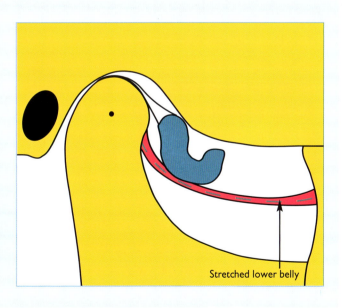

Masseter: superficial layer.

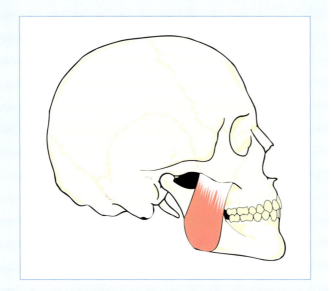

Masseter: deep layer.

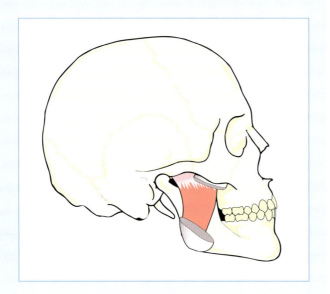

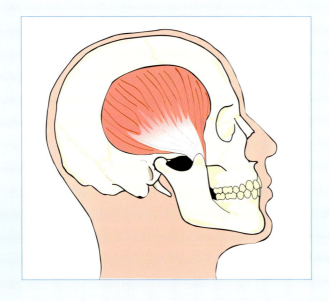

MASSETER

The masseter is a powerful muscle with robust fibers extending from the lower edge of the zygomatic bone to the ramus and body of the rear of the mandible. The superficial layer, inclined downward from the front toward the rear, is active in chewing. The deep layer, inclined downward from the rear forward, elevates the mandible.

TEMPORALIS

This characteristically fan-shaped muscle arises from the temporal fossa and, to a lesser extent, from the parietal and sphenoid bones. All of its bundles (anterior, median, and posterior) converge downward to the coronoid process of the mandible and onto the mandibular ramus. The anterior belly elevates the mandible and, in synergy with the superficial layer of the masseter, is highly active in chewing and grinding food. The median and posterior fibers are more active in mandibular stabilization and retrusion.

Masseter: superficial layer.

MANDIBULAR DEPRESSOR MUSCLES

DIGASTRIC

The digastric muscle consists of two bellies united by an intermediate tendon. The anterior belly arises from the small digastric depression of the mandible and passes to the lateral extremity of the body of the hyoid, where the intermediate tendon is connected to the osseous body by a fibrous loop. The posterior belly arises from the mastoid process of the temporal bone and is attached to the body of the hyoid by the intermediate tendon.

MYLOHYOID

The mylohyoid makes up the floor of the mouth. Its two halves (right and left) originate from the internal surface of the mandible. They are joined medially in a fibrous raphe and then insert posteriorly into the body of the hyoid bone.

Only the posterior fibers lower the corner of the mandible, resulting in condylar distraction.

STYLOHYOID

The stylohyoid is a slender muscle that arises from the styloid process of the temporal bone and then divides into two bundles. It is perforated by the intermediate tendon of the digastric muscle shortly before its point of insertion into the lateral extremity of the hyoid bone.

NECK MUSCLES

STERNOCLEIDOMASTOID

The sternocleidomastoid is a powerful muscle with a medial and lateral head situated in the anterolateral region of the neck. It originates from a sternal head from the manubrium sterni and a from clavicular head from the medial portion of the upper clavicular surface. The two heads join in a thick belly, which enters the mastoid process of the temporal bone. Contraction of the sternocleidomastoid on one side alone causes the head to flex obliquely toward the same side. Simultaneous contraction of both muscles extends the head.

TRAPEZIUS

Lying in the nuchal region and posterior thoracic area, the trapezius muscle is commonly divided into three parts: descending, transversal, and ascending. The descending fibers arise from the superior nuchal line, an external protruberance of the occipital bone and ligamentum nuchae. The transversal portion arises from the spinous processes of the vertebrae from C7 to T3. And the ascending portion arises from the spinous processes of the vertebrae from T2 or T3 to T12. The descending, transversal, and ascending portions insert, respectively, onto the lateral third of the clavicle, the medial margin of the acromion, and the superior lateral margin of the spine of the scapula.

Among its functions, the trapezius elevates and retracts the shoulders and extends the head by rotating it toward the opposite side.

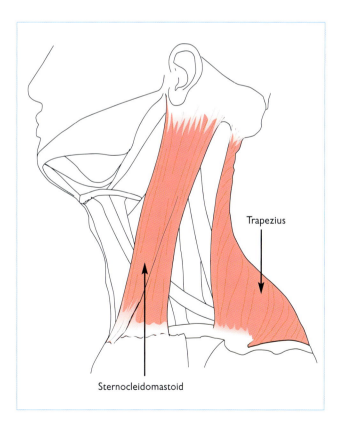

Trapezius

Sternocleidomastoid

AXIAL ALIGNMENT OF JOINT STRUCTURES

Observations suggested by Dr G. C. Coari

An essential condition for correct function of all types of human skeletal joints is the axial alignment of the component parts. The same concept should be applied to TMJs. In normal physiologic conditions, the condyle, disc, and articulating surface should be aligned when still and in motion.

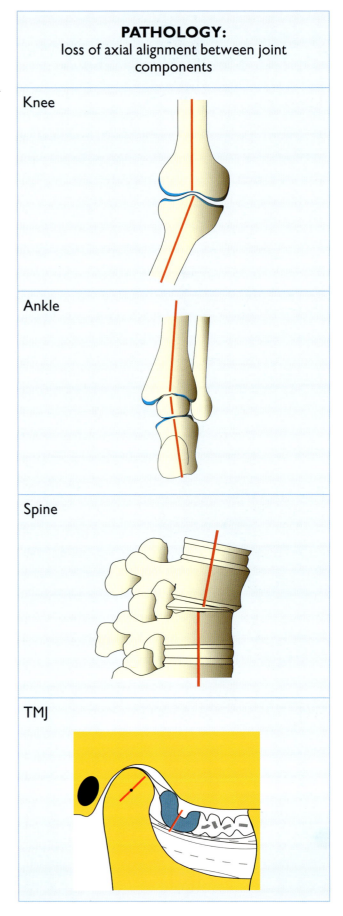

PATHOLOGY:
loss of axial alignment between joint components

Knee

Ankle

Spine

TMJ

THERAPY:
to seek to restore axial alignment
between joint components

RECOVERY:
of axial alignment between joint components

Osteotomy

Articulated joint distraction

Manipulation

ARS

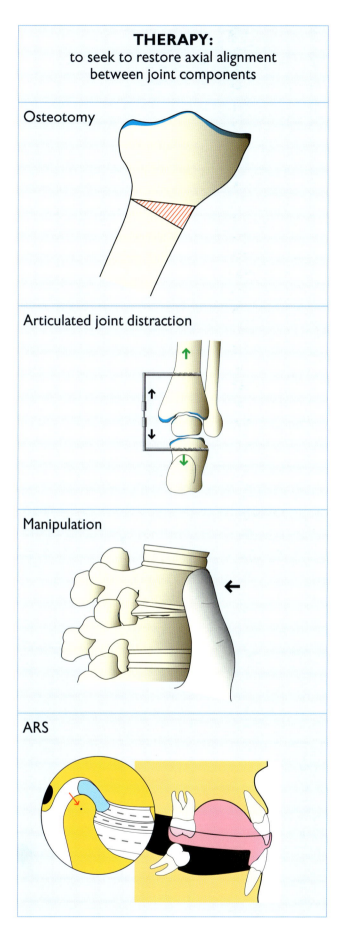

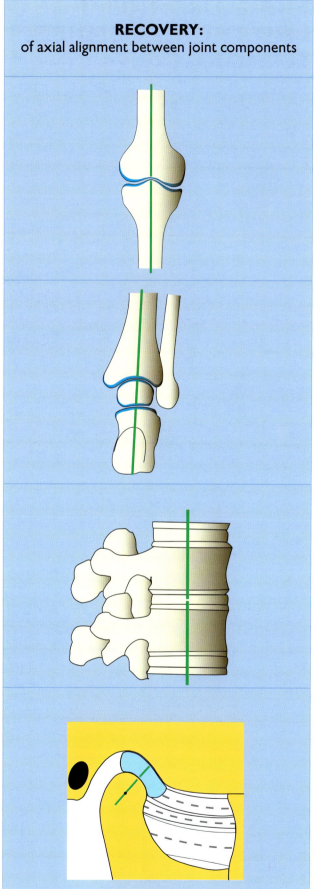

THE OLD CONCEPT OF CENTRIC RELATION AND THE NEW CONCEPT OF AXIAL ALIGNMENT: TERMINOLOGY

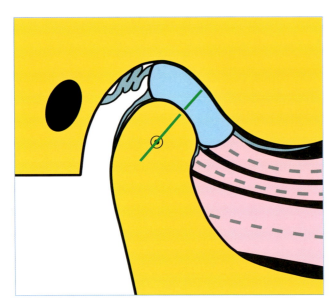

NORMAL FUNCTION (BASELINE)

For normal function, baseline is defined as correct anatomy with axial alignment (geometric centering) and normal muscle length.

During the 1980s, the author, Dawson PE,[4] determined that the ideal correspondence between maximum intercuspation and geometric centric relation (condylar position) should be roughly in the center of the mandibular fossa. He concluded that this correspondence can be obtained only when a person has healthy TMJs and no dentoskeletal discrepancies between the maxilla and mandible.

With the vast majority of patients suffering from dislocation or derangement, the solution is often a compromise. The clinician must seek a correspondence between con-sistent dental occlusion and functional recovery or adaptation, which between them will guarantee axial alignment between the condyle, disc or pseudodisc, and temporal bone counterpart without the need for geometric centering. These conditions also help to restore satisfactory muscle function.

*Note: From a clinical point of view and for simplicity of explanation, **dislocation** without reduction has been grouped together with altered anatomic condylar shape (tissue **destruction**).*

ANOMALOUS POSITION: DISLOCATION WITH REDUCTION

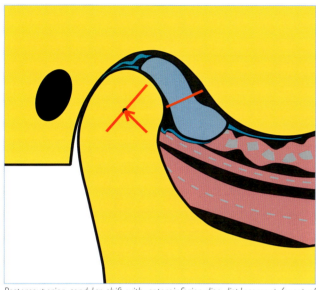

Posterosuperior condylar shift with anteroinferior disc displacement (onset of pathology with axial disalignment) is almost always accompanied by muscle tension and pain with various clicking patterns as the disc is recaptured during jaw opening. This condition is commonly observed during clinical practice.

FOLLOWING ARS THERAPY: FUNCTIONAL RECOVERY

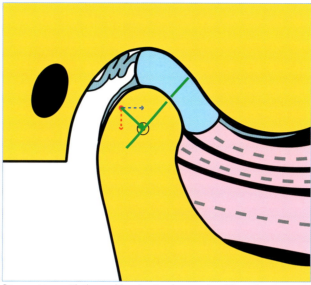

Disc recapture with the condyle returning downward and forward restores correct axial alignment and normal muscle length.

ANOMALOUS POSITION AND SHAPE: DISLOCATION WITHOUT REDUCTION WITH TISSUE

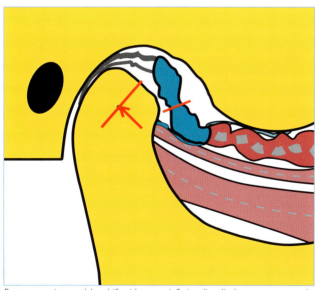

Posterosuperior condylar shift with anteroinferior disc displacement causes derangement of joint structures, especially of the disc, posterior ligament, and bony surfaces.
Acute pathology with axial disalignment.
Mucle tension and pain.

DESTRUCTION FOLLOWING ARS THERAPY: FUNCTIONAL ADAPTATION

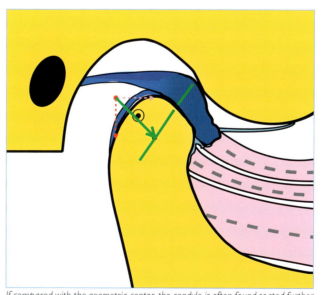

If compared with the geometric center, the condyle is often found seated further downward and forward. Distraction of the osseous components of the TMJ allows them to rearrange with the ligament as a pseudodisc, which leads to improved muscle tone and pain relief. Both functional recovery and functional adaptation can be referred to as functional efficiency (see following chapter and Diagnosis, pages 92 and 93).

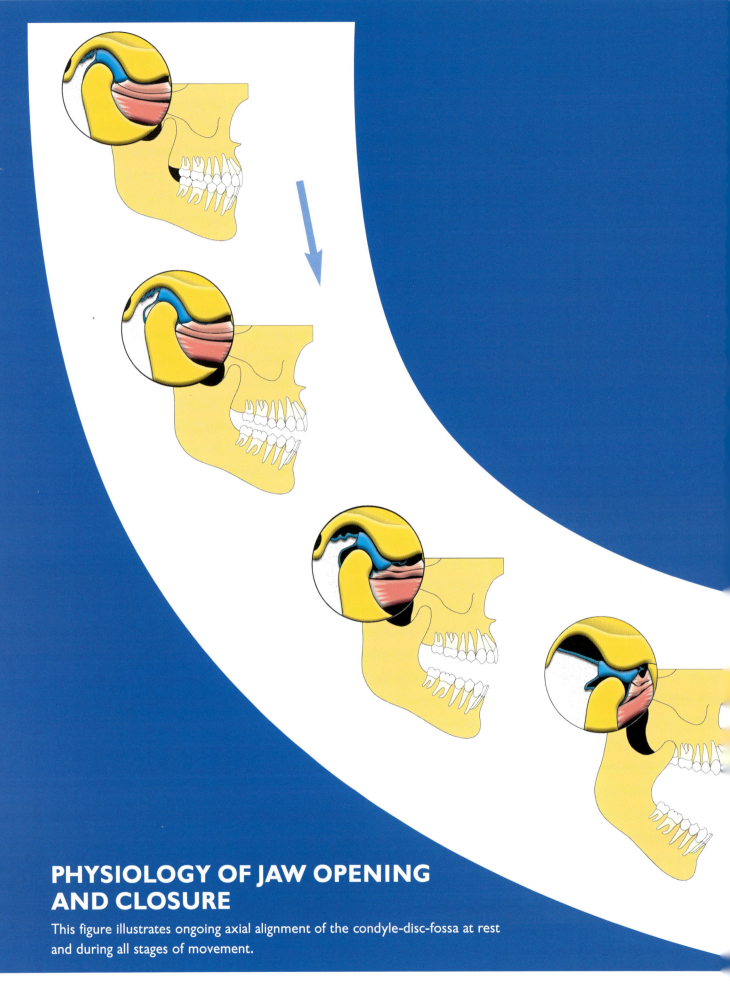

PHYSIOLOGY OF JAW OPENING AND CLOSURE

This figure illustrates ongoing axial alignment of the condyle-disc-fossa at rest and during all stages of movement.

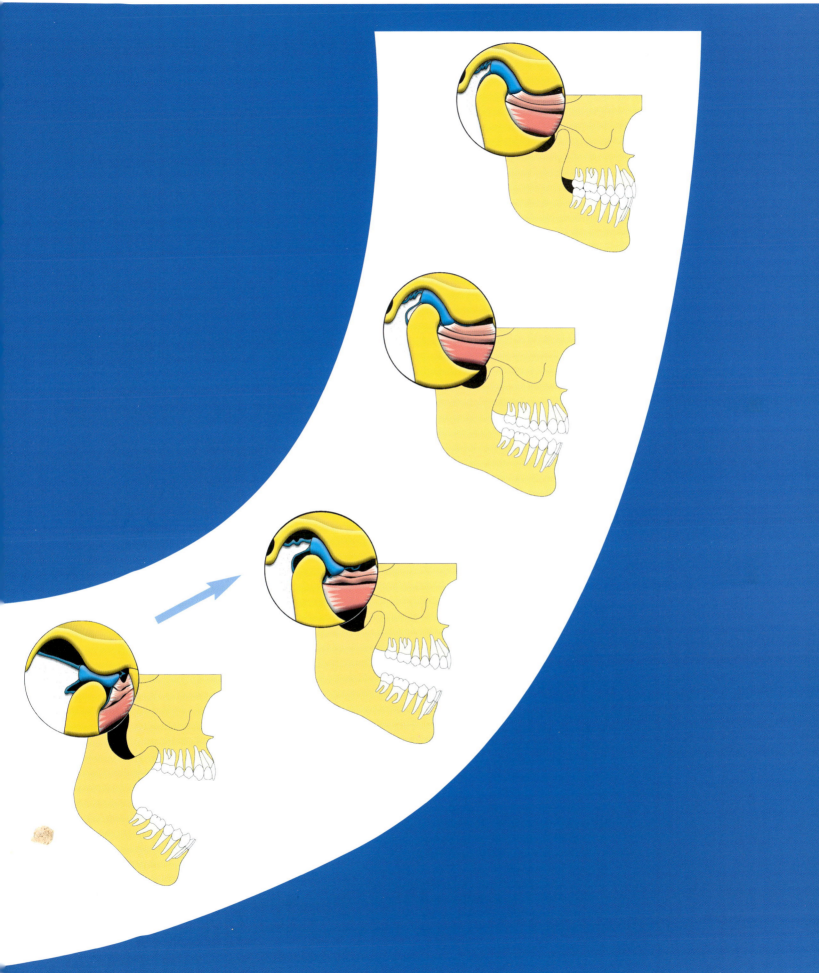

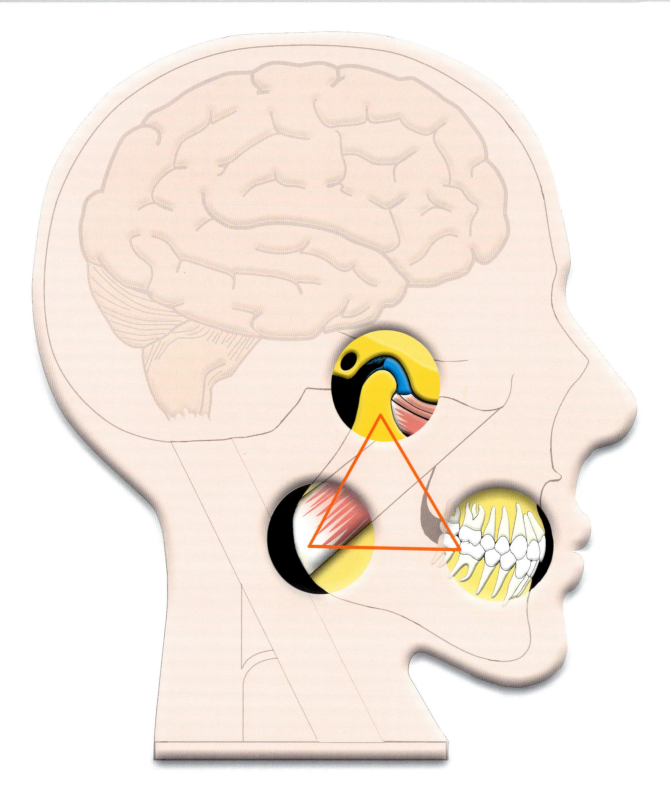

An inseparable unit: The teeth, muscles, and joints are controlled by the central nervous system.

ANATOMICAL PARTS INVOLVED IN MASTICATION

Correct anatomy and functional efficiency are key points of reference in diagnostic assessment and treatment procedures. Contributions from various anatomic parts enable the mouth to perform its numerous functions. These components include the following:

- **Maxilla:** the fixed jaw inserted into the skull.

- **Mandible:** the mobile antagonist with its twin TMJs (among the most complex joints in the human body) that enable the mandible to move in three spatial dimensions.

- **Various muscle pairs:** the muscles that provide movement through integrated agonist-antagonist pulling forces and maintain antigravitational muscle tone.

- **Opposing teeth:** the maxillary and mandibular teeth, which intercuspate simultaneously under normal, nonworking conditions, such as swallowing.

- **Protection systems:**
  - posterior protection: prevents anterior tooth contact,
  - anterior protection: prevents posterior tooth contact (incisal guidance),
  - canine protection: keeps the remaining teeth apart.

- **Nervous system control** of the complex stomatognathic mechanism reflex arches: commanded by pathways 1a and 1b with near-instant integrated neuromotor responses.

Important contributions to successful TMD treatment also include:

- **The patient:** presents a unique combination of genetics, psychology, and behavior.

- **Esthetics:** an essential factor in achieving patient satisfaction and must be considered during diagnosis and treatment planning.

TOOTH DYNAMICS

Posterior protection: with posterior teeth in contact, the anterior teeth are a few microns apart.
This tiny distance is impossible to illustrate on a visible scale.
Mouth closed.
Detail of anterior teeth slightly apart.

Anterior protection: with anterior teeth in contact (incisal guidance), the posterior teeth remain apart.
Detail of anterior teeth on protrusion.

Canine rise: right side
Only the canines are in contact.
Posteriorly, no teeth are in contact on either the working or nonworking side.

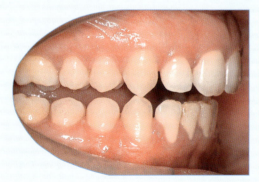 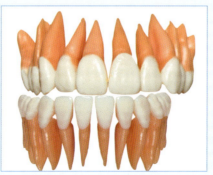 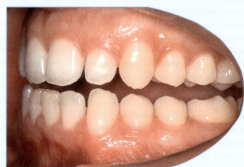

View from right (working side).   *View from left (nonworking side).*

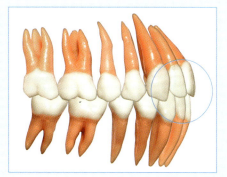

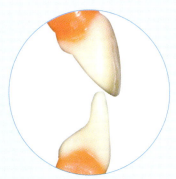

Detail of anterior teeth slightly apart, without contact.

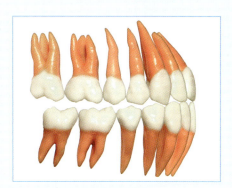

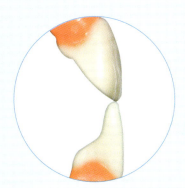

Detail of anterior teeth on protrusion, with contact.

Canine rise: left side

Only the canines are in contact.

Posteriorly, no teeth are in contact on either the working or nonworking side.

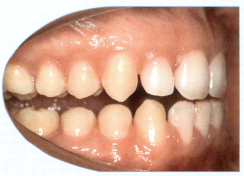

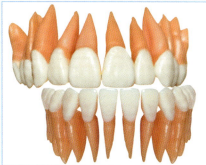

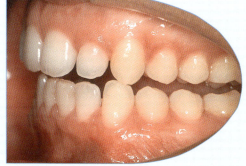

View from right (nonworking side).   *View from left (working side).*

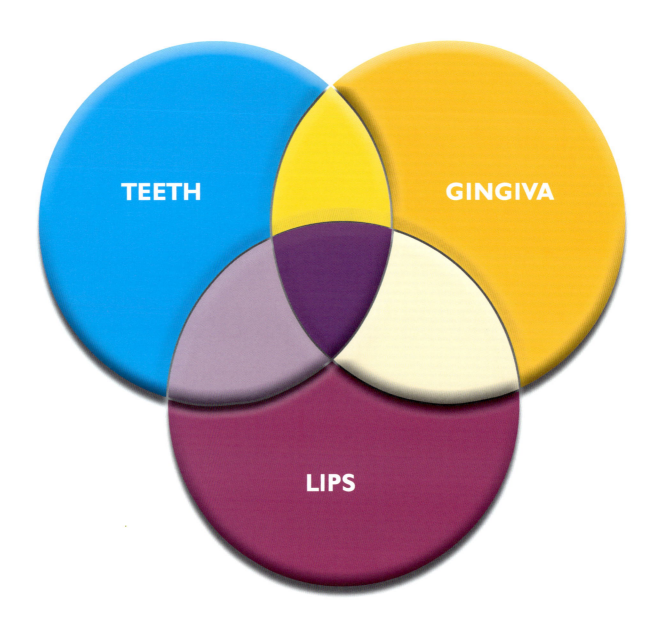

(Illustration by Dr Lorenzo Vanini)

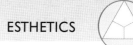

ESTHETICS

During assessment, the appearance of the patient's face and smile must be enhanced.

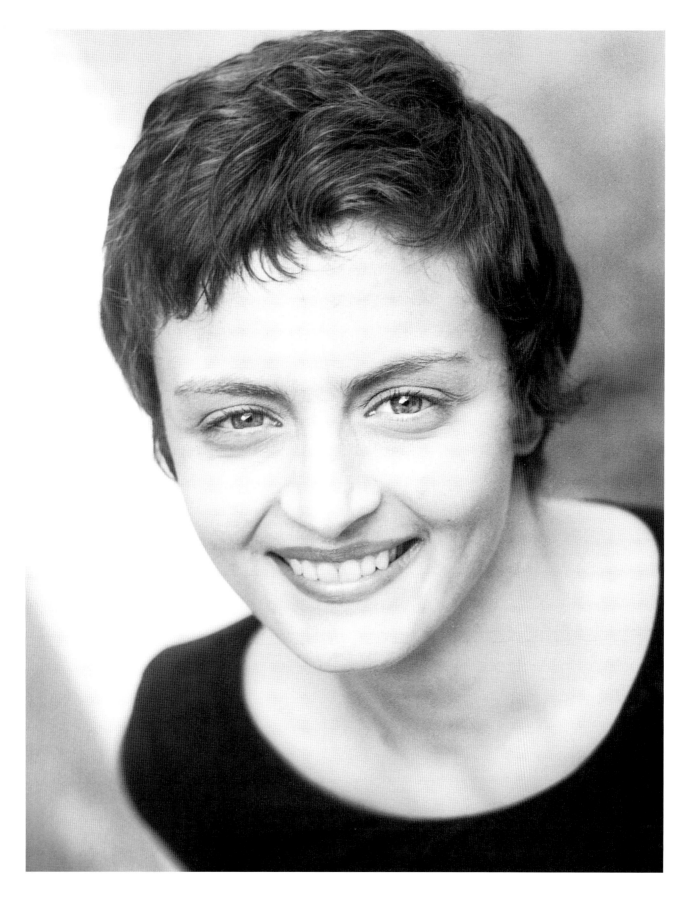

FUNCTION

ESTHETICS

Conventions of esthetics and the smile.

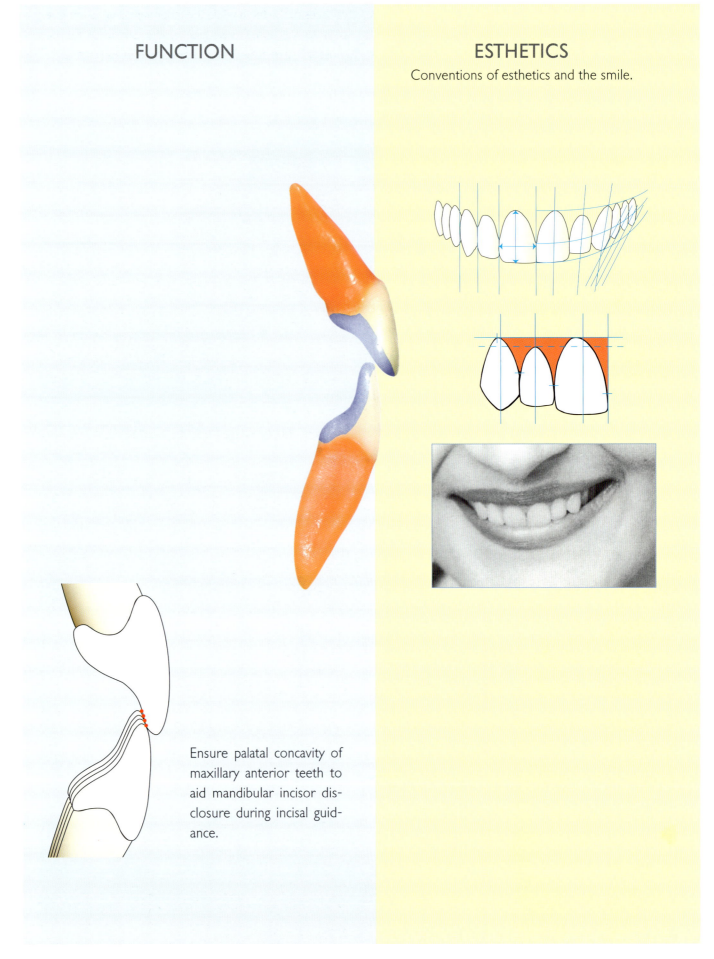

Ensure palatal concavity of maxillary anterior teeth to aid mandibular incisor disclosure during incisal guidance.

When dealing with esthetics in buccal and lingual recontouring of maxillary incisors, care must be taken to ensure incisal guidance functionality. Esthetics affect the outer buccal faces of the teeth while the inner lingual faces are given over to function. Consequently, the search for function must also take esthetics into consideration and vice versa.[5-7]

Esthetic recontouring of maxillary incisors
Coordinated by Dr Lorenzo Vanini

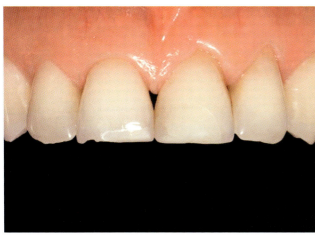

Before.

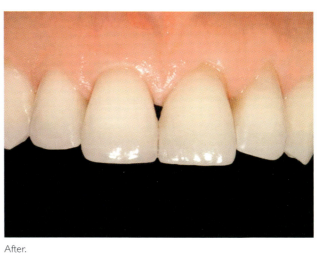

After.

To ensure incisal guidance disclosure, the lingual faces of the four incisors have been recontoured (in this case, with porcelain veneers).

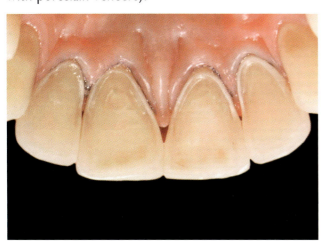

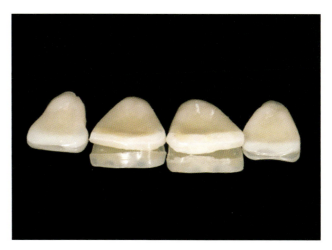

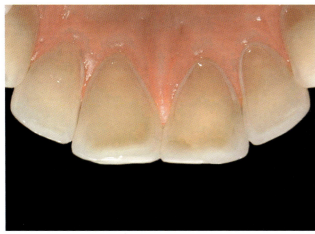

Occlusal view, before.

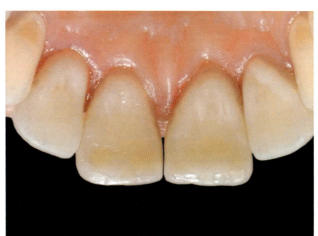

Occlusal view, after.

REFERENCES

1. Testut L, Latarjet A. Anatomia umana. Osteologia Artrologia. Vol 1. 5th ed. Torino: Utet, 1971.
2. Dubrull EL, Miani A, Ferrario VF. Anatomia Orale di Sicher. Milan: Edi-Ermes, 1988.
3. Drace JE, Stuart WY, Enzmann DR. TMJ meniscus and bilaminar zone: MR imaging of the substructure—Diagnostic landmarks and pitfalls of interpretation. Radiology 1990;177:73–76.
4. Dawson PE. Optimum TMJ condyle position in clinical practice. Int J Periodontics Restorative Dent 1985;3:11–31.
5. Vanini L, Mangani F, Klimovskaia O. Il Restauro Conservativo dei Denti Anteriori. Viterbo: ACME sas, 2003.
6. Zachrisson BU. Facial esthetics: Guide to tooth positioning and maxillary incisor display. World J Orthod 2007;8:308–314.
7. Spear FM, Kokich VG. A multidisciplinary approach to esthetic dentistry. Dent Clin North Am 2007;51:487–455.

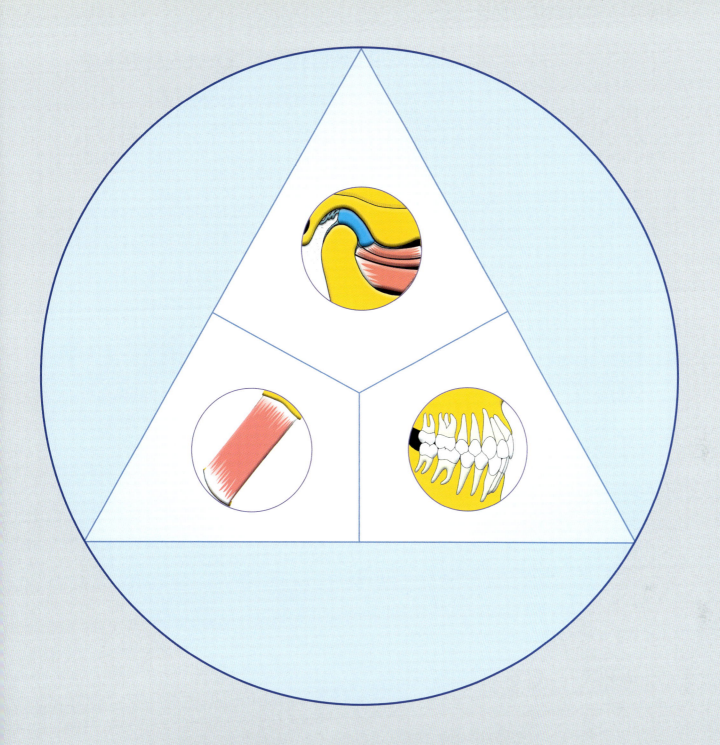

DIAGNOSIS: PATIENT RECORDS

The teeth, muscles, and temporomandibular joints (TMJs) make up an inseparable unit even throughout pathology, therapy, and final outcome. It must be remembered that every proposed treatment for a temporomandibular disorder (TMD) is an attempt to find the best solution for the patient, a human being in discomfort or pain seeking a remedy for what is sometimes a disabling pathology. The clinician must make every effort to combine professionalism with humanity while referring to the most recent guidelines and employing efficient clinical solutions.

Dentists should monitor not only for immediate oral problems, such as caries, gingival recession, and orthodontic and prosthodontic needs, but also for disorders affecting the head and neck muscles and the TMJs, which can have effects ranging from minimal to very complex. **The dentist is primarily responsible for dealing with disorders of the stomatognathic apparatus** unless the case clearly requires the attention of a specialist in some other field such as neurology, otorhinolaryngology, or rheumatology. This is also true of problems related to the muscles of mastication and the TMJs, the treatment of which often differs little from other more general orthopedic procedures.

A thorough diagnosis of the disorder, based on patient history, physical examination, and radiologic imaging, should be completed. The patient should be fully informed about the diagnosis as well as details of the proposed treatment plan.

PATIENT ASSESSMENT

The initial assessment of dysfunction should be kept reasonably brief while taking several key factors into consideration: *(1)* pain (if present, note type and location), *(2)* altered mandible excursions on all three spatial planes, and *(3)* TMJ noise.

The TMJs should be palpated and checked with a stethoscope should during their various movements. A benchmark orthopantomography (OPT) should always be taken on the patient's first appointment, except in children less than 7 years old. This baseline information helps guide the dentist in collecting other data, such as computed tomography (CT), magnetic resonance imaging (MRI), and consultation with other specialists.

In summary, a diagnosis must be based at least on a combination of patient history, physical examination, and radiologic images. These data are complemented as needed by traditional orthodontic records including face and mouth photos, dental stone casts, cephalograms, and additional OPT.

BASIC PATIENT HISTORY

After obtaining the patient's or guardian's consent, a thorough patient history should be acquired, including reason for the appointment, previous illnesses going back to childhood, and any serious infectious diseases, past or present. In children, check specifically for dental-related issues, including tooth changes and accidents or injuries, and orthodontic-related issues, including oral habits and dentoskeletal growth pattern. In adults, pay particular attention to signs of TMD. Symptoms include:

-   Pain and other complaints associated with the stomatognathic apparatus.
-   Tiredness during mastication.
-   Noise when the jaws open and close.
-   Masticatory muscle tension or tiredness on awakening.
-   The onset of complaints after an injury or alteration to the maxillomandibular relationship.
-   Any suspicious pain. Note its location, intensity, onset, and duration. Typical areas of
    -   TMJ-related pain include the ear (due to condylar pressure), forehead, face, neck, and
    -   other parts of the body affected by posture.

CLINICAL RECORDS

A good record should *(1)* provide a comprehensive checklist to gather as much information as possible and ensure that no essential information is overlooked, and *(2)* show all major items at a glance. Therefore, the record should be an A3-size double page with simple visible graphics (see pages 40 to 41). Red is a good color to highlight any pathology for immediate identification. In the areas dealing with muscles and joints, leave room to the side for notes on any problems such as tension, noise or clicks, and lack of TMJ coordination on jaw opening and closure.

The record card used by the authors has a first page for personal information and diagnosis summary followed by blank pages (not shown) for details of all observations, procedures, limitations, and advice given to the patient.

REACHING AN INDIVIDUAL DIAGNOSIS
PHYSICAL EXAMINATION: ESSENTIAL DIAGNOSTIC ELEMENTS

HISTORY: Specific in-depth questions for both children and adults, according to existing or suspected pathology

CRANIOFACIAL UNIT:
- Spatial position of individual teeth
- Arch shape and intercuspation patterns
- 3D relationships:
  - Between maxilla and mandible
  - Maxilla and mandible with the skull
- Symmetry and proportional ratio of the various parts of the face, seen both full-face and in profile
- Smile esthetics
- Oral habits, typically mouth breathing, atypical swallowing, tongue posture, and/or thrust
- With children, assess growth pattern

MANDIBULAR EXCURSIONS:
- Protrusion, right and left lateral movements, maximum opening, extent and type of pathway
- TMJ palpation and auscultation with stethoscope

MUSCLES:
- Palpation of muscles of mastication
- Palpation of muscles of posture

INDENTATIONS OF TONGUE OR INNER CHEEKS:
- Signs of a physiologic "bite"

HYPERMOBILE CONDYLES AND LIGAMENTOUS LAXITY

PERIODONTAL CONDITIONS:
- Hygiene
- Alveolar bone height surrounding each tooth

PSYCHOLOGIC ATTITUDE:
- Normal reaction, minimizes symptoms, or over-reacts

DIAGNOSTIC TESTS:
- Tart with an OPT
  - As appropriate, perform an MRI (preferentially) and/or a CT

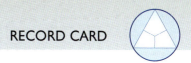

FIRST APPOINTMENT RECORD CARD

DATE _____

PERSONAL DETAILS

Family name _____   First name _____

Place of birth _____   Date of birth _____

Address _____

ZIP code – Town/City _____   Tel _____

Referred by Dr _____   Tel _____

Currently treated by Dr _____   Tel _____

REASON FOR APPOINTMENT: _____

OPT DONE   our office ❐   externally ❐   Date _____

NOTES _____

(DATA PROTECTION NOTICE AND WAIVER)

DETAILS UNDERLYING DIAGNOSIS

Skeletal: _____

Dental: _____   Type of bite _____

Teeth present   8 7 6 5 4 3 2 1 | 1 2 3 4 5 6 7 8   Teeth missing or   8 7 6 5 4 3 2 1 | 1 2 3 4 5 6 7 8
              8 7 6 5 4 3 2 1 | 1 2 3 4 5 6 7 8   requiring extraction 8 7 6 5 4 3 2 1 | 1 2 3 4 5 6 7 8

Development and growth: positive ❐   negative ❐

TMJ dynamics   1) Occlusal surface wear   ❐   4) Muscle problems   ❐

                   2) Loss of alveolar bone height ❐   5) Tongue or cheek indentations   ❐

                   3) TMJ problems   ❐   6) Attitude _____

TMJ and occlusion _____

Any oral habits _____

Esthetics: any drawbacks _____

Worst problem _____   Estimated compliance _____

HYGIENE   Nonexistent ☐
           Poor   ☐
           Good   ☐

ORAL HABITS

Mouth breathing   ☐
Atypical swallowing ☐
_____   ☐

INDENTATIONS
           Tongue   ☐
           Inner cheeks ☐

Ligamentous LAXITY   ☐

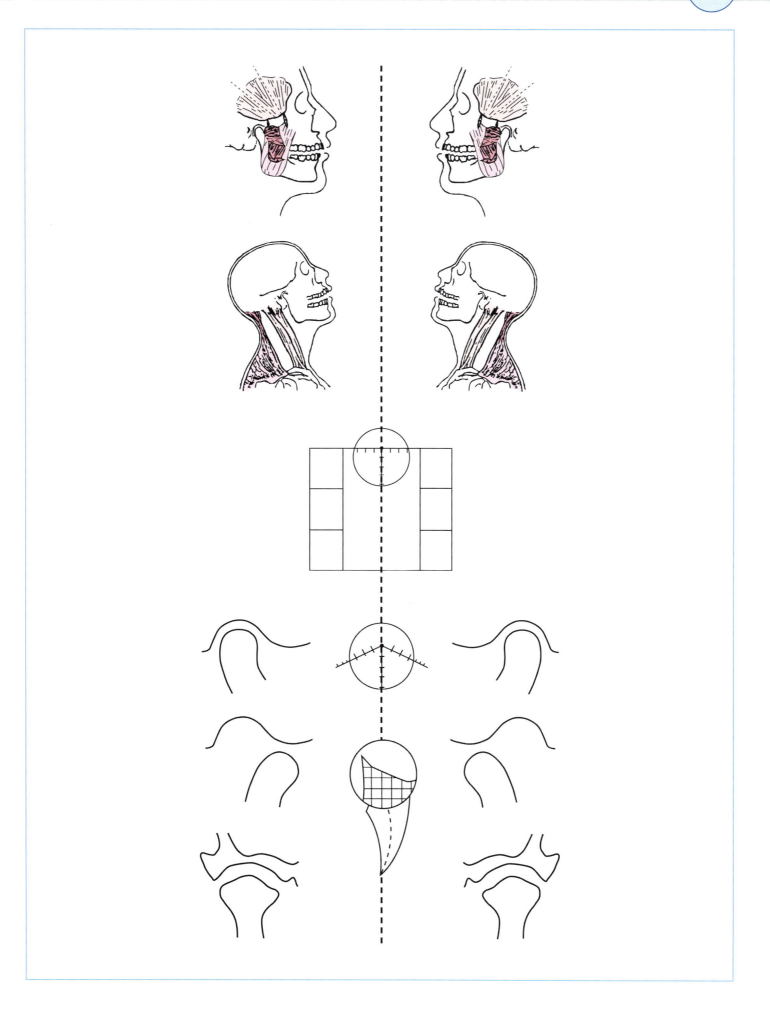

CLINICAL ANALYSIS

EXAMPLES OF OCCLUSAL ALTERATION

ANTEROPOSTERIOR PROBLEMS
- Class II skeletal relationship
- Class III skeletal relationship

TRANSVERSAL PROBLEMS
- Crossbites
- Scissor bites (monolateral or bilateral)

VERTICAL PROBLEMS
- Deep bite
- Open bite

OTHER PROBLEMS
- Missing teeth
- Arch asymmetry
- Tilting or tipping
- Rotation
- Crowding
- Gaps
- Extrusion
- Intrusion
- Posterior collapse due to missing molars

No correlation exists between severity of anatomical damage and functional deterioration.
An example of this is illustrated on the opposite page: In an almost perfect dentition, the edge-to-edge bite between a maxillary second premolar and its antagonist may cause a severe dysfunctional pathology. Conversely, a patient with a poor anatomical situation, including several missing teeth, may have relatively little dysfunctional damage—possibly due to the patient's habit of placing the tongue between the teeth to prevent traumatic contact, as evidenced by indentations on the tongue.

INDICATORS OF DYSFUNCTIONAL PATHOLOGY

ABRADED OCCLUSAL SURFACES
These indicate excessive bruxing between the dental arches with progressive enamel destruction potentially leading to total loss of the occlusal surfaces. A number of factors may be involved, including psychologic causes. It is not uncommon to observe abraded occlusal surfaces in children's primary teeth.

PERIODONTAL CONDITION AND ALVEOLAR BONE HEIGHT
Dysfunctional and orthodontic therapy must always be preceded and accompanied by correct oral hygiene and proper home care. Alveolar bone height should be assessed by probing.

PERIODONTAL FREMITUS
A simple yet telling test is to place the tips of the index, middle, and ring fingers against the labial surfaces of the maxillary incisors during closure to detect any fremitus due to microtrauma-induced dental mobility. If present, fremitus indicates that an eccentric load is being placed on the teeth and is frequently a sign of dual bite.

INDENTATIONS ON THE TONGUE AND INNER CHEEKS
Marks left by the teeth, typically on the tongue but also inside the cheeks, indicate a defense mechanism. The tongue is used to buffer contact between the opposing arches, thereby preventing pain and trauma. Typically, the patient uses this antalgic posture or "natural mouth guard" during the day, but this protective action ceases at night. In the morning, the masticatory muscles feel tired and stiff, and the joints are overloaded.

LIGAMENT TONE
The patient should be checked for ligamentous laxity since slackness often correlates with dysfunctional pathology. Extended movements of the wrist, or even the middle finger alone, indicate a person's general ligament tone.

CLASSIC EXAMPLES

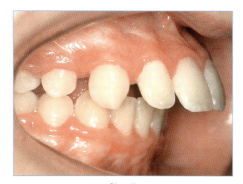

Class II.

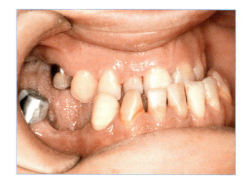

Class III.

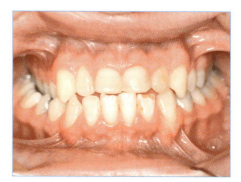

Posterior crossbite.

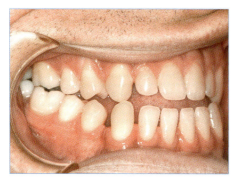

Open bite.

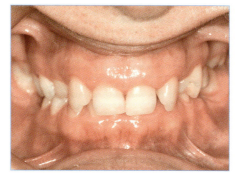

Deep bite.

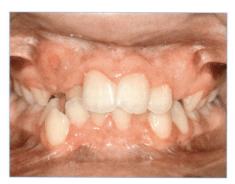

Crowding.

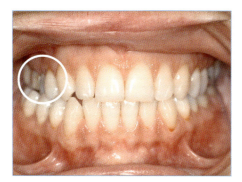

Maxillary second premolar edge-to-edge bite.

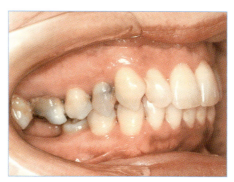

Posterior collapse due to missing antagonist molars.

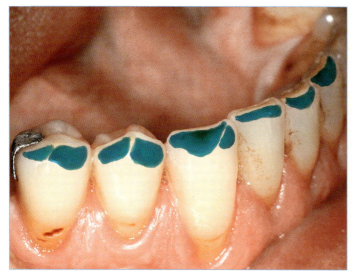

Abraded occlusal surfaces.

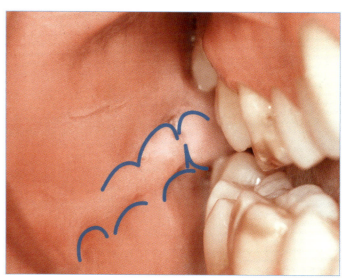

Indentations on inner cheek.

MUSCLE PALPATION

Although an empirical indicator, muscle palpation performed by an experienced dentist with good clinical intuition can provide much useful information.[1] This simple investigation can detect tension and pain affecting the postural and masticatory muscles. For didactic simplicity, this section mentions only the basic muscles, grouped as muscles of mastication and muscles of posture. Recommended reading on this topic includes works by Simons et al[1] Okeson,[2] and Bumann and Lotzmann.[3]

MASTICATORY MUSCLES

The lateral pterygoid should be checked first. Intraoral palpation of the lateral pterygoid area involves placing the little finger on the maxillary tuberosity and exerting slight distal pressure (see illustration) while the patient lateroextrudes the mandible on that side. Despite some controversy, this test is of diagnostic relevance since the lateral pterygoid may be the first muscle affected by the pathology and the last to recover entirely.

Subsequently, the other muscles of mastication are palpated, specifically the temporalis anterior, middle, and posterior bundles and the masseter superior, middle, and anterior bundles.

Lateral pterygoid area.

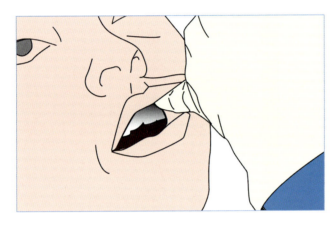

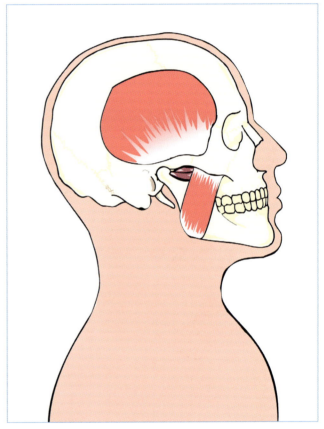

Temporalis (anterior part).

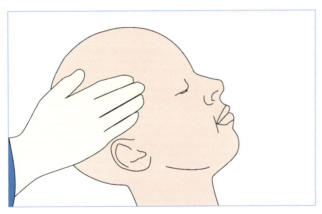

Masseter (middle part).

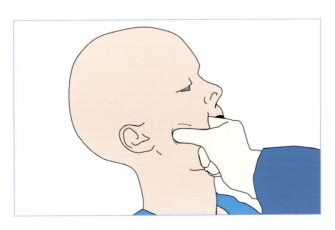

The degree of discomfort caused by muscle palpation can be assessed by the clinician with the aid of feedback from the patient. A simple grading scale such as the following is useful, with the results noted on the patient's chart:

- 0 = no negative effect
- 1 = minor tension and/or pain
- 2 = moderate tension and/or pain
- 3 = high intensity of tension and/or pain

POSTURAL MUSCLES

The dentist should also check for palpation of the occipital, trapezius, and sternocleidomastoid muscles, including the mastoid insertion point of the sternocleidomastoid.

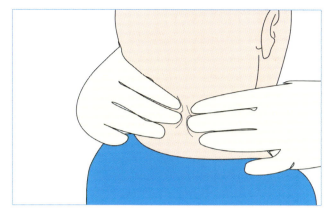

Occipital muscles.

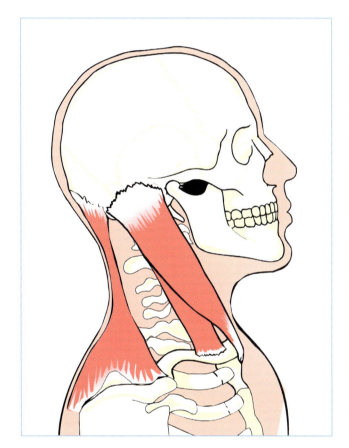

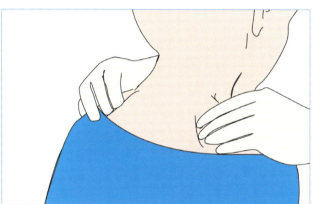

Superior trapezius.

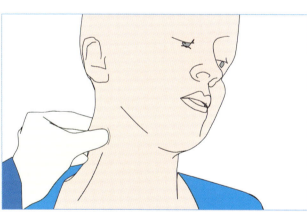

Body of sternocleidomastoid.

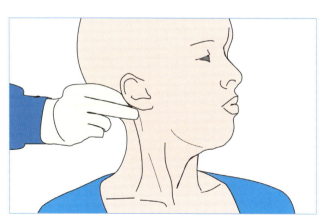

Superior insertion of sternocleidomastoid.

DUAL BITE

The generic expression dual bite refers to an occlusal alteration occurring in the final stage of jaw closure, according to two distinct patterns:

- DENTAL CLOSURE:
  As the patient closes the jaws more tightly, the mandibular cusps slide along the maxillary cusps, reaching maximum intercuspation, which places pressure on the muscles and the TMJs.

- MUSCLE-LED CLOSURE:
  The two arches settle together and stop upon the first dental contacts, no matter how few, without muscle tension.

DUAL BITE	MUSCLE-LED CLOSURE	DENTAL CLOSURE
Other definitions	Centric Normal function Functional efficiency Therapeutic position Centric relation	Habitual Maximum intercuspation Pathologic function Incorrect position Centric occlusion
Contacts between opposing teeth	Very few	Maximum intercuspation
Interarch relations:	Unstable	Stable
Muscle involvement	Normal tension	Stress
Posttreatment outcome	Acceptable or correct	Debatable or negative

Instability of a **MUSCLE-LED BITE** can be checked in a number of ways. These include:

- Initial dental contacts made by guided closure of the patient's jaws
- Psychologic-behavioral training (biofeedback)
- Interposition (possibly subconscious) of the tongue between the teeth, recognizable from visible indentations
- Placement of dental cotton rolls (only for simple immediate checks)
- In very simple cases, selective grinding down of some enamel on a few teeth in a single sitting following articulator study of casts
- In more complex cases, total occlusal restoration, both positive and negative—first done on articulator-mounted casts and then faithfully reproduced on the patient's teeth
- Normal orthodontic treatment to restore correct anatomical and functional relationships
- A six-point splint
- A stabilization splint, which has a positive, albeit a nonspecific, effect
- An anterior repositioning splint (ARS), the most widely used not only to maintain correct condyle-disc-fossa relations but also to rearrange them if necessary

CONSIDERATIONS

- A patient who unknowingly has dental closure is a likely candidate for TMD. All dentists should watch carefully for the warning signs of TMD, no matter what kind of dental checkup is being done.

- In phase II orthodontic occlusal finishing, the choice between dental closure and muscle-led closure is not limited to the pretreatment stage. It must be an ongoing process since gradual tooth movement will create a succession of dual bite patterns requiring attention.

- If muscle-led closure is systematically chosen/preferred, the difference between the two conditions will become gradually less and less, finally disappearing altogether when the teeth have been adapted to the requirements of the muscles and joints, which should be the aim of all dental treatment including orthodontics.

How to proceed

To identify the tooth movements necessary for phase II orthodontic occlusal finishing, patients are asked to reproduce the muscle-led position by removing their ARS and closing their jaws as if the splint were still in place. The clinician notes the extent and location of dental movements required to bring the maxillary and mandibular teeth into a correct intercuspation. The means of accomplishing this differ according to the basic method used. With a removable appliance, the splint is adapted by grinding down the resin and using screws or other additions. With a fixed appliance, movement is achieved with techniques that include, among others, archwire shaping, ligatures, and loops. **It is unthinkable to consider orthodontic treatment completed if the patient still has a dual bite.**
It is important to note that there are patients with stable, muscle-led closure who nevertheless present with muscle and articular complaints. These problems are very likely caused by masticatory parafunction such as bruxism.

Should dual bite always be treated?
The answer is definitely not. A number of factors must be considered in arriving at a decision. If the treatment plan is complex and involves prosthodontic work, surgery, or other significant changes, then the dual bite must be addressed and corrected. In less complicated cases, such as those requiring a simple filling, treatment will probably involve only minor correction techniques. What matters is that the clinician not bend to the patient's wishes without discussing the options and recommending the course of action prompted by professional conscientiousness.

The following double-page illustration shows dual bite documented with cephalography (page 48) and dual bite documented with CT of the left TMJ (volume rendering multilayer spiral CT) (page 49).

DUAL BITE DOCUMENTED WITH CEPHALOGRAPHY
Patient: L. S., age 9 years 5 months

ACCEPTABLE MUSCLE-LED BITE

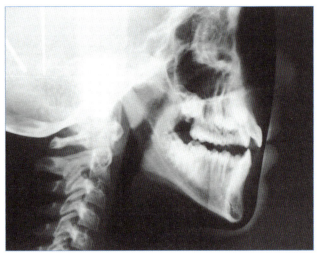

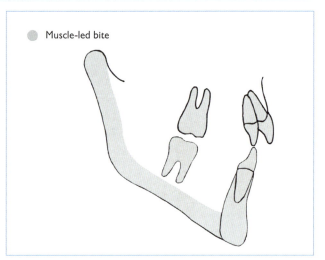

POSITIVE:
- Muscle silence
- Correct anteroposterior relationship
- Correct transversal relationship

DEBATABLE: • Very few dental contacts

NEGATIVE: • Increased vertical height

UNACCEPTABLE DENTAL BITE

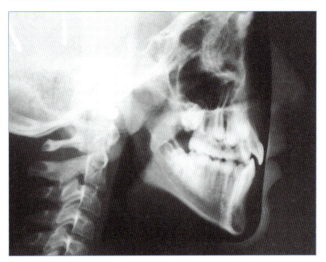

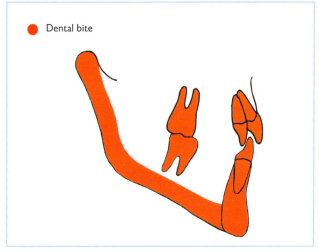

NEGATIVE:
- Muscle stress
- Incorrect anteroposterior relationship
- Incorrect transversal relationship

POSITIVE: • Correct vertical height

It is generally harder to achieve a muscle-led closure in patients with Class II malocclusion, because of the greater skeletal discrepancy, than in patients with Class III malocclusion, whose skeletal discrepancy is less marked than their dental bite discrepancy.[4] As in all aspects of dentistry, correct diagnosis is essential for a successful outcome.

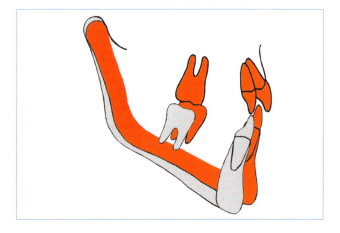

DUAL BITE DOCUMENTED WITH CT OF THE LEFT TMJ (VOLUME RENDERING MULTILAYER SPIRAL CT)

DENTAL-LED BITE	MUSCLE-LED BITE
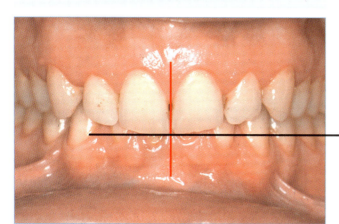	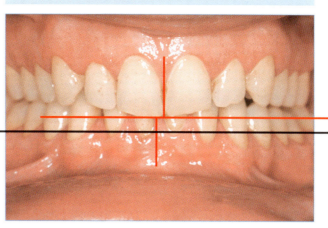
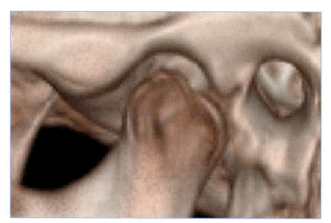	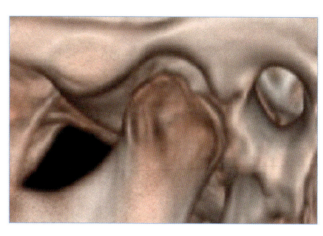

Patient P.F.C.

Left side.

POSITIVE: • In the muscle-led bite, the condyle is seated in an acceptable position within the fossa.

NEGATIVE: • In the dental bite, condylar position within the fossa is unacceptable.

In collaboration with Dr Marialuisa Mandalà, director of Radiology and Imaging Diagnostics Department, City Hospital of Cannizzaro, Italy, and Dr P.F. Carrara.

The patient exhibits a visually evident dual bite, which indicates significant TMJ differences in the different positions. The dislocation is confirmed by volume rendering computerized axial tomography (CAT) scans showing differing condylar head position during maximum intercuspation versus the functionally valid musculoarticular posture. The superimposed outlines further highlight the dislocation.

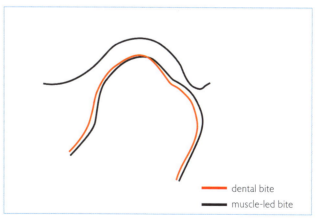

dental bite
muscle-led bite

Superimposed outlines of the condylar head.

MEDICAL IMAGING

TMJ IMAGING DIAGNOSTICS
Section edited by Dr Fabio Ferretti

The information gained from a thorough physical examination can be combined with results of a series of medical tests, coming under the heading of imaging diagnostics, to provide a more accurate diagnosis. The available options include:

1) **OPT** (this page)[5,6]
2) **Oblique transcranial radiography** (facing page)
3) **Conventional tomography** (page 52) (with preliminary axial projection)[7–10]
4) **CT** (page 53)[11]
5) **MRI** (page 56)[12–18]

ORTHOPANTOMOGRAPHY

A dental panoramic radiograph, or OPT, is almost always a first step in the routine examination of stomatognathic pathology and, consequently, in monitoring the TMJs. Proper execution requires a total absence of movement to eliminate artifacts and image distortion. If this is accomplished, the OPT can provide information on:

- Condylar shape
- Condylar osseous structure (with a digital OPT)
- Asymmetry between the two condyles
- Asymmetry between the two mandibular rami

In extreme cases, as when one condyle is clearly less mobile than the other, it may be decided to take an open-mouth OPT to investigate condyle-fossa relationships. And with good skill, particular with positioning and processing techniques, OPT can provide a view of TMJs even in small skulls.

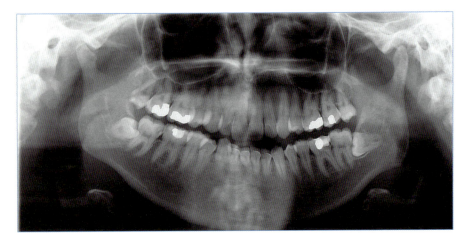

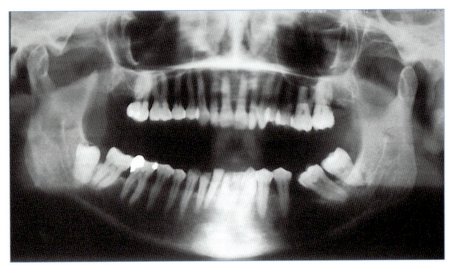

OBLIQUE TRANSCRANIAL RADIOGRAPHY

Craniostat images aid the clinician in diagnosis by giving information on:

- Shape and osseous structure of both condyle and mandibular fossa
- Condyle-fossa articular osseous relations
- TMJ functionality, if comparative images are taken showing the right and left lateral sides of the closed mouth and open mouth.

Right side

Left side

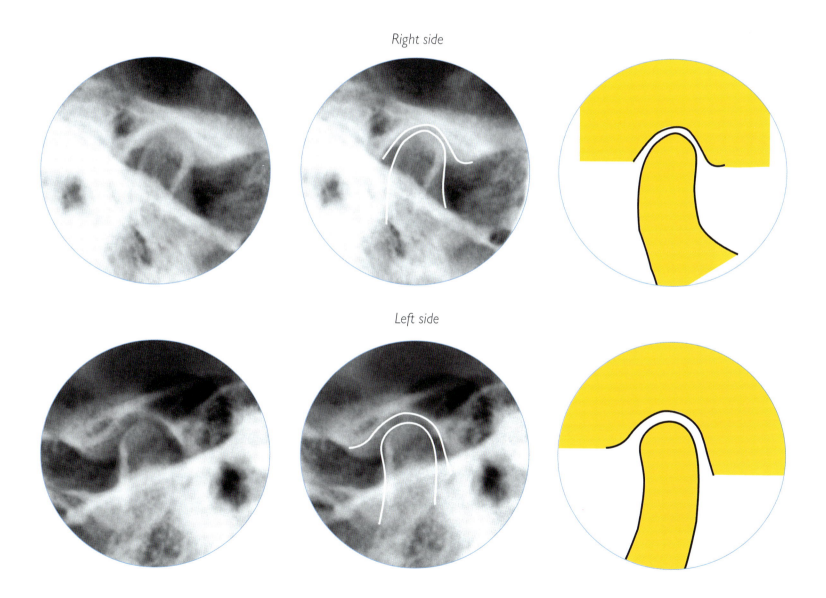

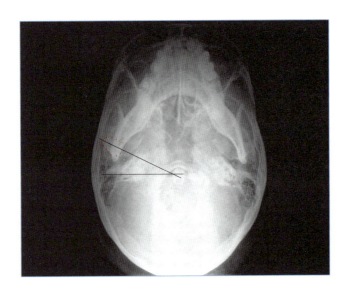

CONVENTIONAL TOMOGRAPHY WITH PRELIMINARY AXIAL PROJECTION

A preliminary submentovertex axial cranial radiograph is useful in establishing condylar position and angle to correctly center the incident beam for the actual tomography. The information provided by tomography is almost identical to that obtained through oblique transcranial radiography with a craniostat. The main drawback of tomography is that the patient receives a greater dose of radiation because of the need for 3 to 4 TMJ projections per side to give both open-mouth and closed-mouth images.

Closed mouth, right side

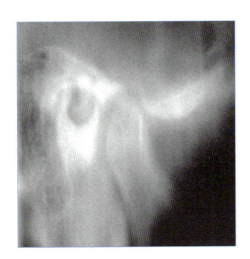 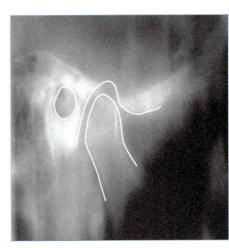 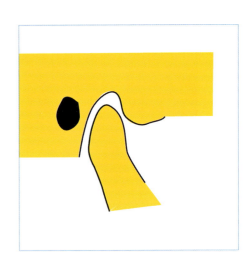

Open mouth, right side

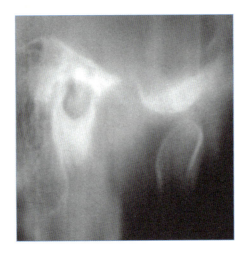 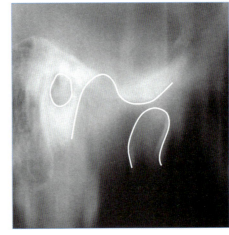 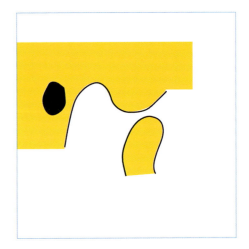

COMPUTED TOMOGRAPHY

Computed Tomography (CT) is a method based on x-ray emission that provides a high-definition scan of the TMJ bony structures. MRI provides better feedback about the soft tissues, specifically the articular disc and muscles. However, well-defined images of TMJ osseous tissue can be obtained with either of the latest-generation CT scanner types: cone beam CT or helical CT.

Cone beam CT scanners include devices designed specifically for the dental office. Dental cone beam CTs gather information from an x-ray beam projected through a "volume" of the maxillofacial region. They provide satisfactory image definition with a relatively low dosage of radiation. In a helical, or spiral, CT, the x-ray beam rotates in a helical trajectory around the maxillofacial region while the patient is moved axially, yielding a spiral scan effect. Another type of CT, computed axial tomography (CAT), also provides axial or transverse images, but stomatologists tend to be less familiar with this type of image.

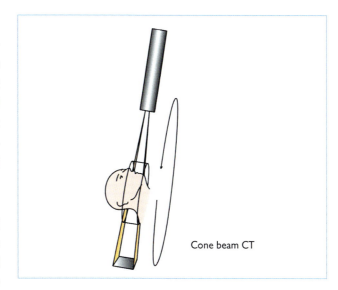

Cone beam CT

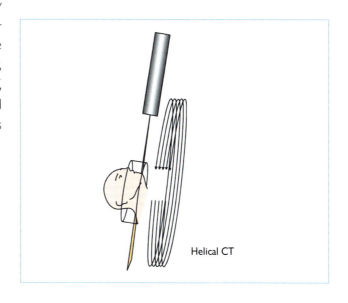

Helical CT

Three-dimensional (3D) reconstruction software programs produce high quality, user-friendly images. The most commonly used projections are oblique sagittal slices, which give a lateral view of the condyle, and oblique coronal slices, which give a front view of the condyle. The usual procedure is to take a series of oblique sagittal slices, left and right and open and closed mouth, followed by a series of oblique coronal slices, also taken left and right and open and closed mouth.

For descriptive simplicity and as a good compromise between test quality and completeness, **a good practice** is to analyze a single left or right TMJ in terms of the **three central slices of each projection** (one closed-mouth sagittal, one open-mouth sagittal and one closed-mouth coronal), as shown bordered in red on the facing page. For even greater simplicity, one may analyze only the central slice (**dual bordered red box**).

Not only does CT aid in the diagnosis of injuries, malformations, and neoplasms, but it is also potentially useful in diagnosing TMDs, including:

- Asymmetric condylar shape
- Bony structure alterations including erosion, flattening, and osteophytes
- Condylar position in relation to the glenoid fossa (closed mouth static study)
- Condylar position in relation to the glenoid fossa (open mouth dynamic study)

While a 3D reconstruction may be useful to provide further clarification into the TMJ anatomic-pathologic state, the general consensus today is that CT is not the imaging technique of choice because of the high dosage of radiation received by the patient.

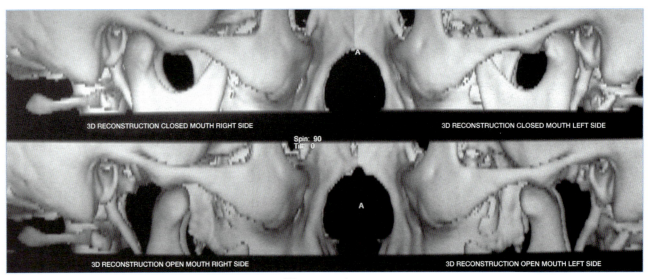

3D reconstruction.

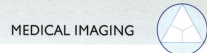

CLOSED-MOUTH SAGITTAL PROJECTIONS
WITH SELECTED SLICES HIGHLIGHTED

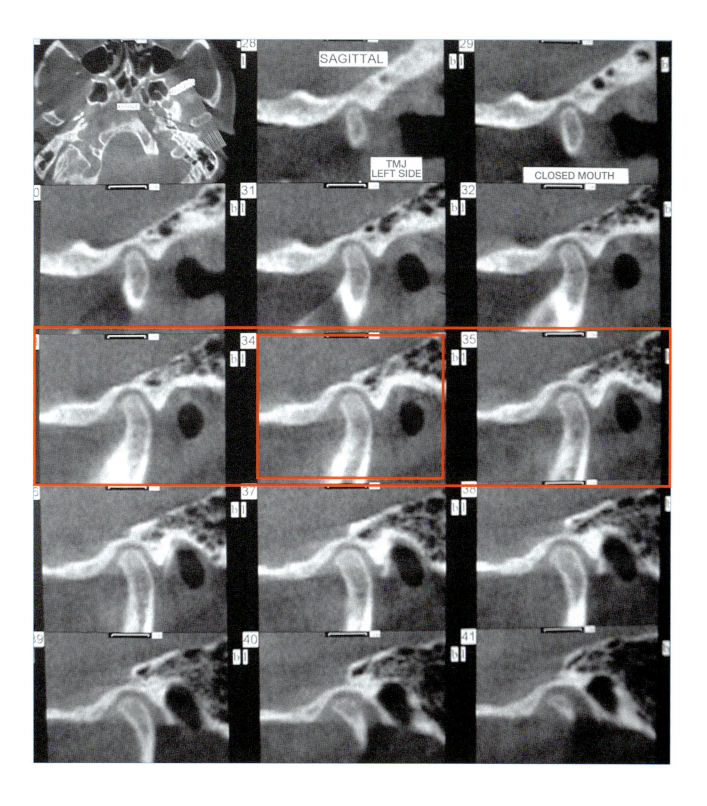

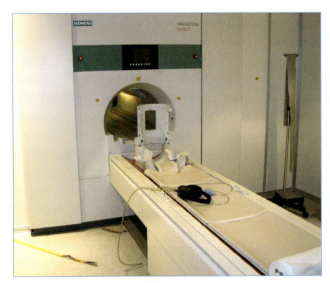

MRI scanner.

is largely its variety of image weighting and relaxation time options, which can be selected according to tissue type whether in normal or pathologic conditions.

Images can be weighted by:

- **T1-relaxation time or the similar proton-density weighting,** which gives predominantly morphologic and dynamic readings
- **T2-relaxation time with fat suppression,** which permits analysis of pathology affecting the **soft tissues** (disc, muscles, bilaminar zone) and **osseous joint structures** (cortical and trabecular bone) and shows any pathologic fluids indicating an inflammatory process such as edema of muscles or trabecular bone or the presence of intracapsular synovial fluid

Fat-suppression techniques are required in T2-weighted sequences to avoid error caused by the resonance frequency similarities of fat and water. By eliminating signals generated by body fat, the technique selects only those coming from pathologic fluids. Failure to suppress these signals would make it impossible to reach a differential diagnosis.

A complete overview of the TMJs requires:

- Closed-mouth sagittal T1-weighted or proton-density–weighted images
- Closed-mouth sagittal fat-suppressed T2-weighted images
- Closed-mouth coronal T1-weighted or proton-density–weighted images
- Open-mouth coronal T1-weighted or proton-density–weighted images

MAGNETIC RESONANCE IMAGING

This medical imaging technique has assumed greater importance in diagnosing TMD because of its reliability and greater safety, having no ionizing radiation. The advent of MRI makes it possible to view not only bony structures but also noncalcified tissue (eg, cartilage)—and thus the disc.

MRI gives information regarding the:

- Condyle, disc, and fossa morphology and relationships
- Presence of intracapsular fluid
- Trophic conditions of the trabecular and cortical bone
- Anatomy and trophic conditions of the peri-articular muscles, especially the lateral pterygoid
- Condition of the bilaminar zone and retrodiscal pad

During MRI, the patient lies for approximately 30 minutes on a table inside a cylindrical tunnel containing a strong magnetic field. This permits good image definition with relatively short scan times, especially if specific receiver coils are used. MRI is contraindicated for patients suffering from claustrophobia or those who have any metal items in their body. An open scanner may be suitable for use with claustrophobic patients, but it has a weaker magnetic field and may give lower quality images.

The advantage of MRI over other imaging techniques

BENEFITS OF MRI FOR PATIENTS WITH TMJ DYSFUNCTION

MRI has become an essential tool in diagnosis and the ongoing clinical management of TMD patients at differing stages. It enables the clinician to:

- Detect an unsuspected pathology
- Confirm a suspected pathology
- Evaluate the stage of pathology
- Assess the effects of treatment

MRI assists with diagnosis, prognosis, treatment, and outcome by helping the clinician to:

- Be aware of any signs indicating muscle involvement or intracapsular fluids (such as those provoked by injury) where there is currently no alteration to the condyle or disc
- Know the exact disc position:
  - Anterior disc dislocation, posterior dislocation being extremely rare
  - Medial or lateral disc dislocation (forms of rotational disc dislocation)
  - Anteromedial or anterolateral dislocation, these being the most common
- Classify open-mouth disc recapture:
  - Dislocation with disc reduction or recapture
  - Dislocation without disc reduction
- Observe any signs of arthopathy (sign of tissue destruction) when the pathology has advanced

These considerations and the certainty of further technologic improvement in image quality make it likely that MRI use will continue to increase, accompanied by greater cooperation between radiologists and dentists.

CONDYLE-DISC-FOSSA MORPHOLOGY AND RELATIONS

MRI oblique sagittal images show the TMJ anatomy in much the same way as conventional radiography. The drumstick-shaped condyle appears to float within the temporal bone depression concavity, bordered anteriorly by the anterior articular eminence and posteriorly by the external auditory meatus. What MRI adds to the picture is the fibrocartilagenous disc, an addition that shows disc position and movement both anteroposteriorly and mediolaterally. When viewed sagitally, a normal articular disc is biconcave in shape, with thicker anterior and posterior regions and a thinner central portion. When the jaws are closed, the posterior segment lies in the 12 o'clock position over the condylar apex.

One of the first structures affected by TMD is the disc, which dislocates from its normal position in the first stages of internal derangement. Initially, only a part of the disc protrudes, producing a clicking or popping sound. Only MRI can establish the exact nature of the dislocation although the usual pattern is disc forward and condyle backward in the fossa. When the mouth is opened, it is possible to see whether the disc is recaptured. As the pathology progresses, the disc shape can also indicate the stage of pathology, becoming progressively more irregular, whether torn, folded over, or biconvex.

INTRACAPSULAR FLUID

Unlike all other currently available imaging techniques, MRI can show the presence of bodily fluids because of its versatility in imaging according to the acquisition parameters applied. The TMJ, like all skeletal joints, reacts to inflammation with exudate, which can be recognized even in small quantities in certain fat-suppressed T2-weighted sequences. Obviously, proof of the presence of intracapsular or pericapsular fluid is of key importance for the clinician, especially if associated with localized pain.

TROPHISM OF TRABECULAR AND CORTICAL BONE

Familiarity with MRI semiotics is fundamental to distinguishing compact cortical bone (extremely low MRI signal intensity; seen as black in both T1- and T2-weighted images) from trabecular bone (seen as white in T1-weighted images and yielding an intermediate appearance in T2-weighted images). Because MRI makes it possible to detect even the slightest sign of fluids, such as edema in the condyle's trabecular portion, this technique may acquire diagnostic importance in the context of an evolving arthropathy causing internal derangement. In such cases, the T2-weighted images of the condylar trabecular bone will give an intense white signal greater than its normal intermediate response. The expected visual signs of TMJ arthropathy—such as flattening of joint extremities, osteophytes, and bone necrosis—that are familiar from traditional radiology are present in MRIs as well.

ANATOMY AND TROPHISM OF LATERAL PTERYGOID MUSCLES

TMDs may be expressed by muscle pathology alone or in association with joint involvement. The muscles of mastication, with the lateral pterygoid foremost, are the primary target of dental malocclusion, which leads in various ways to TMJ functional asymmetry and ultimately affects masticatory muscle tone. Sooner or later, the muscles respond with contraction, inflammation, edema, and altered muscle trophism.

MRI produces an excellent portrait of the lateral pterygoid muscle that distinguishes the superior and inferior bundles, enabling the clinician to detect these initial signs of dysfunction. With MRI, it is also possible to observe *(1)* edema in fat-suppressed T2-weighted images, semiotically viewable as thin white lines of signal hyperintensity between the muscle fiber bundles, and *(2)* areas of atrophy visible as widespread areas of adipose infiltration (intense T1-weighted or proton-density–weighted signal) in the muscle bundles, reduced in height, too.

CONDITION OF THE BILAMINAR ZONE AND RETRODISCAL PAD

The bilaminar zone and retrodiscal pad of the TMJ have undergone recent investigation by a number of authors. Physically, the bilaminar zone extends posteriorly to the posterior disc band and consists of two laminae of dense connective tissue. The superior lamina, a connective tissue rich in elastic fibers, inserts into the posterior wall of the glenoid fossa. The inferior lamina, a fibrous tissue with low elastin content, inserts into the posterior profile of the mandibular condyle. It is less visible in MRI than is the superior lamina. Open-mouth proton-density–weighted MRI has shown that when the jaws are open, the superior lamina stretches and comes into contact with the dome of the glenoid fossa.

When the condyle translates anteriorly, the empty space left in the retrodiscal pad is engorged by venous dilation from the considerable venous plexus present among the fibers and elastin that make up most of the loose connective tissue. The retrodiscal pad is clearly visible in open-mouth, oblique, sagittal T1- or proton-density–weighted images. It presents a brighter signal than the posterior band of the meniscus and bilaminar zone because of its rich adipose tissue pattern and heavy vascularization.

The greater the extent of buccal opening (and hence the greater the extent of anterior condyle translation), the clearer the MRI signal. This is explained by the so-called blood pump function of the retrodiscal area by which anterior translation of the condyle causes the elastic connective tissue to stretch and expand the inner venous plexus spaces, increasing blood supply. Return of the condyle on buccal closure creates pressure that forces blood out of the plexus.

In the early stages of TMJ internal derangement, a secondary effect of the abnormal movement of the disc and, consequently, of the bilaminar zone layers is a state of hyperemia in the retrodiscal tissue. In these cases, especially where the patient complains of articular pain, confirmation is given by increased signal intensity from the retrodiscal tissue in open-mouth T2-weighted sequences.

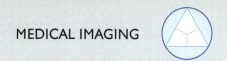

TMJ MAGNETIC RESONANCE SEMIOTICS

Magnetic resonance imaging contrast

	T1	T2
Cortical bone	Low intensity (black)	Low intensity (black)
Trabecular bone	High intensity (white)	Low intensity (black)
Disc	Average intensity (gray)	Average intensity (gray)
Pterygoid muscle	Average intensity (gray)	Low intensity (black)
Pathologic fluids (secretion or edema)	Not always visible	High intensity (white) with fat suppression

MRI SEMIOTICS IN TMJ EVALUATION: A CLINICAL VIEWPOINT

The dense bone of the cortex and glenoid fossa gives a very low signal (black) in all sequences. The same is true of fibrous connective tissue, such as that covering the cortex and fossa, which has a weak signal (black) indistinguishable from that of the dense bone. In contrast, trabecular bone gives an intense, bright white signal with T1- or proton-density–weighted images.

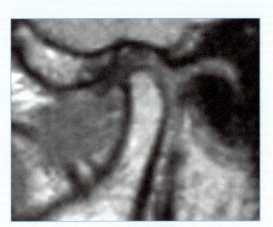

T1 normal TMJ.

The articular disc presents a moderately low signal (varying shades of gray) in all T1- or proton-density–weighted scans.

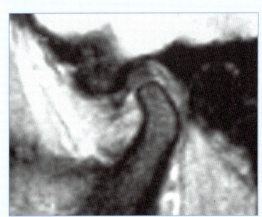

T2 normal TMJ.

The lateral pterygoid muscle is visible as a fan shape with its condylar insertion and two muscle belly (superior and inferior) often separated by a gap corresponding to an intense MRI signal of vascular origin. In healthy conditions, this muscle gives an even, moderately intense signal, weaker than that given by the disc.

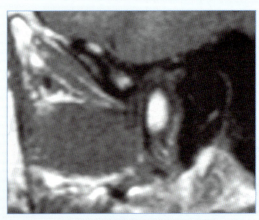

Normal TMJ and pterygoid.

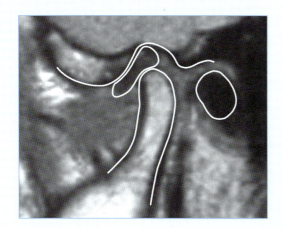

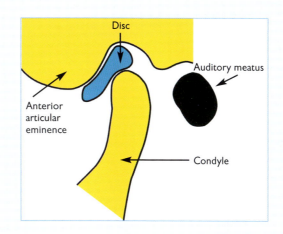

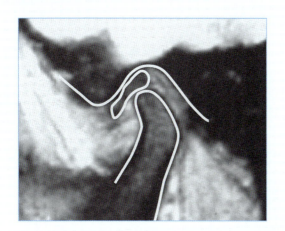

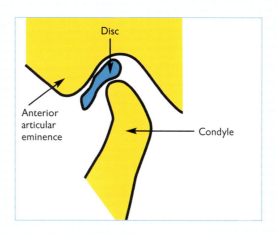

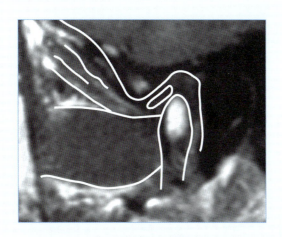

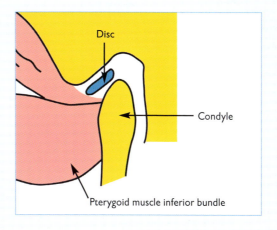

MRI OF SELECTED MUSCLES

T1-weighted coronal cross-section showing medial pterygoid muscle on the inside and masseter on the outside.

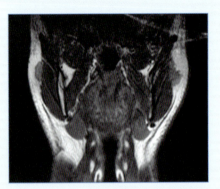

Coronal cross-section of masseter and medial pterygoid.

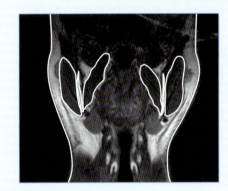

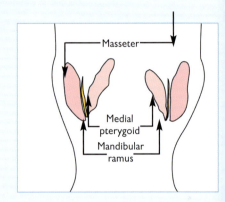

T1-weighted axial cross-section of the neck: The sternocleidomastoid muscle is seen on the outside.

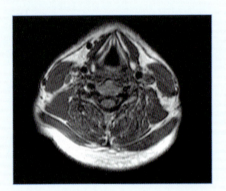

Sternocleidomastoid: axial cross-section.

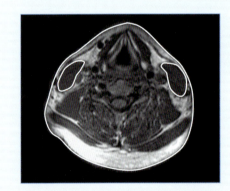

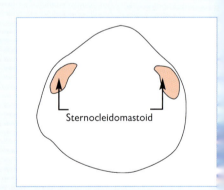

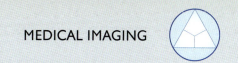

SYNTHESIS OF ADVANTAGES AND DISADVANTAGES OF DIFFERENT TMJ IMAGING TECHNIQUES

Test type	Patient radiation dose	Bony structure definition	Soft tissue definition
OBLIQUE TRANSCRANIAL RADIOGRAPHY	Low	Average	None
CONVENTIONAL CT	High	Good	None
CT CONE BEAM Helical	High Very high	Very good Excellent	Minimal Minimal
MRI	None	Average	Excellent

IMPORTANCE OF CHECKING 3D MANDIBULAR MOVEMENTS
Essential indicators in clinical practice

Testing mandibular dynamics on all three spatial planes is a straightforward process and is of strategic clinical importance at all stages, including diagnosis, treatment, evaluation of final outcome, and subsequent follow-up. Careful observation of hinge, lateral, and translatory movements ensures attention to functional efficiency, especially in cases where medical imaging such as CT and MRI may not be feasible. Assessment of 3D mandibular movement is therefore recommended as part of a routine screening procedure, with results entered in the patient's records as a matter of course. Especially where other diagnostic information is unavailable, it is reasonable to suppose that a good response to mandibular assessment indicates, with clinical validity, a good equilibrium between teeth, muscles, and TMJs.

TEETH

Even with the slightest of jaw movements, the teeth are the point of reference, both in the final stages of closure (dual bite) and in checking 3D mandibular dynamics.

MUSCLES

The muscles are the motors of all orofacial movement including mastication, speech, and posture. Muscle stress may contribute to alterations in mandibular movement with long-term effects on the TMJ.

TEMPOROMANDIBULAR JOINTS

The TMJs are a systematic cause of altered pathways with changes of position and shape in joint anatomic structures.

MANDIBLE

The mandible is a suspended organ hinging on two reciprocating joints that allow it to perform a vast number of movements.

To aid examination of the details, especially at the beginning of each movement, a magnifying glass has been drawn at the point corresponding to the first few millimeters of movement *in each drawing*.

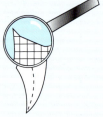

SAGITTAL PLANE:
POSSELT'S ENVELOPE
To assess the extent of sagittal movement, both posteroanterior and vertical.

In clinical practice: This is difficult to apply. Examination of the sagittal plane is very useful in assessing dual bite, which should always be checked.
Not included in the authors' clinical evaluation.

HORIZONTAL PLANE (occlusal surface level): Shows both protrusion (average, 7 mm) and right and left lateral movements (average, 11 mm).

In clinical practice: The horizontal plane is easy to monitor, and this evaluation **should be standard practice.**

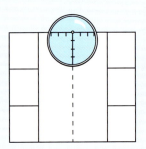

TRANSVERSAL PLANE (front): This is divided vertically into three segments of 15 mm each. The extent of mouth opening, or gape (average, 45 mm), is measured with handheld calipers or a gauge with the clinician facing the patient. If pathology is suspected, the clinician should assess lateral movements by looking from above the patient's head. However, lateral movements should also be checked from the front, ideally every 15 mm.

In clinical practice: Transversal plane assessment **should always be done,** despite a certain degree of subjectivity of interpretation. Any clicks should be noted with details of position and type of noise.

SUMMARY OF 3D TESTS

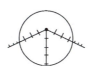

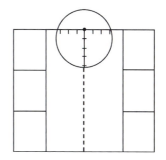

INTERPRETATION: TYPICAL EXAMPLES		

Limited excursions:

Right: healthy condyle
The locked left condyle is unable to orbit to the right toward the healthy condyle.

3   10

Left: locked condyle
The healthy right condyle is able to orbit to the left toward the locked condyle.

Ligamentous laxity
Excursions exceed the normal limits, almost always on both sides, indicating a tendency that most likely affects all joints in the patient's body.

13   14

53 mm

Deflection
Lack of coordination in dual TMJ dynamics. The opening pathway is deflected to one side when the mouth is opened but then returns toward the center at the end of the movement.

Deviation
Prevalent musculoarticular pathology in one condyle. The mandible shifts laterally, often with limited movement, as in this case where it is affected by damage to the right condyle.

Clicking
Sudden deviation due to disc recapture on the damaged side. The disc can sometimes be heard popping out.

click

The 3D images give a clear and complete view of the mouth in isolation, which cannot always be achieved when observing a patient.

PROTRUSION AND LATERAL MOVEMENT   PROTRUSION

NORMAL

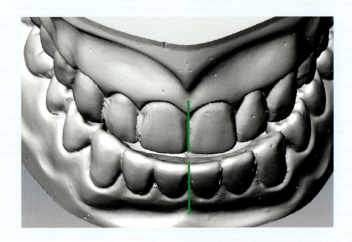

In normal conditions, protrusion should measure approximately 7 mm; left and right lateral movements, approximately 11 mm.

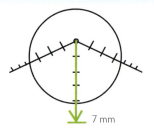

7 mm

PATHOLOGY

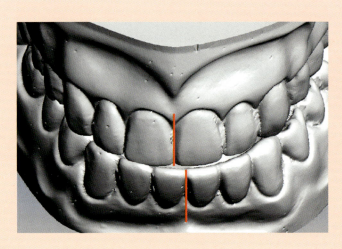

Deviation to the left on protrusion due to pathology of the left condyle.

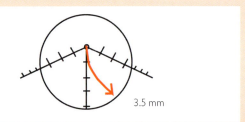

3.5 mm

Right   **LATERAL SHIFT**   left

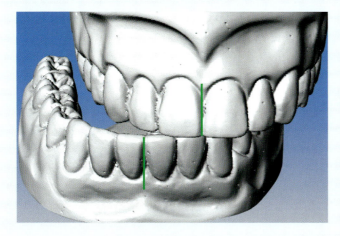

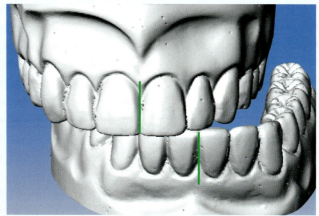

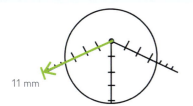

11 mm

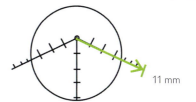

11 mm

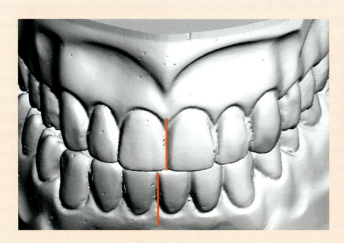

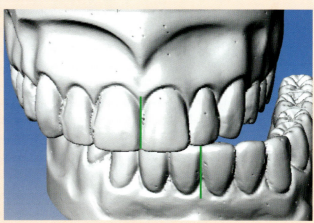

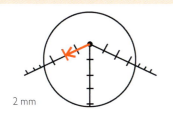

2 mm

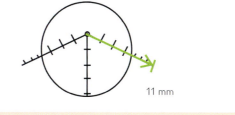

11 mm

Lesser extent of excursion to the right due to damaged left orbiting condyle.

Complete lateral excursion to the left is possible because the damaged condyle is the rotating left condyle.

OPENING AND CLOSURE

Normal mouth opening should measure approximately 45 mm and be free of deviation or deflection on both opening and closing movements. Any altered movements should be investigated to determine the cause. For instance, a monolateral dislocation without reduction (or recapture) may deviate toward the affected side, which is extremely serious. In contrast, a monolateral deflection on the same side may indicate a less serious dislocation with reduction. Clearly, the two cases have a considerably different prognosis.

NORMAL

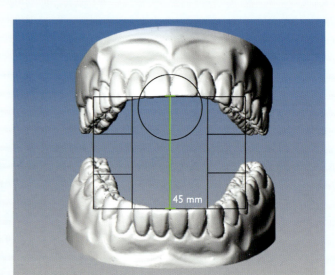

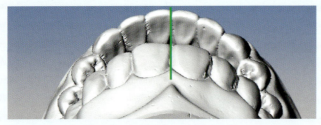

View from behind the patient's head.

PATHOLOGY

Deviation on opening and closure.

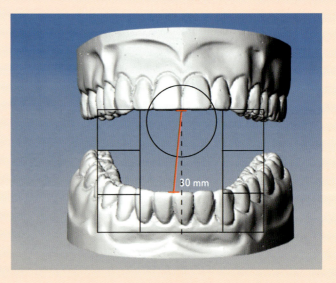

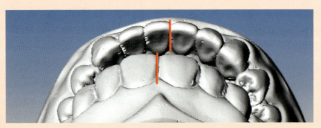

View from behind the patient's head.

The full extent of the patient's gape should be measured with calipers with the clinician facing the patient whereas assessment of opening and closing movements should be done from behind, with the clinician observing the maxillary incisor midline or frenula to note any misalignment with the mandibular incisor midline or frenula.

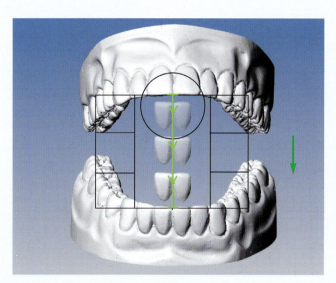

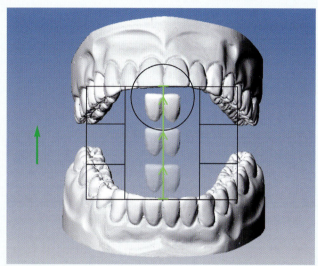

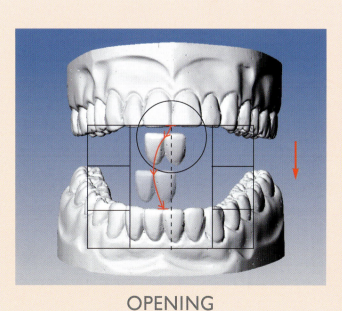

OPENING

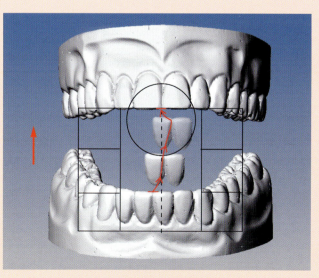

CLOSURE

TMJ PALPATION

TMJ movement and noise are assessed during buccal opening and closure, left and right lateral movements, and protrusion.

Procedure
- To proceed with external palpation, the tips of the index and middle fingers are placed over the TMJs, anterior to the tragus. Both TMJs should be palpated simultaneously as the patient opens and closes the jaws so that any lack of coordination between left and right can be observed. Ask the patient to repeat the movements several times.

The main points to feel for include:

- Excursions: Are they simultaneous or staggered? Are they complete or limited?
- Noises: Are any noises present? If so, what type (eg, clicking, grating) and when do they occur (early, mid-excursion, late, reciprocal, during both opening and closure)?
- Pain: Is the patient experiencing pain? If so, it probably results from both posterior bilaminar zone pressure and involvement of the lateral pterygoid external band.

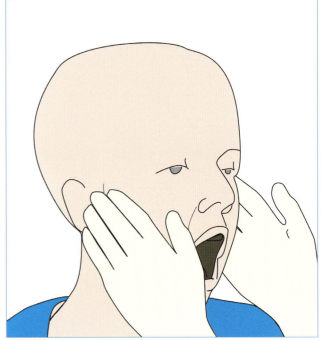

External palpation.

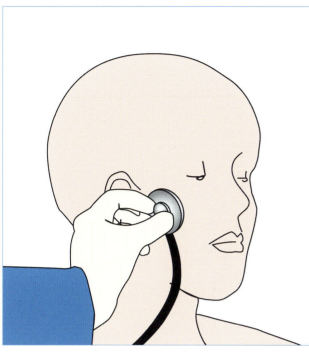
Auscultation with stethoscope.

AUSCULTATON

A stethoscope is valuable for providing additional information during thorough examination of the TMJs. To avoid interference from hair or facial hair, the stethoscope diaphragm should be placed over the zygomatic bone. Auscultation can indicate whether the disc is recaptured and the effects of recapture where there is dislocation with or without reduction. It also gives further details on the sound signal, which can actually be heard with this method, and the different types of noise (eg, snapping, sandy, continuous grating, clicking, popping).

A change in noise can provide useful information about a patient's condition, such as:

- The disappearance of noise on normal opening movements indicates an improvement in articular function.
- A total absence of articular noise associated with reduced gape indicates TMJ or muscular lock.
- The disappearance of a noise previously heard may suggest the forward dislocation of the disc without reduction, indicating deterioration of the pathology.

Manipulation of one or both joints to place the mandible into what is, presumably, its best position (usually forward and downward from where it was) while having the patient open and close the jaws repeatedly in this position may cause the noise to disappear or lessen considerably as the disc itself reduces. However, only a thorough examination of mandibular movements combined with essential MRIs will enable the clinician to clearly distinguish the condition of and relations between the condyle, disc, and articulating surface. It is unlikely that these conditions will remain consistent because of factors such as alterations in TMJ structure, the patient's attitude and behavior, and efficacy of treatment, among others.

DIAGNOSTIC-THERAPEUTIC MANUAL TECHNIQUES

WHAT ARE THEY?

Diagnostic-therapeutic manual techniques are hands-on maneuvers performed by the clinician on the patient for a number of reasons: They may help the clinician assess muscle and TMJ pathology. They may provide some relief for the patient, thus indirectly aiding the teeth as well. For example, diagnostic-therapeutic manual techniques may help to restore teeth, muscles, and joints from a condition of maximum intercuspation (dental closure), which is unacceptable since it creates muscle tension, to a correct, muscle-led musculoarticular relationship, albeit with few interarch dental contacts yet functionally efficient. **Another technique includes taking wax bites and impressions for the subsequent manufacture of splint, which hold the mandible and TMJs in a therapeutic position that serves as a permanent point of reference during treatment (see page 102).** The vast range of solutions allows clinicians to choose different treatment options based on personal preference, but all choices are directed at achieving the same positive outcome.

Manipulation sometimes provides instant relief of symptoms and the underlying pathology, thus contributing noticeably to solving the case. It is often a pleasant surprise to see an apparently simple procedure produce a major benefit, and how rapidly. A key condition of using any manual technique is that it must be performed skilfully, at the right moment, and with the most efficient procedure. A limitation of these techniques is that they are considered difficult to standardize.

ESTABLISHING CORRECT INTERARCH RELATIONSHIPS IN THE FINAL STAGES OF BUCCAL CLOSURE

It should be borne in mind that a dual bite (full intercuspation versus muscle-led closure) may recur during the various stages of orthodontic treatment. Although imaging may be performed in either position, muscle-led closure is the preferred choice, even if there are few dental contacts.

Regardless of the type of specialist dealing with the case, the type of closure must be chosen, and treatment must be concluded with total muscle silence, ie, absence of tension.

In addition, it should be remembered that, whatever the treatment applied, spontaneous changes may occur, for the better or for the worse, thus improving or deteriorating interarch dental relationships.

SUMMARY AND CLINICAL IMPLICATIONS OF DUAL BITE

MUSCLE-LED CLOSURE with normal muscle tone	DENTAL CLOSURE with muscle tension
No deviation when closing the jaws, but few dental contacts (FUNCTIONAL EFFICIENCY).	Deviation in every direction, in final contacts between arches, showing maximum dental intercuspation (or HABITUAL closure).

ANTEROPOSTERIOR RELATIONS

ACCEPTABLE or at least functional.	INCORRECT (often) due to deviation. Class II division1 may in fact be class I. Class III cases may seem worse than they actually are.

TRANSVERSAL RELATIONS

ACCEPTABLE or at least functional.	INCORRECT (often) due to deviation.

VERTICAL RELATIONS

ALTERED as a result of increase.	FUNCTIONAL even if deviated in other relationships.

IN ALL CASES, THE TEETH, MUSCLES,
AND JOINTS FORM AN INSEPARABLE UNIT

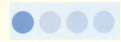

FIRST PROCEDURE:
Guided buccal closure aided by the clinician

PURPOSE: to detect the presence of dual bite
This method should always be used to ascertain whether the patient has a dual bite, specifically:

- A muscle-led bite with few dental contacts and without muscle tension—the reference bite for all therapeutic procedures
- A dental bite in maximum intercuspation (also known as habitual), often accompanied by muscle tension and pain indicating the onset of pathology

1. Ask patients to relax their muscles.
2. Place the fingers of one hand against the lower part of the mandible with the thumb on the dimple.
3. Gently guide mandibular movements; open and close the jaws with the muscles still relaxed.
4. Try to bring the condyles downward and forward with the chin slightly protruded until a final contact position is reached between the teeth in the opposing jaws, even if the contacts are few.

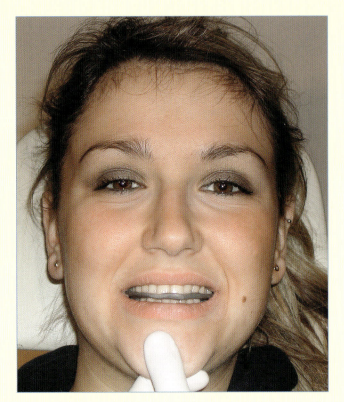

Since the patient's muscle tone is relaxed, the movements and contacts must be consistent. The greater the patient's compliance and the less the degree of damage present, the easier it will be to achieve a repeatable movement. **This manipulation should take place not only at the initial examination but also systematically at every appointment with the patient and at all stages of treatment, whether orthodontic or not.**
A key consideration is that the teeth must adapt to the requirements of the muscles, and not vice versa, to prevent abnormal pressure of the joints, which is likely to lead to pathology. Furthermore, bear in mind that maximum intercuspation may be natural to a particular patient. It is not necessarily a symptom of pathology **unless accompanied by muscle tension.**

FIRST PROCEDURE:
Guided buccal closure aided by the clinician

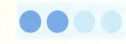

SECOND PROCEDURE:
Dawson's manipulation method[19]

PURPOSE: to detect the presence of dual bite by checking dental contacts in a correct function without muscle tension

This method is more investigative than the previous method, and it is particularly efficient for neuromuscular deprogramming.

1. With the patient lying supine, point the chin upward.
2. Move behind the patient, and hold the patient's head as still as possible.
3. Grasp the lower edge of the mandible bilaterally with the four fingers of each hand on either side.
4. Exert slight pressure on the mental symphysis with the thumbs.

5. Very gently manipulate the mandible to open and close it slowly as it glides automatically in a position of muscle relaxation. Any pressure exerted will cause a periarticular response with greater contraction, making it extremely difficult to find a physiologic relaxed contact between the arches. The purpose of this maneuver is to deprogram muscle tension to obtain a correct mandibular closure path until the first dental contact is achieved with correct muscle tension.

6. Apply upward pressure with the fingers while using the thumbs to press on the symphysis to open the bite. The doctor must maintain this pressure firmly while exercising a rotating movement on the condyles.. If the patient does not present any sign of tension, it may be initially deduced that this is the therapeutic position, which then should be confirmed by medical imaging done in the same position.

THIRD PROCEDURE:
Cotton rolls

PURPOSE: to detect the presence of dual bite

1. Place two cotton rolls, approximately 1.5 cm long, in the posterior quadrants of the patient's mouth. If needed, use support clips during placement. (Remove them once the rolls have been positioned.) The exclusion of occlusal interference makes it possible to confirm whether the patient has a dual bite. If this is the case, only the muscle-led bite will be correct.
2. Ask the patient to walk for several minutes and to swallow as often as possible before sitting down again.
3. Remove the cotton rolls, and guide buccal closure until the first dental interarch contacts are reached in a muscle-led therapeutic position.

The same procedure may be used at various treatment stages for instant monitoring of muscle relaxation.

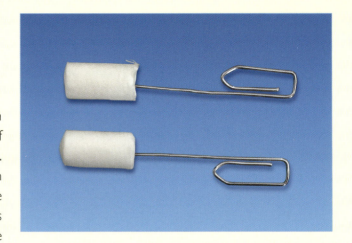

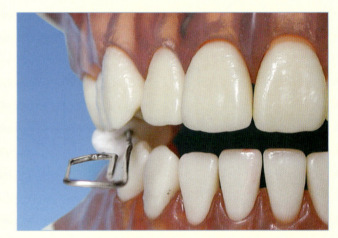

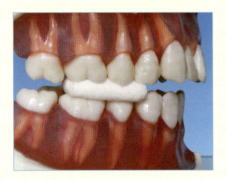

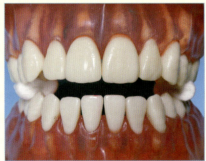

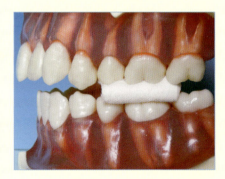

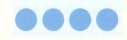

FOURTH PROCEDURE:
Use of cotton rolls to diagnose facial pain and postural disorders

PURPOSE: to relieve facial pain and improve skeletal muscle postural pathology
This procedure is a variation of the third procedure.

FACIAL PAIN
1. Palpate the muscles of mastication and posture, and record the results in terms of intensity.
2. Apply cotton rolls to ascertain, beyond doubt, whether the patient is actually affected by the pathology. If the third method had a positive effect, then this procedure will more clearly indicate the degree of stomatognathic apparatus involvement.

POSTURE
The cotton roll method is used to establish changes in skeletal muscle posture. Observe the same muscles before and after the cotton roll treatment, and note any positive changes.

EMPIRICAL EXPERIENCE
The same techniques used during diagnosis and observation—with and without the cotton rolls—are repeated, as follows:

1. Have the patient stand still, and from behind, observe whether both shoulders are held at the same height.
2. With the patient sitting, palpate the head, neck, and shoulder postural muscles.
3. With the patient lying supine, check the length of both legs.
4. Remove the cotton rolls, and ask the patient to perform protrusive and closure movements, without previously bringing the teeth into contact, until the first contact is reached.

This procedure should be performed last since closing the jaws is likely to return the patient to a position of maximum intercuspation with muscle stress.

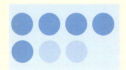

FIFTH PROCEDURE:
HORIZONTAL AND VERTICAL MANIPULATION

CLINICAL APPLICATION: dislocation with disc reduction

Purpose: to obtain axial alignment between condyle, disc, and fossa and make clicking noises disappear by achieving total or partial disc recapture

It should be borne in mind that, typically, condylar excursions are greater than those followed by the disc. In dislocation, the condyle rests in the posterosuperior part of the mandibular fossa while the disc is usually displaced in an anteroinferior or (occasionally) medial position.

MANIPULATION ON THE HORIZONTAL PLANE

1. From a position at the patient's side, place one hand and wrist beneath the mandible, with the thumb in the symphysis.
2. With slight movements that gradually become more active, move the mandible laterally on the horizontal plane, first to one side and then to the other.

MANIPULATION ON THE VERTICAL PLANE

1. From the same position at the patient's side, place the thumb on the mandibular incisor's occlusal faces, with the other fingers under the mandible to distract it anterovertically.
2. If appropriate, intensify the vertical movement by exerting greater thumb pressure on the incisors to rotate the mandible further forward and downward.

In many cases, these manipulations bring about considerable improvement in articular dynamics in all three planes of space because of the (temporary) recapture of the disc and consequent disappearance of the clicking noise. In straightforward cases, manipulation alone may be a definitive solution. Remeasurement of the patient's various mandibular movements often confirms improvement in terms of both extent and correct direction.

This is one of the most commonly indicated types of manipulation and often gives distinctly positive results.

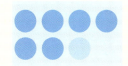

SIXTH PROCEDURE:
HORIZONTAL AND VERTICAL MANIPULATION OF GREATER INTENSITY AND DURATION

PURPOSE: dislocation without reduction of the disc and/or tissue destruction through osteoarthrosis causing changes in shape and position

The clinician should carry out the fifth procedure to treat dislocation with reduction, repeatedly moving the mandible horizontally (both left and right) and vertically. This is done with the aim of rearranging, as far as possible, the partially or totally damaged articular structures.

It is not uncommon to find that postmanipulation measurements confirm considerable improvement, with spontaneous movements becoming wider and following a more normal path. A number of factors, including age, duration of pathology, and extent of progressive deterioration, contribute to the profile. Clearly, the greater the anatomic and functional damage and the more limited the patient's mandibular movement, the less hopeful the prognosis will be.

It should be emphasized that the manipulation should be repeated frequently and with increasing pressure. Ideally, a compliant patient will be taught to do the movements as exercises at home.

LEFT LATERAL MOVEMENT

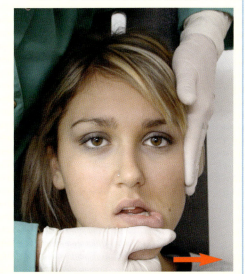

RIGHT LATERAL MOVEMENT

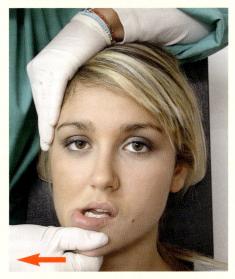

PROTRUSION

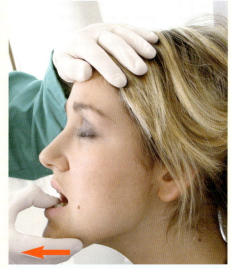

Side view

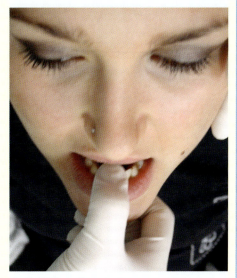

Viewed from above and front

GAPE

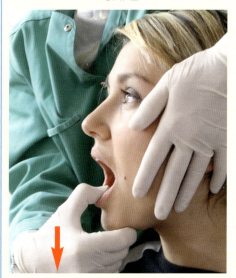

Side view

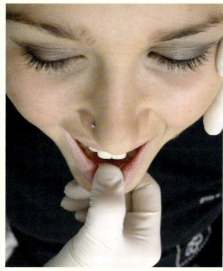

Viewed from above

79

UNLOCKING DOCUMENTED WITH PRE- AND POSTMANIPULATION CT SCANS-CHANGE IN CONDYLAR POSITION AS A RESULT OF MANIPULATION
Edited by Dr Pietro Petroni

Patient D. S., age 21

The patient reported progressive difficulty in opening her mouth properly. Clinical examination confirmed TMJ lock with reduced all-around movement. Her gape was limited to 28 mm with considerable deviation (approximately 12 mm) toward the left side.

CLOSED MOUTH (RIGHT SIDE)

Premanipulation

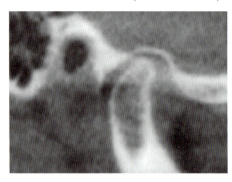

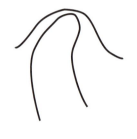

Superimposed pre- and postmanipulation outlines

Postmanipulation

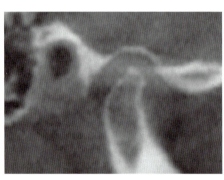

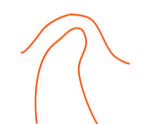

CLOSED MOUTH (LEFT SIDE)

Premanipulation

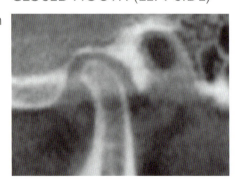

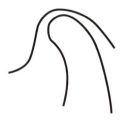

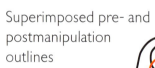

Superimposed pre- and postmanipulation outlines

Postmanipulation

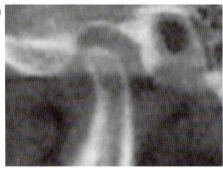

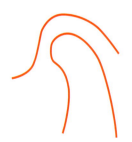

Unlocking exercises almost immediately produced a gape of 50 mm in an almost straight line. The startling changes were also documented through CT scans taken only minutes apart during the same appointment in both closed-mouth and open-mouth positions.

INCREASE IN CONDYLAR TRANSLATION POSTMANIPULATION
(pre- and post-CT scans taken the same day)

OPEN MOUTH (RIGHT SIDE)

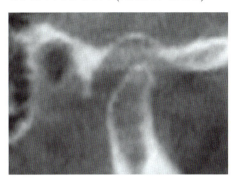

Premanipulation

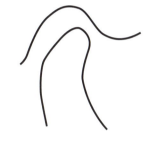

Superimposed pre- and postmanipulation outlines

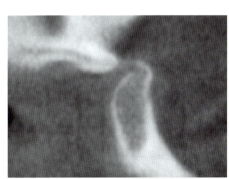

Postmanipulation

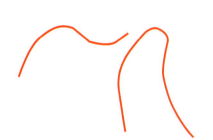

OPEN MOUTH (LEFT SIDE)

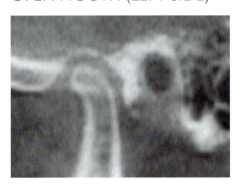

Premanipulation

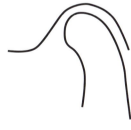

Superimposed pre- and postmanipulation outlines

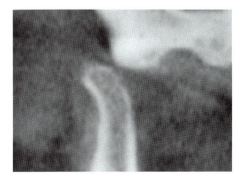

Postmanipulation

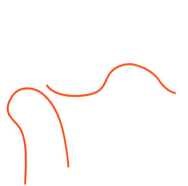

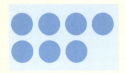

SEVENTH PROCEDURE. UNLOCKING MOVEMENTS

PURPOSE: to reduce TMJ lock of one or both joints (also referred to on page 183)

The **TMJs are manipulated** using the techniques described for the fifth and sixth procedures. Multiple factors determine success, including the patient's age, anatomic alteration, and length of time the pathology has persisted.

In cases of **acute TMJ lock**, a mere few movements may produce an extremely positive effect, giving intense satisfaction not only to the patient, most of whose immediate symptoms seem to miraculously disappear, but also to the clinician, whose diagnosis is confirmed and whose treatment is seen to have worked. As in the other cases, it is advisable to measure results by recording pre- and postmanipulation movement widths. Patients with acute cases of TMJ lock may see an increase in gape ranging from about 20 mm to as much as 40 mm or more in the course of a few minutes. In its turn, this improvement leads to considerable improvement in muscle tone and pain relief. An ARS is immediately recommended as a means to maintain a therapeutic position (once this has been confirmed), following appropriate psychologic briefing of the patient.

In cases of chronic TMJ lock, manipulation may fail to produce the desired effect. Additional efforts may be necessary:

1. With both thumbs on the left and right mandibular molars and the remaining fingers under the mandible, press down and forward to lower the condyles and protrude the mandible. If the lock is monolateral, apply the procedure only to the side affected.

2. Place a firm wedge (such as a saliva ejector tube) approximately 5 to 6 cm long between the patient's molars, as far back as possible. This should separate the molars on one or both sides according to the type of TMJ lock. With one hand on the top of the patient's head and the other holding the patient's chin from beneath, apply firm pressure to the skull and chin in an attempt to lower the condyles and free them from the fossa. This may be done several times. In severe cases, encourage the patient to repeat the exercises at home before returning to the office to have the clinician repeat the exercises the following day.

ARS AS JOINT DISTRACTION DEVICE

Should these attempts fail to resolve the pathology or provide significant improvement, a dedicated ARS should be prepared with two wedges corresponding to the left and right maxillary first molars. By indentingwith the mandibular antagonist cusps, these should create a permanent posterior separation between the posterior quadrants, thereby holding the condyles away from the fossa articulating surface. By wearing this splint for a number of days while trying to keep the jaws firmly closed, the patient should succeed in lowering the condyles.

Once a more correct therapeutic position has been achieved with a considerable increase in buccal opening, a cast should be taken so that a traditional ARS can be prepared to maintain this outcome.

If all methods fails, the last resort may be surgery (see page 195 onward).

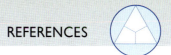

REFERENCES

1. Simons DG, Travel JG, Simons LS. Myofascial Pain and Dysfunction: A Trigger Point Manual. Baltimore: Lippincott Williams and Wilkins, 1998

2. Okeson JP. Il Trattamento delle Disfunzioni dell'Occlusione e dei Disordini Temporomandibolari, ed 3. Bologna: Martina, 1993.

3. Bumann A, Lotzmann U. Diagnostica Funzionale e Terapia, ed 1. Milano: Masson, 2000.

4. Cozzani G, Martignoni M. Diagnosi in occlusione abituale e in occlusione centrica. Mondo Ortod 1976;4:1–12.

5. Bumann A, Lotzmann U, Mah J. TMJ Disorders and Orofacial Pain: The Role of Dentistry in a Multidisciplinary Approach (Color Atlas of Dental Medicine). New York: Thieme, 2002.

6. Sfondrini G, Gandini P, Fraticelli D. Ortognatodonzia: Diagnosi. Milan: Masson, 1997.

7. Pasler FA. Radiology (Color Atlas of Dental Medicine): Thieme, 1992

8. Moller TB, Reif E. Pocket Atlas of Radiographic Positioning: Thieme, 1996.

9. Etter LE, Cross LC. Normal and pathologic roentgen anatomy of the middle ear and mastoid process. Am J Roentgenol Radium Ther Nucl Med 1963;90:1143–1155.

10. Mongini F, Preti G. La Radiologia dell'ATM nel Trattamento delle Occlusopatie. Torino: Cortina, 1980.

11. Fanfani F, Pierazzini A. Diagnostica per Immagini in Odontostomatologia. Torino: Utet, 2003.

12. Sano T. Recent developments in understanding temporomandibular joint disorders. Part 1: Bone marrow abnormalities of the mandibular condyle. Dentomaxillofac Radiol 2000;29:7–10.

13. Sano T. Recent developments in understanding temporomandibular joint disorders. Part 2: Changes in the retrodiscal tissue. Dentomaxillofac Radiol 2000;29:260–263.

14. Milano V, Desiate A, Bellino R, Garofalo T. Magnetic resonance imaging of temporomandibular disorders: Classification, prevalence and interpretation of disc displacement and deformation. Dentomaxillofacial Radiology 2000; 29:352–361.

15. Tanaka T, Morimoto Y, Masumi S, Tominaga K, Ohba T. Utility of frequency-selective fat saturation T2-weighted MR images for the detection of joint effusion in the temporomandibular joint. Dentomaxillofac Radiol 2002;31:305–312.

16. Hollender L, Barclay P, Maravilla K, Terry V. The depiction of the bilaminar zone of the temporomandibular joint by magnetic resonance imaging. Dentomaxillofac Radiol 1998;27:45–47.

17. Westesson PL, Brooks SL. Temporomandibular joint: Relationship between MR evidence of effusion and the presence of pain and disc displacement. AJR Am J Roentgenol 1992;159:559–563.

18. Manzione JV, Tallents RH. "Pseudomeniscus" sign: Potential indicator of repair or remodeling in temporomandibular joints with internal derangements [abstract]. Radiology 1992;185:175.

19. Dawson PE. Optimum TMJ condyle position in clinical practice. Int J Periodontics Restorative Dent 1985;3:11–31.

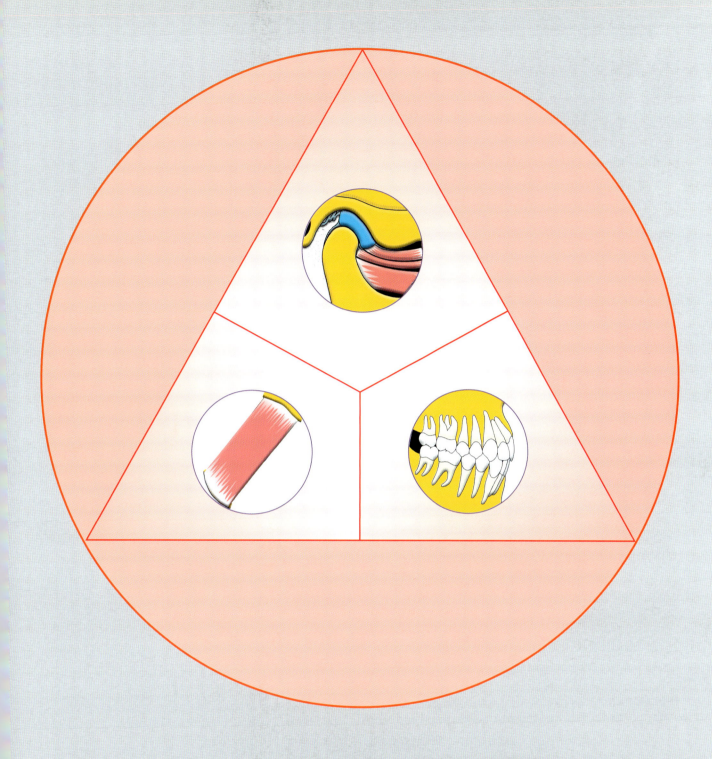

CHAPTER III

PHASE I: MUSCULOARTICULAR THERAPY

After all examinations and tests have been completed, the clinician should be able to reach a clear diagnosis and plan. This can be achieved by:

- Assessing and classifying the symptoms and input from the patient.
- Identifying whether the pathology lies solely within the stomatognathic apparatus (albeit with some effect on other parts of the body) or arises from other sources. Treatment proceeds differently, of course, in each of these situations.
- Determining the extent and severity of dental, skeletal, and musculoarticular damage. Detrimental psychologic effects, if present, also affect the treatment outcome and should be dealt with during this stage.
- Establishing a treatment plan that includes selected procedures, including manipulation and splint selection,[1] based on the severity of damage.
- Integrating the therapy with other forms of help such as medication, exercise, or physiotherapy.
- Allowing the diagnosis and treatment to achieve a positive outcome in straightforward cases. Seeking the most effective procedures and counting on the patient's positive cooperation to reach the best possible compromise in more severe cases.

The primary aim of treatment is to obtain and maintain **normal function** in straightforward cases, **functional recovery** in challenging cases, and **functional adaptation** in very challenging cases. Regardless of the details of a case, some kind of **functional efficiency** should be achieved (see table on pages 92 and 93). The terms functional recovery and functional adaptation are proposed here for the first time. They highlight a dynamic concept of treatment as opposed to the search for a static geometric position proposed by traditional gnathology.

Finally, two practical factors need to be addressed prior to commencing musculoarticular rehabilitation therapy:

Observation of legal and ethical requirements
- Obtain a statement from the patient or guardian concerning any preexisting medical conditions, including infectious diseases.
- Obtain written informed consent accepting the therapeutic procedures.

Clinical and practical issues
- The patient must display positive motivation for treatment.
- Treatment should commence only when hygiene is excellent and may be suspended if hygiene is neglected during treatment.
- There must be no coexisting oral pathologies such as caries, periodontal disease, abscesses, and/or other endodontic risks.

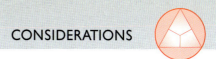
CONSIDERATIONS

COMPROMISE IN THE OUTCOME

The word compromise infers a middle-of-the-road solution with both parties giving way to some extent. In biology, it may be considered an intermediate solution between an anatomo-functional ideal and the initial pathologic situation, with the treatment plan aiming to reach the best possible result, often the best compromise obtainable. The treatment plan is also influenced by the individuality of each patient, which should be considered during diagnosis and treatment, and the patient's attitude toward understanding and resolving his or her problems. Posttreatment success also depends on patients' continuing compliance, including ongoing hygiene and presenting for regular checkups.

ADAPTABILITY TO DIFFERENT CONDITIONS

Adaptability implies a process by which living organisms mutate to conform to their habitat or the changes that occur therein. Specifically, adaptation takes place when a change of some sort is necessary to survive where an original condition no longer exists. In terms of apparatus functionality, pathology arises when the adaptation fails to "survive".

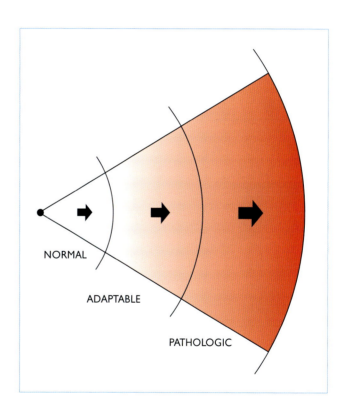

PROGRESSION OF DAMAGE

Altered interarch relationships are frequently associated with musculoarticular pathology.

PHYSIOLOGIC EQUILIBRIUM

EQUILIBRIUM upset by dental derangement

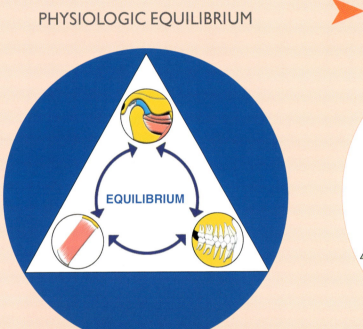
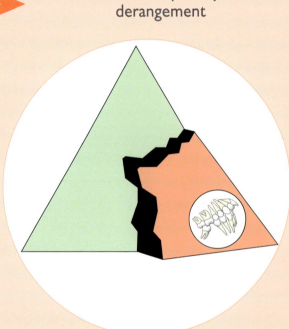

Muscle tension

Articular damage

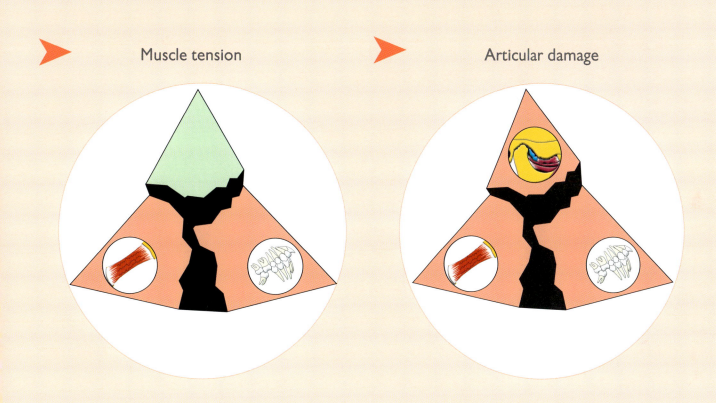

PROGRESSION OF RECOVERY

With rare exceptions, rehabilitation of musculoarticular damage must precede orthodontic occlusal finishing (see page 220).

FIRST PROCEDURE:
Musculoarticular rehabilitation with the ARS worn constantly

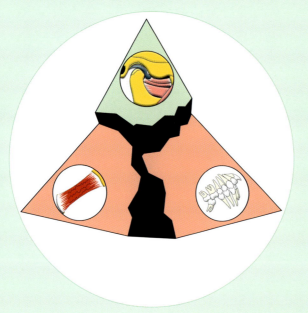
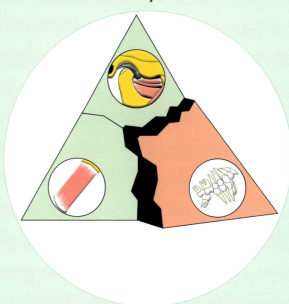

Remember the following considerations:
- It would be illogical to first rearrange the teeth and then the TMJs since second-stage musculoarticular rearrangement would make it necessary to then rearrange the teeth a second time.

- Correct TMJ structure relationships established during the primary rehabilitation procedure must be maintained without further changes for the entire treatment program, including orthodontic occlusal finishing and prosthodontic work if planned.

SUBSEQUENTLY:
Orthodontic occlusal finishing with
the ARS worn constantly

EQUILIBRIUM REESTABLISHED

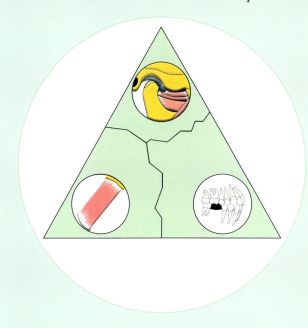

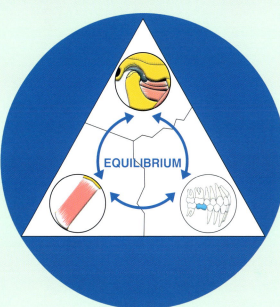

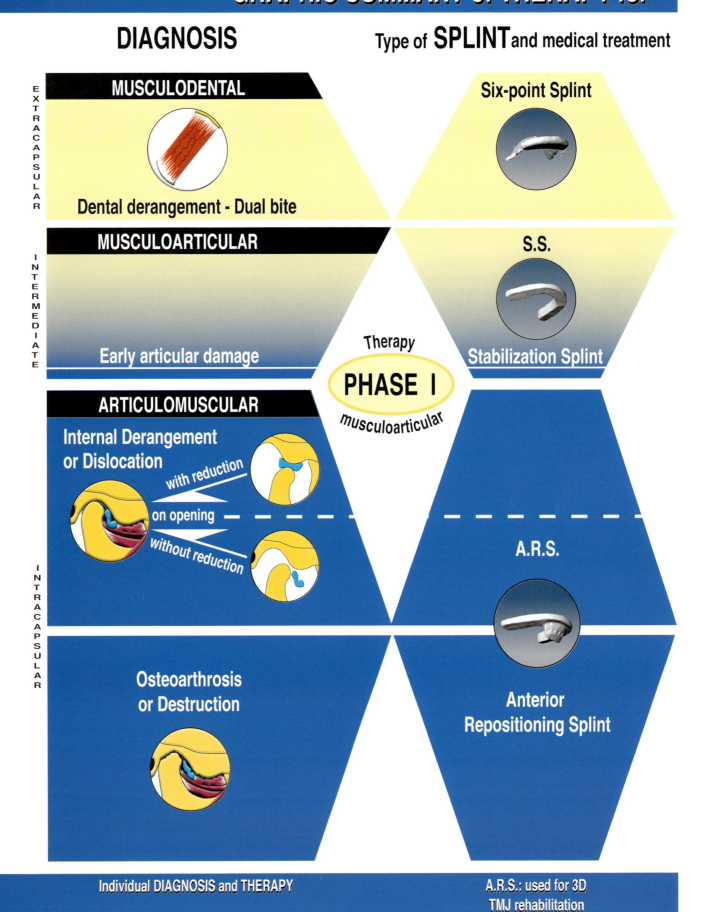

GRAPHIC SUMMARY of THERAPY for

DIAGNOSIS

Type of SPLINT and medical treatment

EXTRACAPSULAR

MUSCULODENTAL

Dental derangement - Dual bite

Six-point Splint

INTERMEDIATE

MUSCULOARTICULAR

Early articular damage

S.S.

Stabilization Splint

Therapy

PHASE I

musculoarticular

INTRACAPSULAR

ARTICULOMUSCULAR

Internal Derangement or Dislocation

with reduction

on opening

without reduction

Osteoarthrosis or Destruction

A.R.S.

Anterior Repositioning Splint

Individual DIAGNOSIS and THERAPY

A.R.S.: used for 3D TMJ rehabilitation

TEETH, MUSCLES, and JOINTS

RESULTS with pain reduction and muscle relaxation

Type of **FUNCTION**

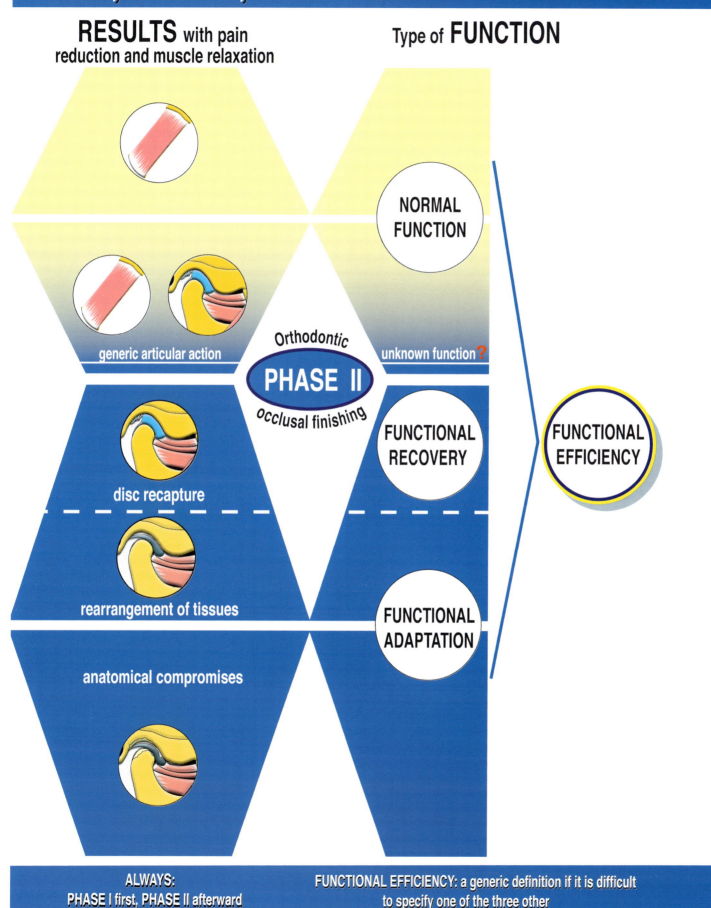

generic articular action

Orthodontic
PHASE II
occlusal finishing

unknown function**?**

NORMAL FUNCTION

disc recapture

rearrangement of tissues

anatomical compromises

FUNCTIONAL RECOVERY

FUNCTIONAL ADAPTATION

FUNCTIONAL EFFICIENCY

ALWAYS:
PHASE I first, PHASE II afterward

FUNCTIONAL EFFICIENCY: a generic definition if it is difficult to specify one of the three other

COORDINATION BETWEEN ARTICULAR EMINENCE INCLINATION, CUSP INCLINATION, AND INCISAL GUIDANCE

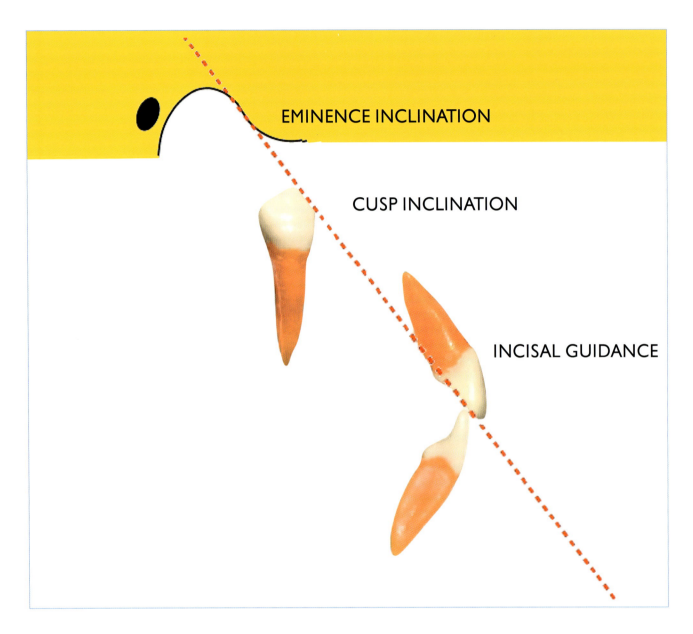

Anatomy and function:

- Articular eminence inclination, incisal guidance, and tooth cusp inclination are parallel with each other.
- The posterior ligament slows condylar advance, which lowers it.
- Many other factors help to determine the relationships between the condyle, disc, and fossa.

The infinite number of relationships that exist between these components can be narrowed down to the following patterns:

- Tending toward the horizontal (typical of Class III)
- Average
- Tending toward the vertical (typical of Class II/division 2)

CONSIDERATIONS: DOES THE DEGREE OF EMINENCE INCLINATION AFFECT THE POSITION OF THE REHABILITATED CONDYLE-DISC UNIT?

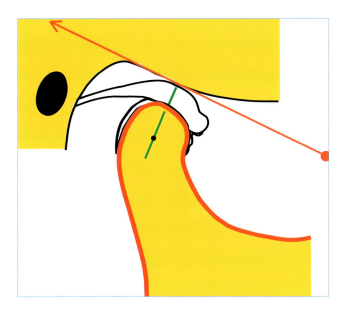

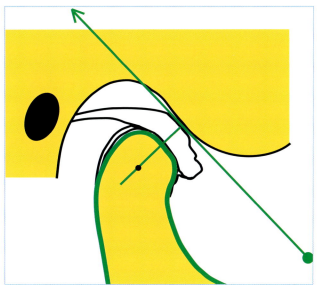

A purely geometrical hypothesis in three different conditions:

- Condylar position in the fossa
- Disc position
- Therapeutic repositioning of the condyle-disc relationship with an anterior repositioning splint (ARS)

Note: *Since many factors contribute to resolution of the pathology, geometric considerations are not the only elements involved.*

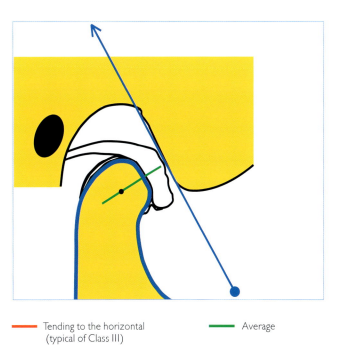

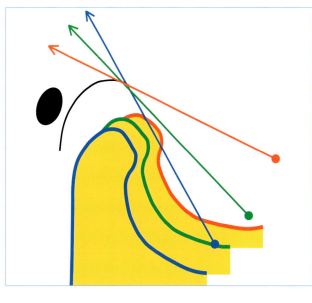

— Tending to the horizontal (typical of Class III)   — Average   — Vertical (typical of Class II/division 2)

ASSESSMENT OF CHANGES IN PRETREATMENT AND POSTTREATMENT CONDYLAR POSITION

This study, led by Dr Emanuele Crudo, investigated three areas:

- Posttreatment condylar position with partial reference to articular eminence inclination
- Amount of posttreatment condylar advance
- Amount of posttreatment condylar lowering

Materials and methods

The study included 9 patients, ages 13 to 59, with a total of 18 temporomandibular joints (TMJs) affected by temporomandibular disorders (TMDs) (pretreatment tests). Pretreatment multilayer computed tomogaphy (CT) images were taken with a cone beam apparatus (MaxiScan, Autel). Patients then underwent ARS musculoarticular therapy and orthodontic occlusal finishing before the second sets of posttreatment images were taken.

The same radiology clinic was used for pretreatment and posttreatment imaging, and the same radiologic technologist performed the work at all sessions. Furthermore, during the posttreatment session, the technician was given the pretreatment records in order to reproduce, as closely as possible, the same position. A strict procedure was followed to center the skull in the gantry and achieve a constant volume. Both closed-mouth left and right oblique sagittal slices were taken.

The multilayer images (gap, 0.5 mm) were reformatted perpendicular to the condylar long axis. The most significant pretreatment cranial images and the corresponding posttreatment images were chosen. Outlines of the fixed parts (skull base, auditory meatus, and fossa) and the mobile part (condyle), covering an area of approximately 12 x 6 cm, were traced on an acetate sheet in an attempt to reproduce the cephalometric superimposition technique used with cranial teleradiography. Red lines show pretreatment baseline findings; yellow lines show posttreatment results.

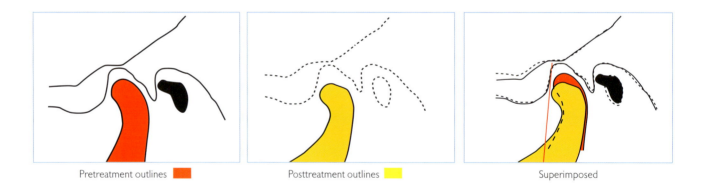

Pretreatment outlines   Posttreatment outlines   Superimposed

RESULTS

The postreatment changes achieved in this study were corroborated by objective improvement assessed clinically as well as by subjective relief reported by patients. A minimal margin of error, similar to that calculated for cephalometry, must be allowed for in interpreting the data. Far from being centered within the fossa (the gold standard of classic gnathology), the condyle was seen in a variety of positions in relation to the fossa (the true articulating surface), each position being different for each patient and TMJ.

Of particular interest is the case of patient M. R., age 31, whose left and right articular eminences had a considerable difference in inclination. The right was almost vertical, with the condyle prevalently lowered posttreatment. The left was almost horizontal, with the postreatment condylar position further forward.

M. R.   Age 31

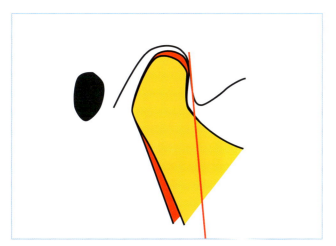

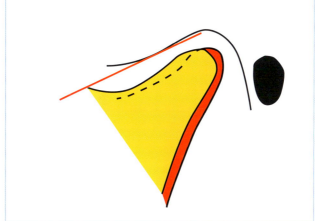

Right: The articular eminence is almost vertical with the posttreatment condyle prevalently lowered.

Left: The articular eminence is almost horizontal with the posttreatment condylar position moved prevalently forward.

CONCLUSIONS

This clinical investigation has highlighted the uniquely individual position of each condyle in relation to the true articulating surface. The infinite variety of patterns into which the damaged structures rearrange themselves—as suggested by comparisons of pretreatment and posttreatment images—warrants further investigation. As an experimental survey, this study justifies research with a greater number of patients and greater attention to detail.

POSTTREATMENT CONDYLAR POSITION IN RELATION TO ARTICULAR EMINENCE INCLINATION

Red lines show articular eminence inclination.

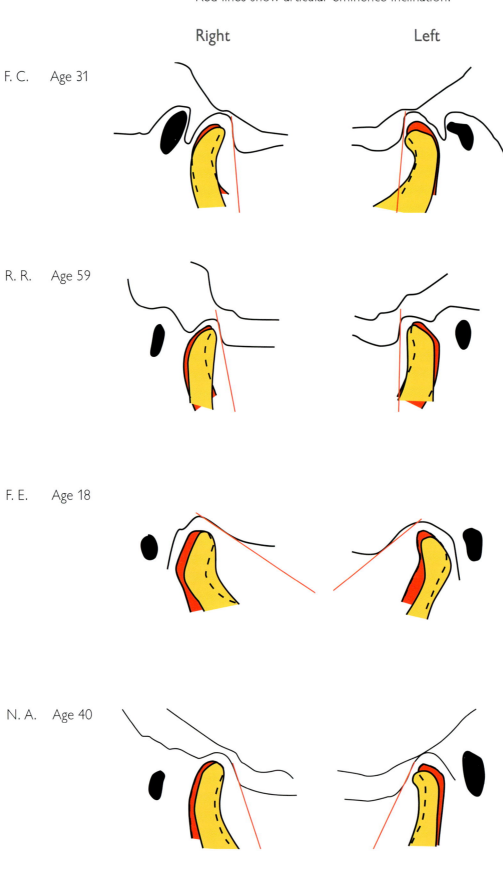

Right · Left

F. C.   Age 31

R. R.   Age 59

F. E.   Age 18

N. A.   Age 40

■ PRETREATMENT   ■ POSTTREATMENT

Red lines show articular eminence inclination.

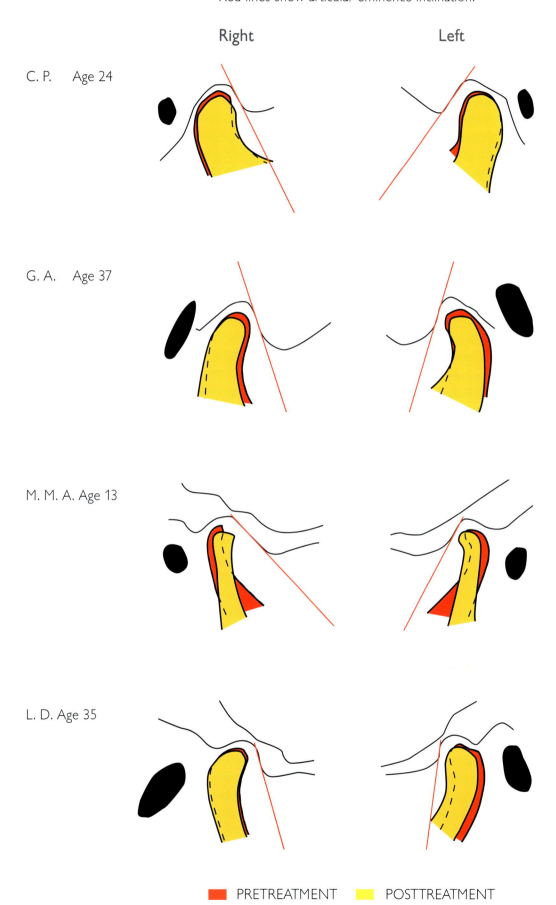

Right   Left

C. P.   Age 24

G. A.   Age 37

M. M. A. Age 13

L. D. Age 35

■ PRETREATMENT   ■ POSTTREATMENT

AMOUNT OF POSTTREATMENT CONDYLAR **ADVANCE**

The immediate practical implications of this clinical investigation are that posttreatment condylar changes tend to be both downward and forward with an average similar amount in both directions, an important factor to bear in mind when taking bite registrations of individual patients.

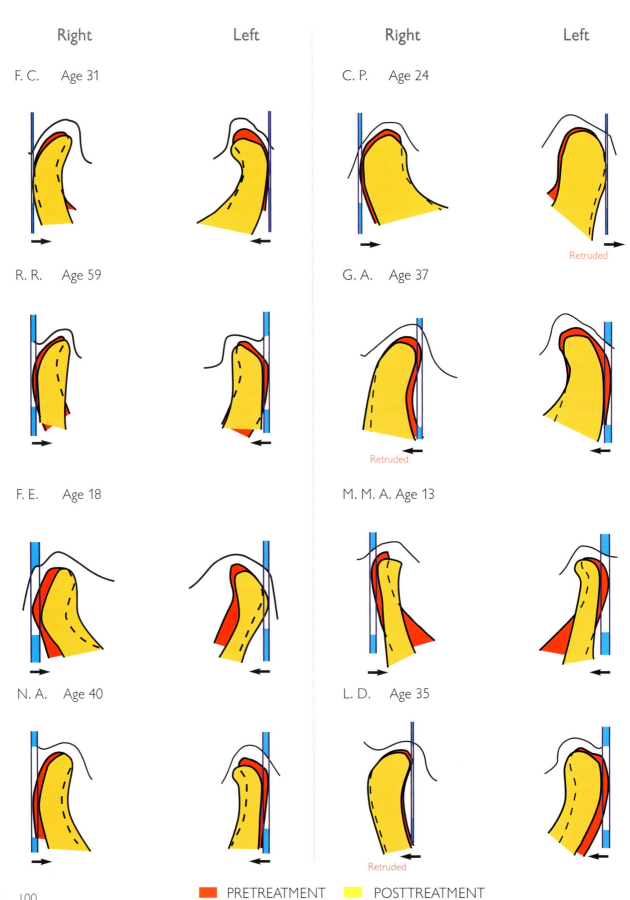

Right	Left	Right	Left

F. C.　Age 31　　　　　　　　　　　　C. P.　Age 24

Retruded

R. R.　Age 59　　　　　　　　　　　　G. A.　Age 37

Retruded

F. E.　Age 18　　　　　　　　　　　　M. M. A. Age 13

N. A.　Age 40　　　　　　　　　　　　L. D.　Age 35

Retruded

🟥 PRETREATMENT　　🟨 POSTTREATMENT

AMOUNT OF POSTTREATMENT CONDYLAR **LOWERING**

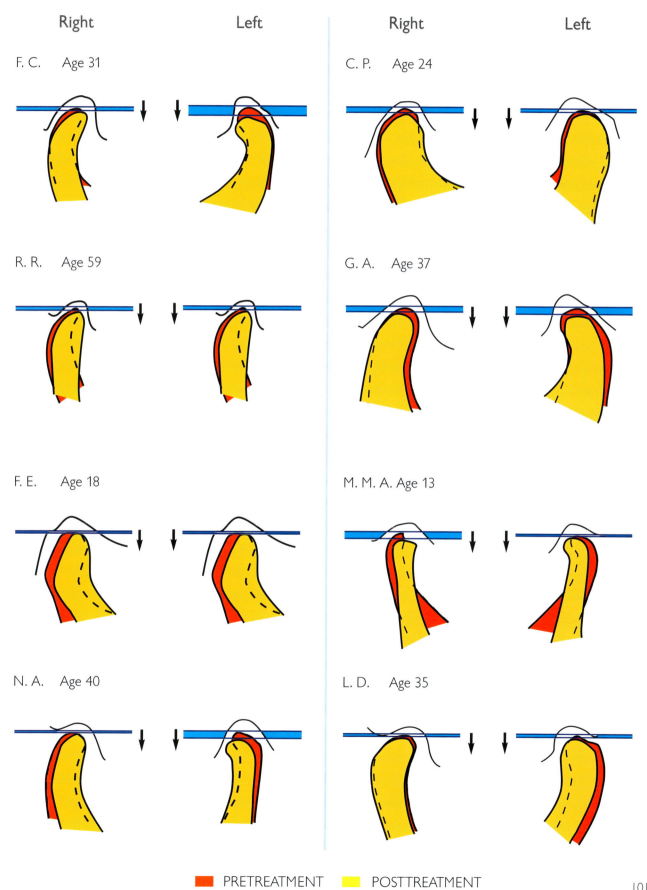

PRETREATMENT   POSTTREATMENT

BITE REGISTRATION: A COMMON FIRST STEP FOR ALL SPLINTS

Regardless of the type of splint manufactured, a wax bite must be made to record the patient's therapeutic occlusion. If properly taken, the bite registration meets several requirements, including ease of use, correct thickness, and stability. The authors normally use Alminax (Kemdent), a material that contains a high percentage of aluminium. Because of its composition, Alminax offers satisfactory heat conductivity and softens within the necessary timeframe, at around 45°C.

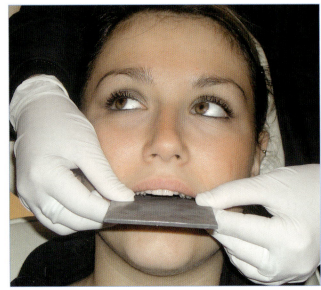

1. The wax is heated over a flame until it is suitably malleable to be fitted on the maxillary teeth.

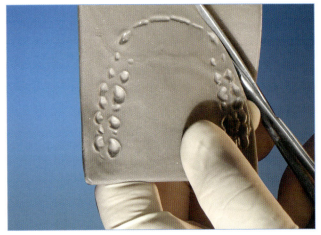

2. A working base is cut out to fit the patient's dentition.

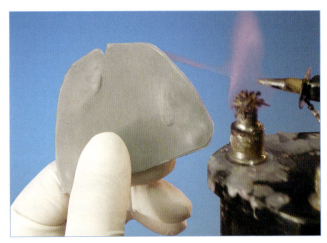

3. The wax is heated again and indented firmly onto the patient's maxillary arch.

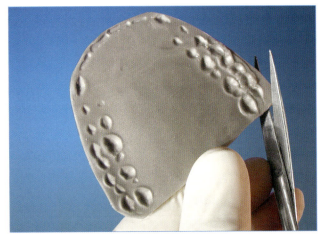

4. The wax is removed from the patient's mouth, and the buccal surfaces of all the teeth are trimmed to come as close as possible to the actual dental arch. The posterior corners are trimmed to remove any retromolar discomfort.

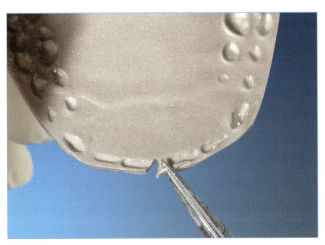

5. A midline interincisor notch is cut to facilitate accurate repositioning in the patient's mouth. Although functional efficiency is an aim common to all splint treatments (see following pages), from this point onward, specific techniques are used for different splints.

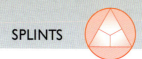

SPLINTS

TYPE	PURPOSE

DIAGNOSTIC

- Six-point splint (page 114)

- Extracapsular (musculodental) pathology

DIAGNOSTIC-THERAPEUTIC

- Stabilization splint (SS) (page 126)

- Intermediate (musculoarticular) pathology

Integration: Michigan plate (of particular interest for prosthodontists) (page 132)

THERAPEUTIC

- ARS (page 144)

- Intracapsular (articulomuscular) pathology
  - Dislocation with or without reduction
  - Destruction

  - Mandibular ARS (page 180)

- Principally provides maintenance without causing loss of therapeutic position (see integration A) or interfering with the patient's social life

  - Distractor with posterior wedges (page 182)

- For cases of TMJ lock

  - Maintenance splint (page 188)

- For patients with hypermobile ligaments, has the opposite effect of an ARS, which is contraindicated (see integration B)

New proposals:
- ARS integration "A": see page 405
- ARS integration "B": see page 406

THERAPEUTIC PROCEDURE SEQUENCE

PHASE I   MUSCULOARTICULAR THERAPY

AIMS: to restore a physiologic distance between bony tissues and, consequently, to:
- Eliminate muscle stress and pain
- Axially align the condyle, disc, and articulating surface, regardless of whether the condyle is geometrically centered in the fossa
- Rearrange the deteriorated or damaged anatomical structures

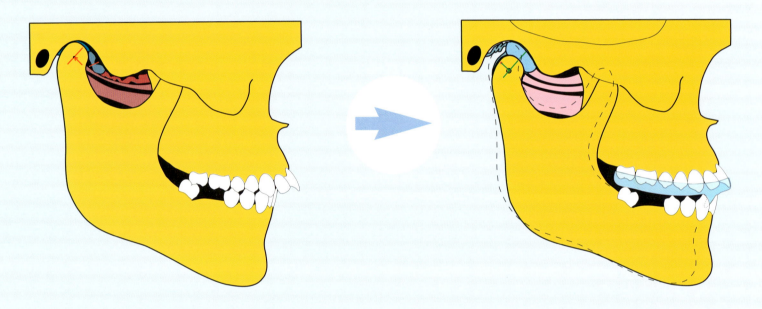

METHODS: application of an ARS to obtain the best 3D relationships and position of TMJ structures and the mandible, and to keep this position stable throughout treatment and afterward.

This is illustrated more thoroughly on pages 92 and 93.

PHASE II ORTHODONTIC OCCLUSAL FINISHING

AIMS: specific orthodontic treatment of both dental arches to obtain correct reciprocal anatomical-functional relationships and intercuspation. The teeth are adapted to the requirements of the muscles and TMJs while respecting esthetic considerations. Innovative procedures are covered in detail in chapter 4 (page 204 onward) with a series of options illustrating the importance of a personalized treatment plan for each patient.

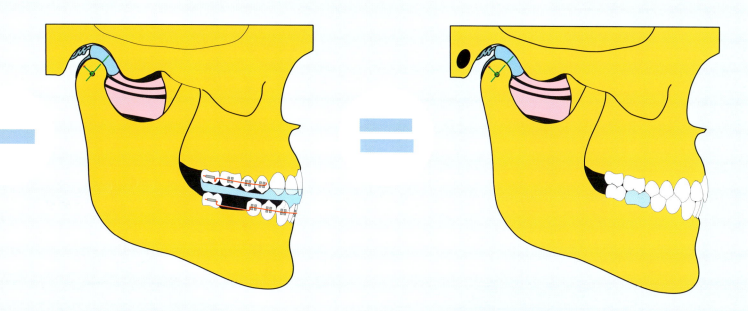

METHODS: selective orthodontics to create alternating areas of tooth anchorage and movement in a step-by-step sequence based on the principle of continuous forces and careful 3D root control.

PRACTICAL LIMITATIONS:
- The ARS precludes the use of lingual brackets.
- Class II and III elastics are ruled out to eliminate the risk of interference with the correct musculoarticular and mandibular therapeutic position. Vertical elastics may be acceptable under certain conditions.
- EOT/headgear should not be considered.

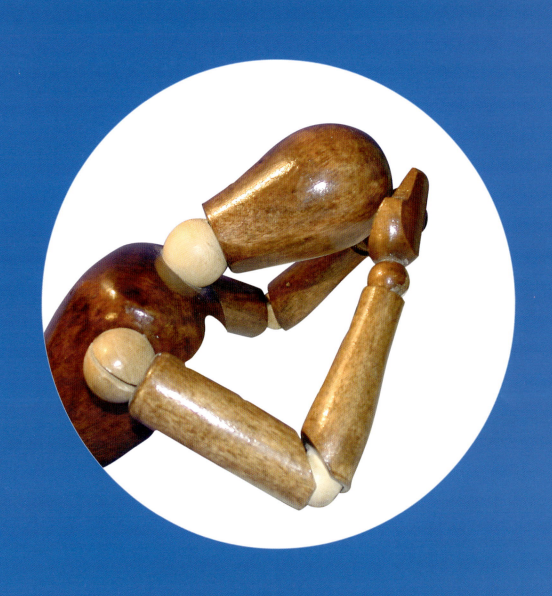

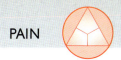

PAIN

A BRIEF INTRODUCTION TO THE PAIN MECHANISM
Coordinated by Prof. Piergiorgio Strata

Pain originates from the stimulation of receptors located in the skin and other tissues. When activated, the impulse travels along the A-δ and C afferent nerves to the brain, where it is interpreted as pain, that is, as a threat to the integrity of the organism that could cause permanent damage. Unlike the majority of other sensations, pain does not attenuate as the signal continues; rather, it persists. The continuing signal helps the organism to survive by motivating it to remove the cause of damage. If this doesn't happen, the stimulus causes the pain to become more and more intense.

Pain amplification is caused by several mechanisms, including:

- Products of local inflammation increasing the sensitivity of nociceptor nerve endings to the stimulus
- Products of local inflammation acting on nerve endings in surrounding areas
- Amplification of central nervous system synaptic transmission

This third mechanism is a memory-related phenomenon responsible for pain lingering (chronic pain) well after the initial stimulus has been removed. In other words, continued pain stimulation "teaches" the central synapses to transmit pain more efficiently.

In response to pain, the body's movements are programmed to reduce strain on the injured part. The altered movements, often of a postural nature, may place strain on other joints, resulting in lesions that become another source of pain. As these new movements are acquired and memorized, they may persist long-term, even when the origin of the pain has disappeared. To heal the resulting pathologic movements or postural habits, it is necessary to remove any residual pain with appropriate motor rehabilitation aimed at "unlearning" the abnormal posture and movements.

FACIAL PAIN

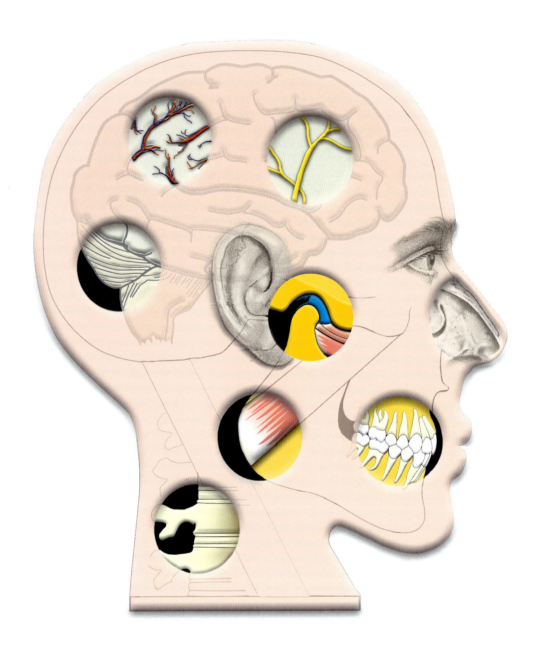

TMDs are part of the group of painful syndromes affecting the head and neck region that cause facial pain.[2,3]

Assessment of any pain is a necessary diagnostic step to differentiate the type of pathology and ensure that the correct solution is used. Normal diagnostic and thera-peutic procedures can exclude or confirm the suspicion of TMD. Dentists should be able to establish whether a patient needs to be examined by another colleague such as a neurologist, otorhinolaryngologist, or ortho-pedic specialist.

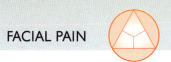

PAIN SYNDROMES AFFECTING THE HEAD AND NECK AREA

Sinusitis

Nervous system alterations

Migraine

Psychologic disorders

Tension type headaches

Cluster headaches

Myofascial pain syndrome

Atypical facial pain

Cephalalgia

TMD

Trigeminal nerve pain

Earache

Postherpetic neuralgia

Facial nerve pain

Other

Dentists are not expected to be thoroughly familiar with the entire field of facial pain. Nevertheless, they should be able to establish with reasonable certainty whether the stomatognathic apparatus is affected.

TMD and POSTURAL DISORDERS

Coordinated by Prof. Felice Festa and Dr Fabio Ciuffolo

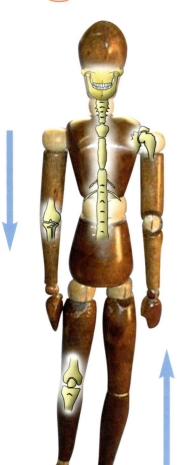

When a patient presents with TMD, due consideration must be given to possible involvement of the musculoskeletal neck area[4,5] and the entire bodily posture[6–9] because of neurologic and fascial connections. The correlation between the stomatognathic apparatus and bodily posture has been the subject of increased attention in the literature, leading to greater awareness not only among the general public, with patients being better informed, but above all among orthopedic and medical practitioners. It is therefore not unusual to receive patients referred by colleagues in other specialties who suspect dental involvement in a patient's postural disorder.

That said, it is by no means easy to clearly establish cause and effect in patients who have a combination of postural disorder and TMD. The safest and most logical approach is, first, to establish that the clinical profile involves more than one somatic area and to decide which area is the treatment priority. Treatment of a single area leaves room for the subsequent treatment of areas that have not benefited from previous therapy. Once the symptoms have been resolved, the next step is to proceed with rehabilitation with the aim of establishing correct asymptomatic bodily posture.

As this discussion makes clear, it is very important to obtain a detailed clinical and imaging profile of the TMD patient to reach an accurate, thorough diagnosis and ascertain whether there is need for further specialist consultation.

OCCLUSION, POSTURE, AND MAGNETIC RESONANCE IMAGING

Coordinated by Dr Lorenzo Vanini and Dr Fabio Ferretti

Cross-bite malocclusions may cause mandibular deviation, which is frequently associated with contracture of the masticatory muscles on the same side. Clinical evidence suggests that postural muscles, too, may become involved in the patient's overall disorder.[6–9] In this context, medical imaging, especially magnetic resonance imaging (MRI), has become a key tool in assessing these muscle groups. Specifically, it has

been possible to observe a frequent correlation between malocclusion, TMD, and hypertonicity of the trapezius and psoas major muscles on the same side. Future development in this area are likely to provide even greater assistance in assessing objective data for purposes of both diagnosis and prognosis.

The MRIs on the opposite page have been overlaid with blue squares marking measurement start and end points. The left-hand MRI shows the trapezius muscles, with the measurements D1 and D2 giving readings, respectively, of 5.3 cm and 4.6 cm. The right-hand MRI illustrates the psoas major muscles. Six measurements—three per side—were taken: (1) muscle length, (2) upper transversal width, and (3) maximum transversal (muscle belly) width. These measurements help to show differences in muscle volume between the left and right sides.

The first assessment recommended by the authors is based on the static STABILOMETRY PRINCIPLE. Static balance platforms are now found in many dental offices. The platform enables the clinician to ascertain objectively whether the stomatognathic apparatus has a destabilizing effect on bodily posture. The platform measures the oscillations that occur under the soles of the feet when a person stands upright and uses these data to plot the person's Romberg sway area, or sway path.

Length and width are the fundamental variables in the sway area, and they vary according to different input signals received by the body. For example, if the variables diminish with the patient's eyes closed as opposed to when the eyes are open, this indicates that the destabilizing influence is visual whereas opposite results indicate a normal situation. Similarly, if maxillomandibular interference (in the form of a splint, bite roll, or cotton rolls) reduces the length and width of the sway path compared with habitual mandibular posture, it may be inferred that the stomatognathic function has a destabilizing effect on bodily posture.

Clearly, when the effects of nonvisual input are being measured, patients must be asked to keep their eyes closed. Sway analysis therefore permits evaluation of the buccal area influence on parts of the body that are, theoretically, unrelated.

The illustrations show an example of sway path measurement and a static balance platform, in addition to the trapezius and psoas major measurements described on the previous page. The clinical case study of a professional soccer player (see page 330 in the chapter on orthodontic occlusal finishing) provides further insight

into this area, and additional reading on this subject is recommended among the specific literature.

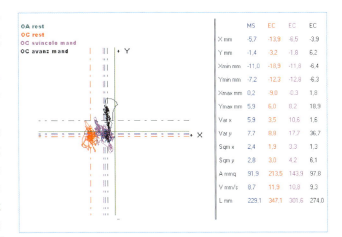

Sway path plot chart.

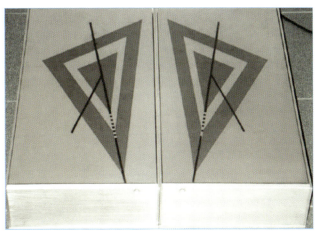

The photo above shows one type of static balance platform. Note the black lines, which help standardize foot position in a repeatable manner.

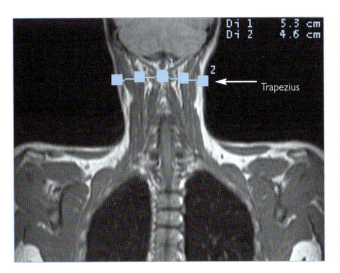

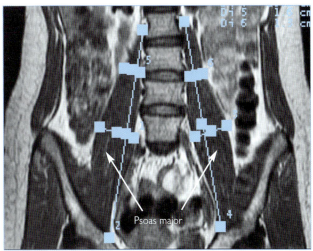

This procedure can prove useful as long as its use is strictly standardized.

MUSCULODENTAL EXTRACAPSULAR PATHOLOGY

This section focuses on patients who complain of interarch dental alterations with consequent muscle-related disorders apparently unaffected by TMJ problems.

DIAGNOSIS

A distinction must be made to determine whether the origin of the muscular pathology lies strictly within the realm of medicine (eg, inflammatory, degenerative, or genetic) or dentistry (muscle tension with pain caused by dental disorder).

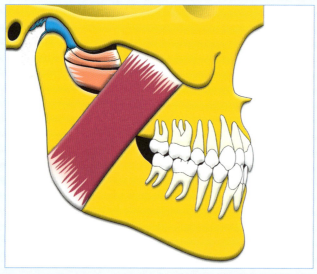

Maximum intercuspation dental closure with muscle tension.

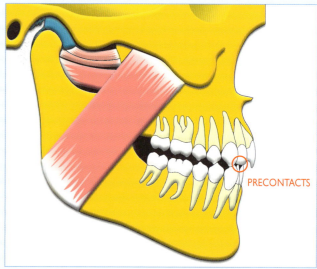

PRECONTACTS

Muscle-led closure in a therapeutic position with few dental contacts and, more importantly, no muscle tension.

In these cases, the initial patient examination should include:

-   Guided buccal closure until minimum initial contacts occur, to seek a point of muscle-led closure.
-   Placement of the fingertips on the labial surfaces of the maxillary incisor to feel for fremitus at the moment of first contact. In normal conditions, a single decisive contact is felt when all the teeth close simultaneously.
-   Palpation of masticatory and postural muscles to confirm the patient's sensation of undefined muscle pain in the region of the head, neck, and shoulders.
-   Indentations on inner cheeks and especially the tongue, which are commonly found in cases of dual bite. (See the summary of dual bite on page 46.)

VIRTUAL DIAGNOSTIC PROCEDURE

A six-point splint is the device indicated to best hold the mandible in correct position in relation to the maxilla, which improves muscle tone and eliminates occlusal interferences. In more challenging cases, the six-point splint may only be a first step toward the preparation of a more efficient and more complete stabilization splint.

The patient's bite should be checked every few days with articulating paper, and as necessary, the occlusal surface of the six-point splint should be ground with a bur in correspondence with the precontacts observed. Because of the risk of condylar upward shift due to the lack of posterior support, this type of splint should not be worn for more than a few weeks.

This procedure should be widely used in dentistry as well as in orthodontics since it ensures that the correct functional conditions needed in all procedures involving the occlusal mechanism are observed. Although other procedures exist (see page 46), a six-point splint prevents the risk of operating in pathologic conditions favoring the onset of muscle tension and pain. On a historical note, it can be likened to the Lucia jig, mainly used by prosthodontists, or to a leaf gauge.

PROGNOSIS

A positive prognosis is to be expected. To achieve this, teeth must be adapted to the requirements of the muscles and joints. Failure to address this critical detail will cause the system to operate in maximum intercuspation, resulting in muscle tension and ultimately setting in motion procedures that will progressively worsen an already negative condition.

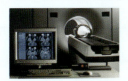

MUSCLE PATHOLOGY IN MRI

MRI enables clinicians to detect edema and atrophy in the superior and inferior bundles of the external pterygoid. Edema in fat-suppressed T2-weighted slices is semiotically visible as pale thin strips of signal hyperintensity between the muscle fibers. Atrophied areas are reduced in volume. They are visible as intense signals of adipose infiltration in T1-or proton-density weighed images of the muscle extremities.

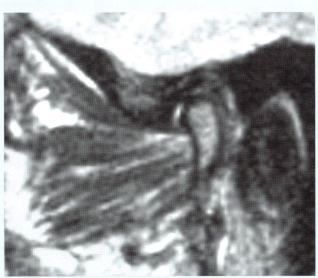

PTERYGOID EDEMA in fat-suppressed T2-weighted slice.

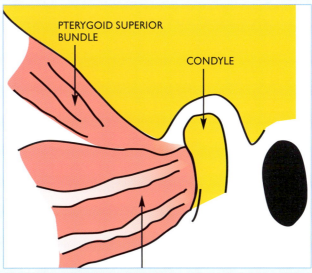

PTERYGOID INFERIOR BUNDLE: Bright bands typical of edema suffusion stand out amid muscle fibers displaying normal signal intensity.

MUSCULODENTAL EXTRACAPSULAR PATHOLOGY: DIAGNOSTIC SIX-POINT SPLINT

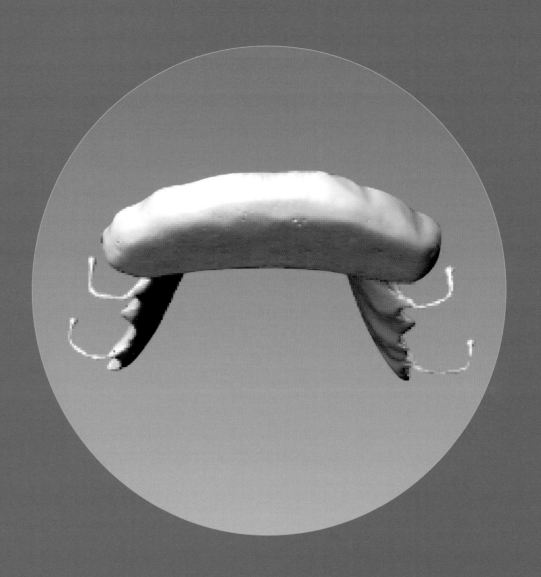

DESCRIPTION

This intraoral splint is worn in the maxillary arch following occlusal preparation on the basis of a wax bite registration taken in the correct functional position. It consists of an acrylic resin shell that fits the anterolateral palatal area and is held in place by 0.7- to 0.8-mm wire hooks. The resin must be as thin as possible. The anterior plane of the splint is parallel to the occlusal table. It fits against the mandibular incisor and canine group simultaneously and smoothly and with a good number of contacts. There are no areas of depression or prominence, and its thickness permits lateral and protrusive movements without contact between the maxillary and mandibular posterior teeth.

BITE REGISTRATION

Proper procedures must be followed to ensure that impressions are taken in muscle-led closure (see page 74 onward and page 102).

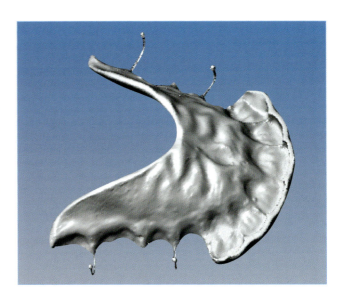

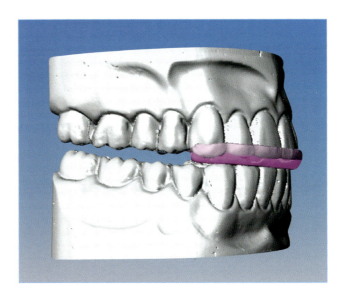

MANUFACTURE OF A SIX-POINT SPLINT

(courtesy of dental technician Andrea Bertelli, La Spezia, Italy).

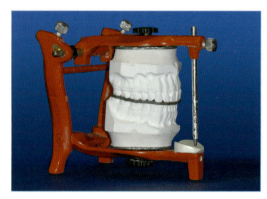

1. Occlusor mounted dental casts with wax bite inserted.

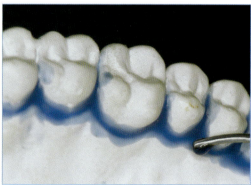

2. Undercuts blocked out with wax.

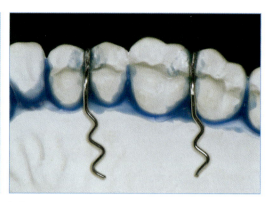

3. Positioning of buccal clasps to hold splint in place when worn.

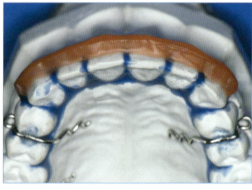

4. Cast boxed with wax to simplify resin finishing stages.

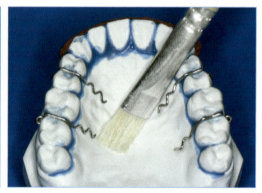

5. Spreading the stone-acrylic separator.

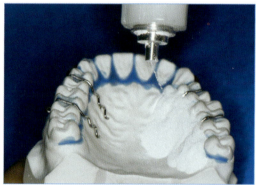

6. SALT-AND-PEPPER TECHNIQUE for splint fabrication: First, the polymer is added.

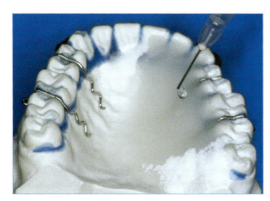

7. Next, the monomer is added.

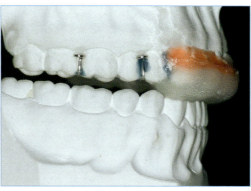

8. Indentation of opposing teeth shapes on anteroinferior contact surface.

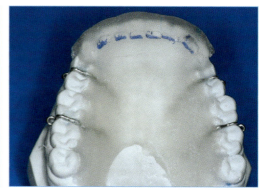

9. Contact points marked with colored crayon to simplify lab setup and smooth the contact surface for the mandibular incisors and canines.

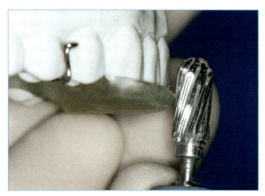

10. Rough modeling.

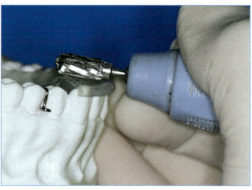

11. The anterior contact plane must be parallel to the occlusal table and touch the mandibular incisors and canines simultaneously.

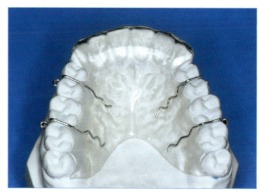

12. Metal bur finishing and silicone bur polishing.

SIX-POINT SPLINT

HOW IT WORKS

The six-point splint is used to relax the muscles by freeing the mandible from occlusal interference. It is important to understand that the anterior dental contact area must be at least 1.5 mm thick. Once a stable consistent position of mandibular closure has been found, a wax bite is taken to work on the occlusal setup.

Key points to remember:

- Patients might be uncomfortable during the first 2 to 3 days of wear since increased vertical height stimulates stretch reflexes.
- Patients with articular compression symptomatology should not be treated with this type of splint because of the risk of further deterioration. Instead, directly fit these patients with a stabilization splint that has an inferior plane in contact with all the mandibular teeth including posterior districts.

A six-point splint may be used as the first step in treating cases where it is difficult to establish an acceptable therapeutic position. The initial splint may be converted into a stabilization splint (SS) by adding resin in the posterior quadrants to extend the contact area to the entire arch. This can be done chairside or in the lab with an occlusor following another impression (see page 128 for advantages and disadvantages). If needed, the SS may be converted into an ARS (page 150).

PRACTICAL EXAMPLE OF DUAL BITE: PATIENT A. S.

Without splint: pathologic centric occlusion (or dental occlusion)

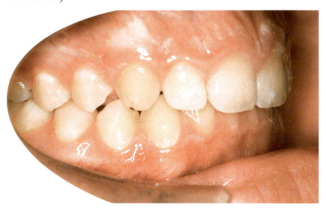

With a six-point splint: muscle-led closure achieved with muscle relaxation and minimum precontacts

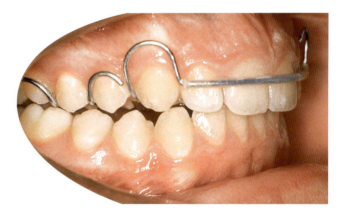

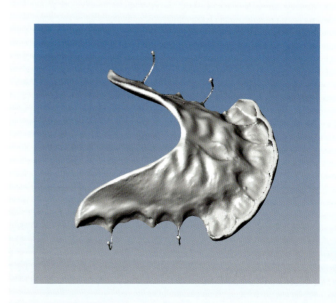

CT SCANS TAKEN SAME DAY WITHOUT (TOP) AND WITH (BOTTOM) A SIX-POINT SPLINT

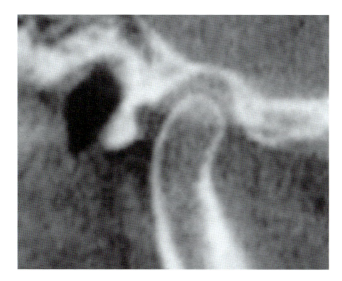

Without splint

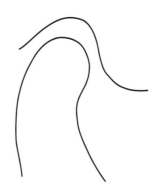

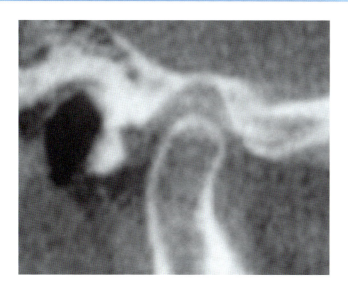

With splint

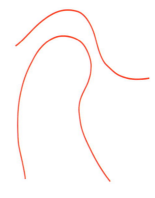

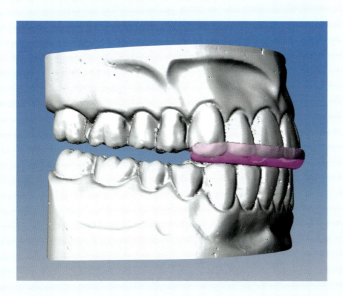

As expected, a six-point splint acts predominantly on the muscles, but there is a slight effect on the TMJ as a result of condylar shift downward and forward.

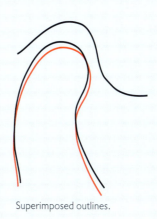

Superimposed outlines.

MUSCLE PAIN IN THE HEAD AND NECK REGION

Coordinated by Prof. Felice Festa and Dr Fabio Ciuffolo

TMDs are frequently associated with discomfort in the muscles of the craniocervical mandibular complex. With the approval of the American Academy of Orofacial Pain, they are classified as myofascial pain, myositis, spasm, protective splinting, and muscular contracture.[2] The symptom most commonly encountered with these disorders is pain. Myositis pain is triggered by flogogenous substances released locally[10] while in the remaining pathologies the pain is created principally by an accumulation of catabolytes and lactic acid.[11]

TMD etiology is multifactorial.[12] Chief risk factors include masticatory parafunction, emotional state, and being a woman. Other contributing factors may include sleep disorders, sociofinancial state, smoking, diet insufficiencies, and work-related incorrect postural habits, all of which appear to underlie this class of disorder.[13-17] However, masticatory parafunction (clenching, grinding, and other habits) is the risk factor most emphasized in literature.[18] It is assumed that repeated, stereotyped movements create a condition of abuse and abnormal pressure on the motor system that, in turn, leads to chronic muscle tension and thence to fatigue and the accumulation of pain-producing substances.

Myofascial pain is frequent in patients with pathology affecting the teeth, muscles, and joints. It is described as dull and deep and may be accompanied by other symptoms of a sensorial, motor, and autonomic nature. A diagnosis of myofascial pain can generally be reached with a simple clinical examination that includes a patient history questionnaire and physical examination. Patient histories provide useful input for initial differentiation as to the nature of the pain, but alone, they are insufficient for a differential diagnosis. Experimental criteria have established the minimum acceptable requisites for objective ascertainment of myofascial pain through palpation. These criteria require solid expertise, technique, and hands-on ability. They are:

-   The presence of a taut, hyperirritable muscle band
-   Localized sensitivity in the form of a tender point and/or remote trigger point (see illustrations)
-   Subjective acknowledgement of the pain evoked[11]

Surface electromyography integrates the information gathered during the clinical examination by revealing increased muscle responsivity and fatigue and diminished recovery capacity.[19]

Treatment of the symptoms and control of the contributing risk factors are the basis for maintaining health long-term. Physical therapy is used to reduce the symptoms (symptomatic phase) and reeducate the individual to acquire correct muscle function (rehabilitation phase).

Treatment of symptoms typically involves the **"spray-and-stretch"** technique,[11] with massage, moist heat application, and the use of a TENS units (muscle stimulation) as optional additions. The rehabilitation stage comprises motivational counseling, behavioral therapy, selected postural exercises, a neuromuscular biofeedback program, and induction of a subjective conscious promoting awareness and control of the associated risk factors.

The spray-and-stretch technique is performed as follows:

1. Ask the patient to sit or lie (supine) in a relaxed position.
2. Hold one of the muscle extremities taut.
3. Spray the skin with a topical vapocoolant—preferably with an ethyl chloride base—according to the direction of the pain and beyond the anatomical limits of the muscle involved.
4. Stretch the muscle. The patient may be passive or actively involved.
5. Repeat the stretch two or three times until significant improvement is noted in the patient's range of motion—specifically, an increase in gape in cases of muscle lock.

The mechanism responsible for relief of symptoms is not so much the anesthetizing effect of the spray as it is that the perception threshold is lower in the cutaneous receptors than in the muscle nociceptors. Stimulation of the thermoreceptors inhibits the perception of pain and consequently interrupts the flinch reflex (muscle pain = protective contracture) that supports muscle pain and reduces the patient's range of motion.

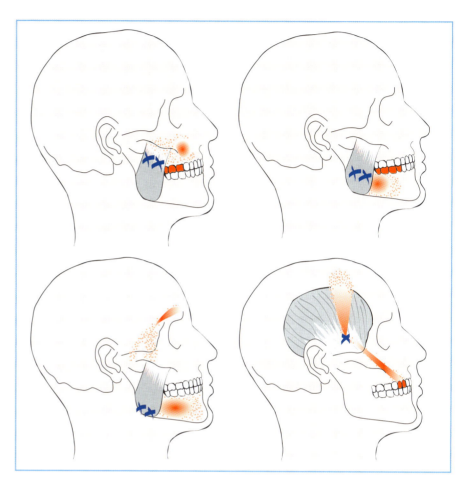

Masseter and temporalis trigger points.

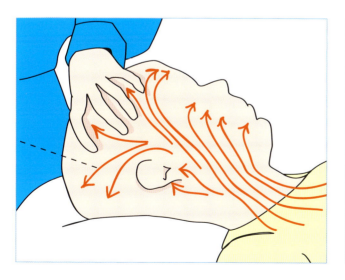

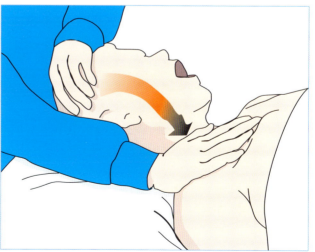

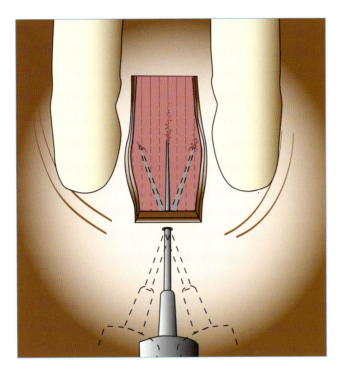

The **injection technique** involves a preparatory phase followed afterward by the actual injection stage.

Preparation

1. Ask the patient to lie supine.
2. Select a 22- to 27-gauge needle, long enough to reach the trigger point but short enough to stay within the anatomical limits of certain areas, such as the neck.
3. Disinfect the skin properly with a common antiseptic.
4. Reduce the discomfort of needle penetration, especially with phobic patients, by applying local skin cryoanesthesia.
5. For patients with a very low pain threshold, block the nociceptor sensitivity of the tissues with a 0.5% procaine anesthetic solution (low myotoxicity and rapid recovery of sensation).

Injection stage

Once the trigger point has been identified and the patient prepared, the muscle is loosened. Move the needle to and fro with changes in inclination in all directions to unwind the muscle band. During this operation, maintain a degree of manual pressure on the area to encourage hemostasis and to fix the point requiring loosening. The mechanism responsible for elimination of the pain appears to be of a mechanical nature, due to movement of the needle, rather than of a chemical nature, due to the local anesthetic.

Injections are contraindicated in patients on anticoagulant medication and phobic individuals.

Electromyography biofeedback is an excellent method to help patients learn correct muscle function, take greater control of masticatory parafunction and incorrect mandibular posture, and maintain a state of muscle relaxation.[20]

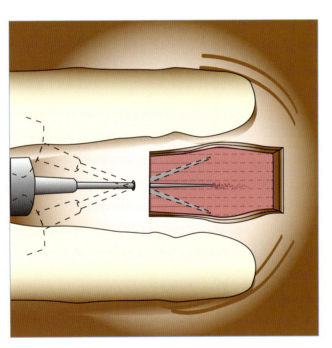

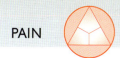

PAIN CONTROL WITH ACUPUNCTURE

Coordinated by Prof. Claudio Maioli

The number of controlled studies into the analgesic effects of acupuncture in the field of dentistry is relatively low, especially if one considers only research based on good methodologic criteria. There is generally widespread agreement that the efficacy of acupuncture is superior to that of placebos or sham treatment in applications such as toothache, postoperative pain (especially following extraction of third molars), facial pain, and TMDs. With one exception, all work published on the subject concurs that acupuncture raises the dental pain threshold and induces an analgesic effect on postoperative pain. The only negative case study reports an unexpected increase in pain following extraction of a third molar with the patient consequently taking greater doses of pain relief medication. The reasons for this discrepancy remain unclear.

Despite overall general agreement concerning the efficacy of acupuncture, there is some justifiable doubt as to its practical value as an analgesic in traditional dentistry. Today's range of analgesic products are economical and easy to take, have minimal collateral effects, and work within a matter of minutes. By contrast, acupuncture is more difficult to administer, less reliable in action, and takes 20 to 30 minutes before its effects are felt.

Acupuncture appears to have far more promise in its effect on TMDs and facial pain of muscular origin. Despite some methodologic shortcomings, all studies published to date on the subject—including six randomized clinical trials—concur that acupuncture is an effective means of treatment. In particular, substantial equivalence has been suggested between the results of acupuncture and occlusal splints in reducing the pain symptoms of TMD.

Compared with splints, which must be worn for a relatively long time before giving therapeutic benefit, acupuncture treatment is simple and economical, often taking effect after a few sessions. A general consensus has been reached that acupuncture may be considered a valid alternative to more conventional forms of treatment for TMDs and facial pain of muscular origin.

APPLICATION OF LASER BIOSTIMULATION IN TMJ THERAPY

Coordinated by Prof. Gianfranco Franchi

Laser treatment applied to the field of orthodontics and TMJ pathology has proven to be valuable. There is ample literature on the subject, ranging from publications in the late 1990s by Pinheiro and Conti to more recent contributions by Bjordal and Kulekcioglu. Low-intensity—or "soft"—lasers act through biostimulating mechanisms and are the most commonly used lasers. They have produced good results with both intracapsular and extracapsular pathology, and in select cases of chronic TMJ lock.

In extracapsular disorders, muscle tension is a determining factor. Low-level laser therapy first "deprograms" mandibular posture ruined by incorrect dental occlusion, thereby contributing to the effect of suitable splints (six-point or alternatively stabilization splints). It also helps to prevent relapse during the maintenance stage.

For intracapsular disorders involving condyle-disc-fossa dysfunction, the usual treatment involves orthopedic action with an ARS. In these cases, laser biostimulation improves tissue healing, reduces pain and muscle stress, and (probably) accelerates the tissue remodeling mechanism.

Laser therapy can also help provide relief for patients with chronic TMJ lock. In cases involving lesions of the disc and other cartilage affected by arthrogenous phenomena, the pain symptoms become an unbearable constant presence. Regular courses of laser therapy noticeably reduce the inflammation and, consequently, the pain.

INTERMEDIATE PATHOLOGY (ONSET OF ARTICULAR DAMAGE AND COMPRESSION OF THE BILAMINAR ZONE)

VIRTUAL DIAGNOSTIC PROCEDURE

The distinction between muscle pathology and articular pathology is unclear since both areas are affected, albeit in a different manner.

DIAGNOSIS

Intermediate musculoarticular pathology may be recognized through muscle tension, pain, and initial general derangement, with the condyle shifting superoposteriorly and the disc shifting inferoanteriorly.

TREATMENT PLAN

An SS,[1] indented onto the maxilla and with a smooth plane touching all the mandibular teeth, is able to eliminate occlusal interferences, thus leading to muscle relaxation and pain relief for the patient, in addition to having a generic action on the TMJ.

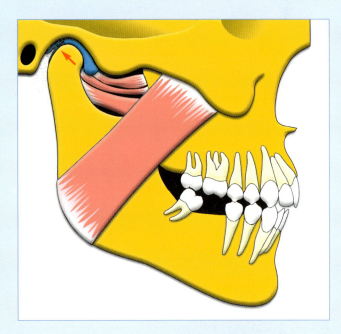

THERAPY

An SS benefits both the patient, who often perceives pain relief and improved function, and the clinician, who is able to work in more favorable conditions. A well-manufactured splint, systematically checked and ground to remove signs of occlusal interference, has an important effect on the muscles. Unlike the six-point splint, an SS can be worn for an unlimited amount of time. Generally, it lowers the condyles in the anteroposterior and transversal directions, unless designed with a more selective purpose in mind. Where the extent of damage is moderate, an SS may aid some recovery although, again, in a nonspecific manner. In more severe cases, it can be a first step in preparing a subsequent bite registration to manufacture a more specific ARS. For all these reasons, the SS is probably the splint most commonly used in treating TMDs.[21]

PROGNOSIS

The outcome is expected to be unequivocally positive in generic cases with prevalently muscular symptoms. Conversely, the use of an SS is debatable and often unacceptable when the seriousness of a case calls for individual specific musculoarticular therapy. In circumstances such as these, however, adaptability and compromise play an important role as does the patient's decision to decline more challenging treatment and to settle for a simpler treatment giving pain relief.

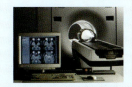

INTERMEDIATE PATHOLOGY IN MRI

CONDITIONS OF THE BILAMINAR ZONE AND RETRODISCAL TISSUE

Anomalous movement of the TMJ disc and consequently of the laminae creates a state of hyperemia in the retrodiscal tissues. In addition to the pain usually associated with it, the increase in blood is seen on open-mouth T2-weighted slices with increased signal intensity.

RETRODISCAL AREA showing T2 signal hyperintensity, indicating inflammation.

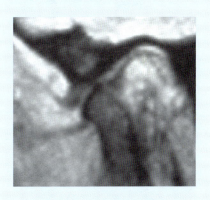

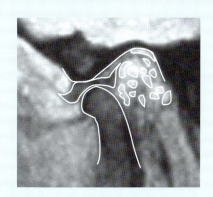

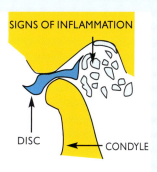

FLUID ON THE JOINT

MRI is an ideal diagnostic tool for detecting fluid buildup because of its high affinity for bodily fluids and versatility of imaging based on the acquisition parameters used. Like all other joints of the body, the TMJ responds to injury with phlogosis, including increased exudates that are recognizable, even in small quantities, in fat-suppressed T2-weighted images.

FLUID ON THE JOINT

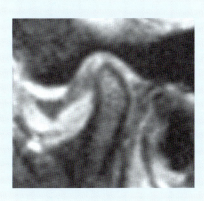

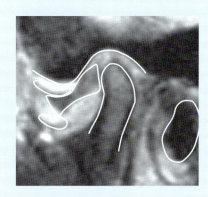

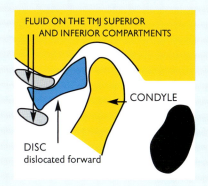

INTERMEDIATE PATHOLOGY: DIAGNOSTIC-THERAPEUTIC STABILIZATION SPLINT

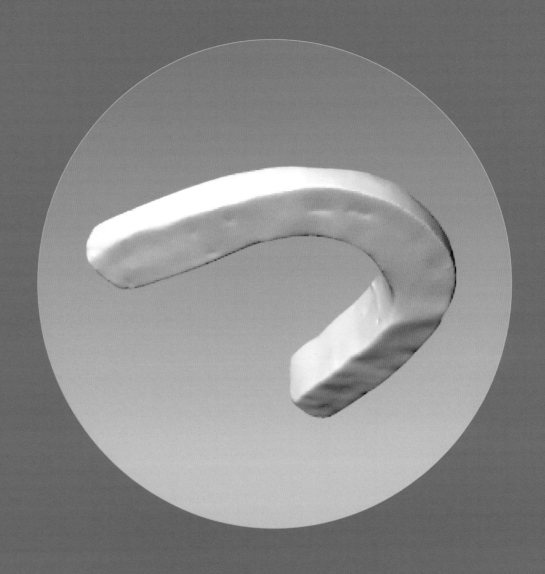

DESCRIPTION

A stabilization splint is prepared on an occlusor or, preferably, on an articulator using the patient's therapeutic bite registration wax impression.
Key features:

- Made of acrylic resin, preferably without metal clasps unless necessary to better hold it in place
- Fully indented on all maxillary teeth to ensure close fit
- Full-arch smooth inferior plane preventing occlusal interference between the two arches

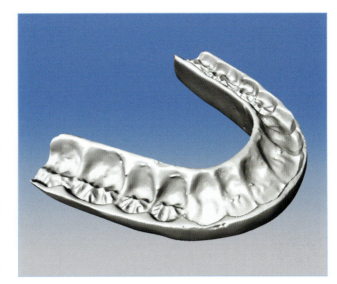

With its smooth inferior surface contacting the greatest possible number of mandibular teeth, an SS performs a dual diagnostic and therapeutic role. As a diagnostic aid, it is ideal to prevent occlusal interference, thereby relaxing the muscles and reducing tension and pain. As a therapeutic aid, it contributes to the general rearrangement of joint structures by acting on the transversal and anteroposterior planes in addition to specific vertical action from the posterior wedge.

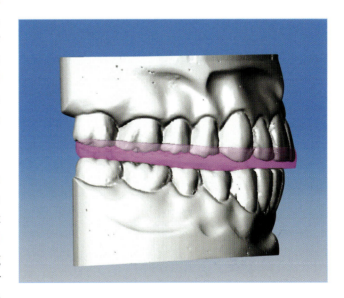

Both these features are advantageous. In straightforward cases, the splint indicates the diagnosis and solves the pathology. In more complicated cases, it improves but cannot resolve the dysfunctional pathology. In these latter cases involving differing degrees of articular tissue damage, an ARS is better indicated. For this reason, some reservations are expressed in the table (pages 92 to 93) summarizing the classifications of imperfect function.

BITE REGISTRATION

Bite registration (see page 102) should be done after the various procedures indicated on pages 74 onward to loosen the muscles and obtain correct muscular centric relation.

CONVERSION OF A SIX-POINT SPLINT INTO A STABILIZATION SPLINT

Conversion can be done either chairside, with the patient present for the fitting, or indirectly in the laboratory. Both procedures have their respective advantages and drawbacks.

DIRECT CHAIRSIDE TECHNIQUE

1. Use colored articulating paper to ascertain the presence of six contact points on the splint's anterior plane and a total absence of precontacts in the posterior quadrants.
2. Next, using a handheld tungsten carbide bur, rough grind the splint surface corresponding to the premolar and molar areas on both sides to improve the adhesion of new resin.
3. Mix new resin, and roll two cylinders approximately 7 to 8 mm in diameter and 20 to 25 mm in length.
4. Add these resin cylinders to the roughened premolar and molar splint surfaces, and fit the altered splint to the patient's maxillary arch.
5. Have the patient close her or his jaws. Remove the splint, and use scissors to trim excess soft resin.
6. Repeat insertion, removal, and trimming until the fit is satisfactory.
7. When the new resin has set, finish the adjusted splint with a cylindrical bur to eliminate all precontacts.
8. Take the splint to the laboratory for normal finishing and polishing.

ADVANTAGES AND DISADVANTAGES OF THE DIRECT CHAIRSIDE TECHNIQUE

ADVANTAGES	DISADVANTAGES
• *Speed of work* • *Lower cost*	• *Lack of necessary skills among some operators* • *Risk of resin infiltration of foreign matter* • *Slight discomfort for patient (odor and temperature of soft warm resin)*

INDIRECT LABORATORY TECHNIQUE

The indirect laboratory technique is outlined in the figures on the facing page. Preparation includes taking both a maxillary impression (with the splint fitted) and a mandibular impression, for cast molding, and a wax bite registration in the therapeutic, or muscular, position. The laboratory work involves pouring and trimming the casts and placing them in an occlusor or articulator.

Next, the old splint's surfaces are rough ground as necessary and boxed with wax before progressive "salt-and-pepper" addition of the monomer and polymer. The splint is then fitted to the maxillary cast, and the articulator is tightened and tied closed to indent the posterior quadrants. The resin is left to set at a temperature of approximately 50°C and a pressure of 2 atm before being finished in the normal manner.

ADVANTAGES AND DISADVANTAGES OF THE INDIRECT LABORATORY TECHNIQUE

ADVANTAGES	DISADVANTAGES
• *Better resin quality* • *Less bother for the patient* • *No hurry*	• *Longer time to prepare* • *Probable higher cost*

PREPARATION OF THE SS

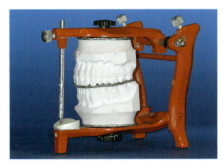

1. Casts mounted in occlusor with wax bite.

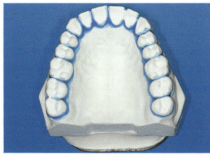

2. Undercuts blocked out on both labial and palatal sides.

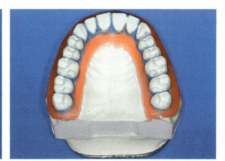

3. Boxing.

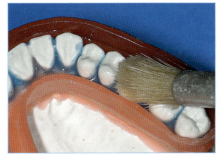

4. Acrylic separator added before mixing liquid and powder.

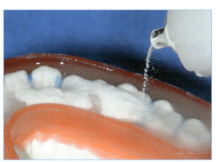

5. SALT-AND-PEPPER monomer-polymer mixing.

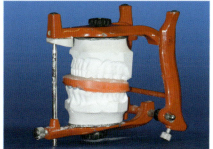

6. Occlusor turned upside when pressure setting the resin to prevent resin from running.

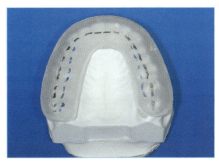

7. Antagonist cusps marked with cast still on occlusor.

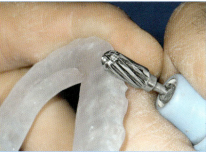
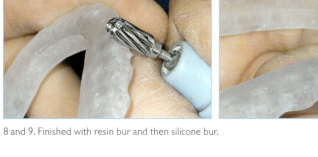

8 and 9. Finished with resin bur and then silicone bur.

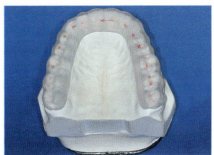

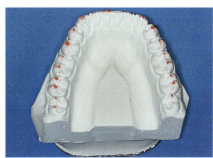

10. Contact points checked on splint with articulating paper.

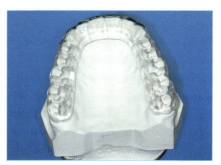

Final polish.

HOW AN SS WORKS

The SS has a dual action:

- It relaxes the muscles and prevents deviating or traumatic dental contacts.
- It exerts a nonprogrammable, nonselective generic orthopedic action that lowers the condyles, as shown by the tomograms on the facing page (taken on the same day without and with the splint).

As described on page 128, the SS may also be fabricated on an existing six-point splint, either chairside or in the laboratory.

PRACTICAL EXAMPLE: PATIENT E. M.

Without the splint

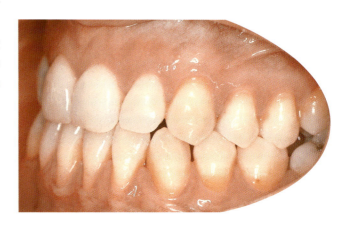

With the fitted splint

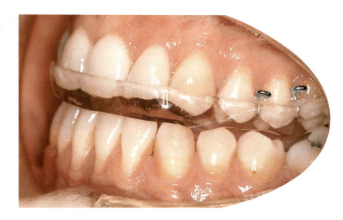

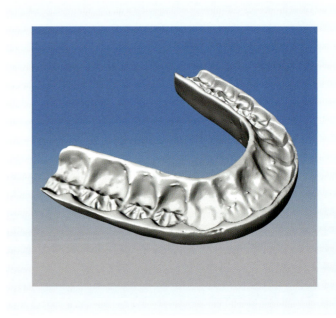

TOMOGRAMS SHOWING CONDYLAR POSITION ON THE SAME DAY WITHOUT AND SUBSEQUENTLY WITH THE SS (courtesy of Dr G. F. Franchi, Leghorn, Italy)

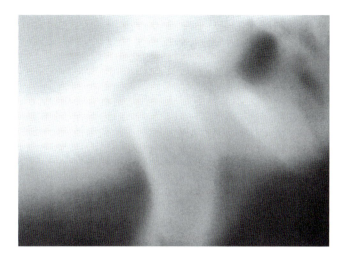

Without the splint

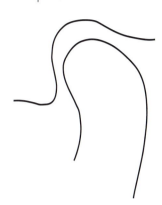

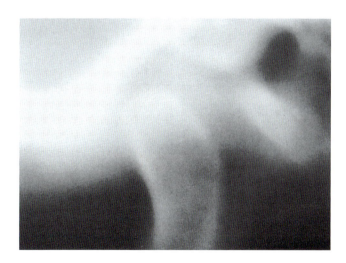

With the fitted splint

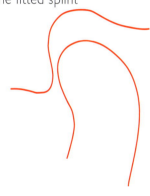

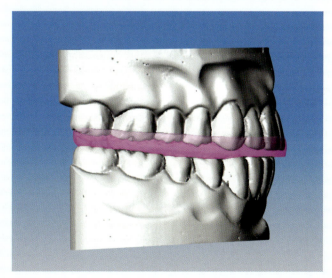

In addition to acting on the muscles, the superimposed outlines show how the SS has produced an orthopedic action on the patient's condyles. Tests on a number of patients give similar results.

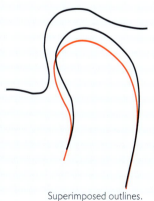

Superimposed outlines.

MICHIGAN PLATE

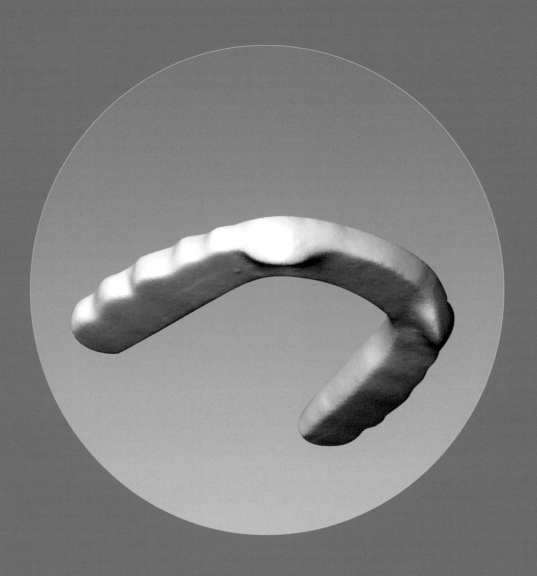

CONVERTING AN SS INTO A MICHIGAN PLATE

An SS (or all-point splint) becomes a Michigan plate with the addition of incisal guidance and cuspid protection. Care must be taken with these dynamic disclosure functions since their application is unsuitable if correct TMJ function has not first been established.

CHAIRSIDE

1. To model incisal guidance, add soft resin to the anterior splint area while guiding the patient's mandible a few millimeters into protrusion.
2. Use scissors to trim excess resin while it is still soft, a little at a time.
3. Once a satisfactory dynamic result has been achieved, cure and finish the resin.
4. Fine tune the dynamic function by checking the amount of movement again and relieving resin as necessary.
6. Place blue articulating paper between the maxillary splint and mandibular teeth. Ask the patient to occlude, and then observe the marks left on the splint. All the mandibular incisors and canines must show maxillary splint contact.

LABORATORY

1. To model incisal guidance, place the casts in an articulator with average settings and proceed as outlined above. This procedure is more easily done in the lab than chairside, especially where cuspid protection is concerned.
2. To create canine rise, with the casts still in the articulator, add two resin pyramids masking the shape of the cuspids at a point that corresponds to the labial face of the mandibular canines.
3. Using oil to insulate the fingertips, mold the resin as it hardens.
4. Finally, grind the cuspid rises to the correct height to give disclosionary lift in left and right lateral excursions. Ensure that the posterior teeth do not come into contact with the splint.

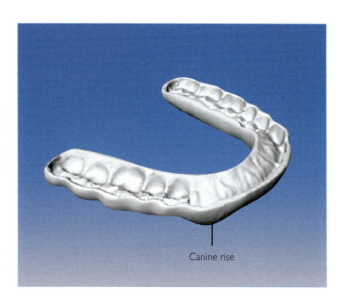

Canine rise

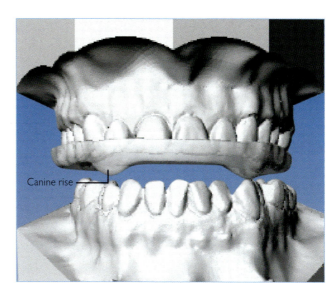

Canine rise

INTRACAPSULAR PATHOLOGY: DISLOCATION WITH AND WITHOUT REDUCTION (ALTERED POSITION)

VIRTUAL DIAGNOSTIC PROCEDURE

DIAGNOSIS

This section deals with patients whose complaint involves TMJ internal derangement with the condyle posteriorized and the disc anteriorized. If the disc is recaptured when the jaws are opened, the phenomenon is classified as dislocation with reduction (or recapture). Conversely, dislocation without reduction occurs when the disc fails to be recaptured and results in TMJ axial disalignment (see table on pages 92 and 93).

Clinical examination reveals evident anomaly in mandibular movements. Disclosure, closure, and protrusion are affected by deflection and deviation in dislocation with and without reduction, respectively. Lateral excursions are also irregular, and there is usually joint noise, the most common being clicks signaling disc loss and recapture in cases of dislocation with reduction.

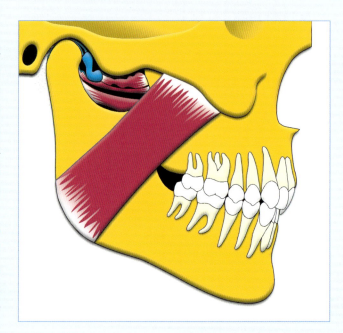

TREATMENT PLAN

The primary aim is to normalize axial alignment of the condyle, disc (or pseudodisc), and articulating surface during both static and dynamic relationships. This will automatically help the muscles to relax and will therefore reduce or eliminate pain.

THERAPY

Although well-executed manipulation can contribute significantly to rehabilitation of TMJ function, the majority of patients will require an intraoral splint (ARS) to lower and anteriorize the mandible.[1,22–25] The ARS must be worn almost constantly—approximately 22 hours per day excepting mealtimes and hygiene—for 8 to 10 months until stable, correct articular relationships have been restored. This therapeutic position frequently causes the mandible to rotate downward slightly, opening the bite and increasing vertical height, a consequence that is addressed as necessary during subsequent orthodontic work.

PROGNOSIS

Any prognosis is affected by:

- The degree of pathology
- The patient's age (the younger, the better)
- The length of time since the onset of pathology (the shorter the time, the better the outcome)
- The patient's compliance in wearing the splint
- Correct condyle-disc-articulating surface axial realignment, both static and dynamic

The presence of several positive factors indicates a greater likelihood of successful outcome.

DEBATE: IS CLICKING ALWAYS A SIGN OF PATHOLOGY?

A typical TMJ click is a clear decisive sound of differing intensity. It may be heard—not only by the patient but also by other people at times—during lateral excursions and protrusion. Clicking may be associated with articular pain, but it may also be asymptomatic, in which case doubt arises as to whether treatment is necessary. Since there are conflicting opinions on the subject, it is useful to reflect on several practical considerations:

- Patient history should be examined carefully. Parafunctional habits such as clenching or grinding undeniably contribute to TMD and its deterioration.
- The patient's interest in the problem and motivation to resolve it partially or more in depth must be determined.
- Whenever possible, medical imaging is recommended to complete the diagnosis. CTs and MRIs (preferred) give a fuller picture of both closed-mouth and open-mouth condyle-disc-articulating surface alignment, TMJ osseous conditions, and the external pterygoid muscle. A fuller diagnosis permits a more accurate prognosis.

Evaluation of all these elements can help the patient and clinician decide whether and how the click should be treated. Remember that prevention is better than a cure, so overtreatment must be avoided. As a general rule, professional ethics indicate that no irreversible procedures such as prosthodontics, surgery, or orthodontics should be performed without fully informing the patient. Likewise, articular dysfunction should always be resolved before dealing with dental issues. A Class II patient will always benefit from occlusal splint therapy leading to posteroanterior skeletal improvement, regardless of the clicks. Lastly, it goes without saying that unless major oral rehabilitation is essential, the patient—properly informed—has the last word.

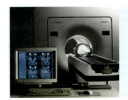

DISLOCATION WITH REDUCTION VIEWED WITH MRI

TMJ dysfunction is caused by abnormal disc position with the cartilage displaced anteriorly, resulting in the loss of its protective function. During the early stages of dislocation, part of the disc may begin to protrude medially or laterally without dislocating entirely. MRI is the only form of imaging that can provide advance warning and greater detail regarding the condition of the cartilage.

The extent and direction of dislocation is revealed by MRI slice selection, with oblique sagittal images showing the disc slipping anterior to the condyle as opposed to the medial or lateral protrusion shown on coronal sequences. As the pathology deteriorates, the disc anteriorizes further and remains dislocated forward, with or without medial or lateral co-protrusion. If this is the case, MRI permits a kinetic analysis by comparing open-mouth sequences that show whether the disc is recaptured, depending on the degree of pathology.

Disc shape also indicates the degree of pathology. While a healthy meniscus viewed laterally presents a biconcave profile, dysfunctional movements will cause it to become shredded, buckled, or biconvex as a result of anterior dislocation and alteration to its other support structures.

KEY FEATURES

- Excursions are within a biologically normal range (maximum mouth opening, 35 to 45 mm; lateral excursions and protrusion, 7 to 10 mm).
- Excursions follow an irregular path and present deflection on opening, closure, and protrusion. Deflections can take many different shapes. They reflect a lateral mandible shift during these movements, with the path becoming straight again toward the end (see page 65).

- Dull noises of differing intensity are heard, ranging from the simplest click to a complex variety of sounds in one or both TMJs, on opening or closure alone, on both opening and closure, and/or during lateral excursions and protrusion.

ANTERIOR DISLOCATION, mouth closed

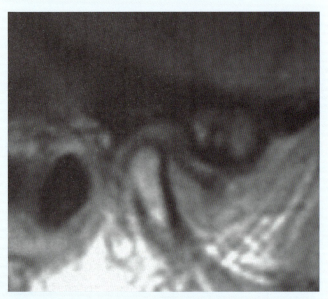

DISC RECAPTURE, mouth open

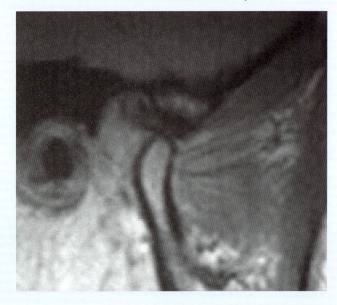

- Classically, a click on opening is interpreted as reduction, or recapture, of the dislocated disc, and this sound occurs in the early stages of opening. When the disc dislocates late in the course of jaw closure, the sound is defined as a late click. This may be particularly loud and heard from some distance.
- The area of the external pterygoid is almost always painful on palpation.

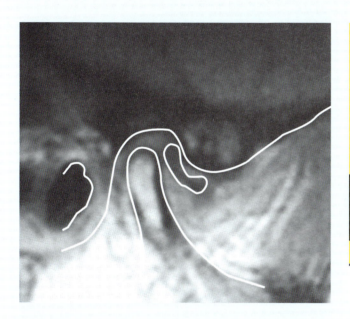

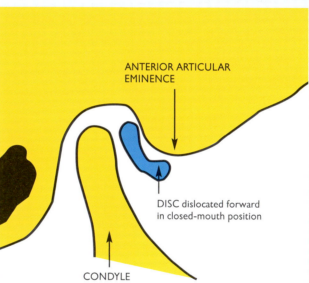

ANTERIOR ARTICULAR EMINENCE

DISC dislocated forward in closed-mouth position

CONDYLE

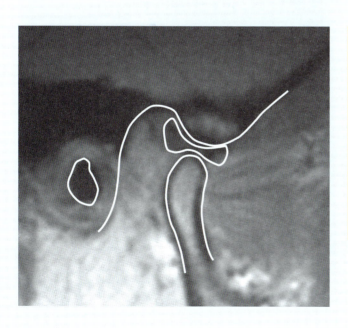

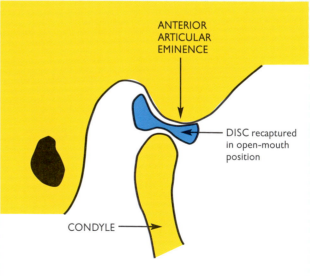

ANTERIOR ARTICULAR EMINENCE

DISC recaptured in open-mouth position

CONDYLE

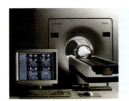

DISLOCATION WITHOUT REDUCTION VIEWED WITH MRI

- Movements are generally limited to less than the normal range (maximum mouth opening, 25 to 30 mm).
- If one condyle is in worse condition than the other, a homolateral mandibular deviation is observed in the late stage of opening along with significant reduction of the contralateral lateral excursion.
- The noises generally sound less like clicks and more like car wheels rolling over rough ground.
- The area of the external pterygoid is almost always painful on palpation.

(See the table on pages 92 and 93.)

ANTERIOR DISLOCATION,
mouth closed with disc crumpled

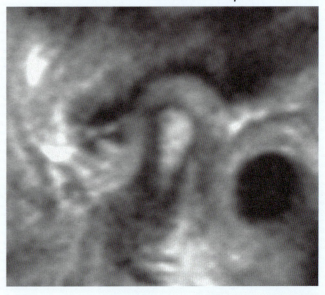

WITHOUT RECAPTURE,
disc crumpled forward but not recaptured

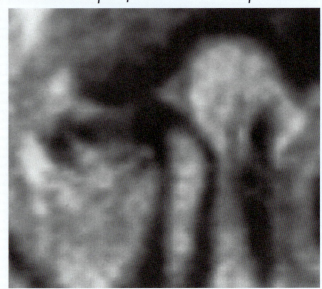

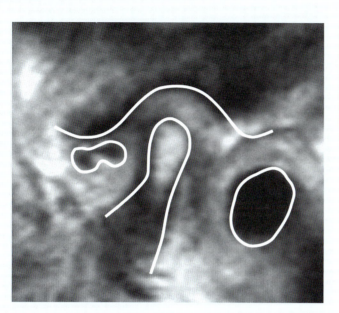

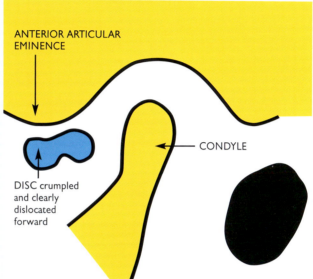

ANTERIOR ARTICULAR
EMINENCE

CONDYLE

DISC crumpled
and clearly
dislocated
forward

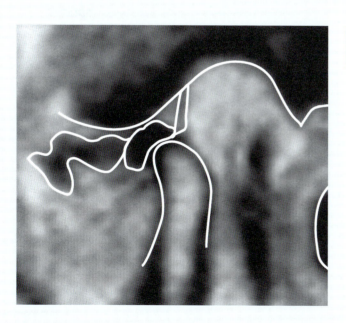

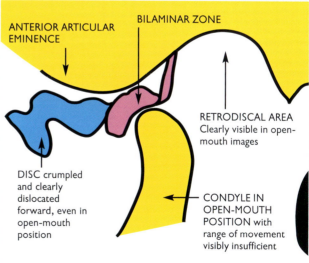

ANTERIOR ARTICULAR
EMINENCE

BILAMINAR ZONE

RETRODISCAL AREA
Clearly visible in open-
mouth images

DISC crumpled
and clearly
dislocated
forward, even in
open-mouth
position

CONDYLE IN
OPEN-MOUTH
POSITION with
range of movement
visibly insufficient

INTRACAPSULAR PATHOLOGY: DESTRUCTION (ALTERATIONS TO POSITION AND SHAPE)

VIRTUAL DIAGNOSTIC PROCEDURE

DIAGNOSIS

The symptomatology is complex as a result of damage done over years or even decades of ongoing deterioration. Limitation of excursions in all three directions is an ever-present feature. The clicks have ceased since the disc is permanently anteriorized, and the joint noise resembles that of car wheels crunching over stony ground. The disc is almost always totally dislocated forward, incapable of reduction, and largely destroyed. Direct friction between the condylar and articular eminence tissues has left them altered, usually flattened, in a variety of shapes, with craters and bone spurs often noted (see pages 92 and 93).

Patients' complaints at this stage of TMJ internal derangement vary enormously. Some report intense pain while others find it minimal, as if a progressive adaptation process has occurred since the least pain is usually associated with the worst conditions (including TMJ lock).

In this context, it is essential to distinguish clearly between **TMJ lock** and **muscle lock**. Although both cause limited disclosure, **muscle lock** does not affect lateral excursion or protrusion. In contrast, **articular lock** limits contralateral excursions on the opposite side and causes deviations on protrusion and on disclosure on the same side as the affected TMJ (illustrated on page 66).

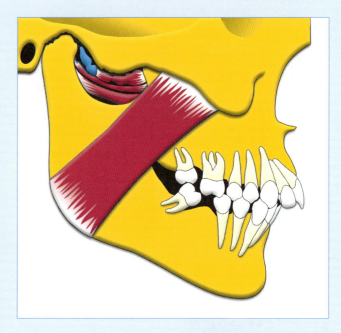

TREATMENT AIMS

Regular manipulation is indicated, and if necessary, the highly sophisticated manual unlocking techniques should be used. Particularly obstinate cases may require a splint (see page 183) with selective ramps for the posterior teeth on one or both sides as necessary. Clearly, in cases such as these, the outcome will always be a compromise since functional adaptation is the most that can be hoped for. Where manipulation, splints, and medication fail to be of benefit, the only remaining option is surgery, as discussed at the end of this chapter.

THERAPY

Several key requirements must be observed during therapy:

- Condylar repositioning must be maintained with the ARS restoring the best possible axial alignment with the disc (or what remains of it) and eminence, in an attempt to achieve some degree of success.
- Muscle tone must be improved to relieve the pain.
- The ARS must be worn at all times, excepting mealtimes and hygiene, for a number of months, the average time being more than a year.

PROGNOSIS

The prognosis may be considered hopeful if the following conditions have been met:

- Therapeutic stability of the restored occlusal relationships obtained with the splint is maintained in both static and dynamic conditions.
- If anatomical rearrangement has been successful, the posterior ligament functions as a pseudodisc.

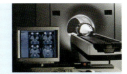

TISSUE DESTRUCTION VIEWED WITH MRI

TMJ internal derangement and its accompanying damage are seen with the following signs:
- Flattened TMJ osseous tissues
- Bone spurs
- Osseous necrosis
- Arthrosis
- Possible inflammation

FLATTENING of TMJ osseous tissues

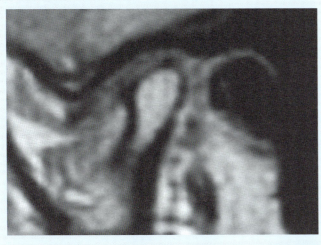
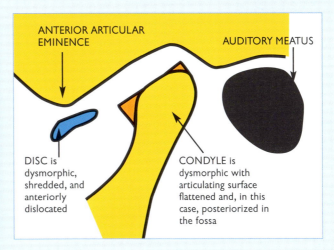

ANTERIOR ARTICULAR EMINENCE

AUDITORY MEATUS

DISC is dysmorphic, shredded, and anteriorly dislocated

CONDYLE is dysmorphic with articulating surface flattened and, in this case, posteriorized in the fossa

BONE SPUR at condylar apex (open-mouth T2-weighted sequence)

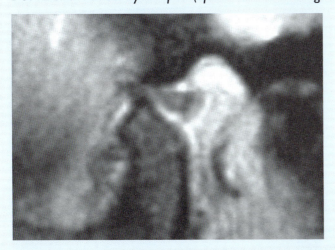
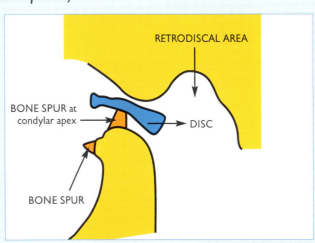

RETRODISCAL AREA

BONE SPUR at condylar apex

DISC

BONE SPUR

CONDYLAR OSTEONECROSIS

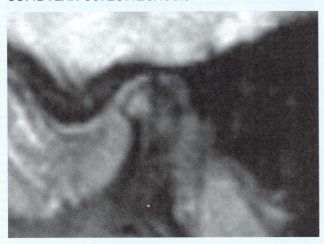
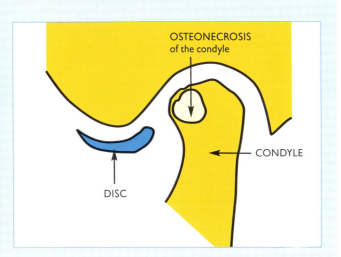

OSTEONECROSIS of the condyle

CONDYLE

DISC

COMMON FEATURES OF DISLOCATION AND TISSUE DESTRUCTION

MAXIMUM EXCURSION PATHWAYS

Where one condyle is more damaged than the other, deviation on opening occurs on the affected side. In lateral excursions, the side opposite the damaged condyle is more limited, since the damaged condyle is unable to orbit, while lateral mandibular excursion is easier to the side of the damaged condyle (see page 67).

PAIN

Both dislocation and destruction are usually characterized by constant pain on palpation of the lateral pterygoid, this being one of the telling symptoms of TMJ pathology even when other muscles are free of pain. Lateral pterygoid tenderness may linger posttreatment as a residual effect of inflammation and muscle involvement.

An investigation of patient history should include inquiries about early morning muscle stiffness with increased tension and pain. This is a sign of subconscious nighttime action, which occurs unimpeded and results in pain. During the day, patients relieve pain by preventing dental contact. Typically, they use the tongue as a bite plane, which leaves visible scallops on the tongue and ridges on the cheeks. These indications should be noted and assigned empirical intensity values: 0, 1, 2, or 3.

Complaints of earache are another sign of musculoarticular pathology. Earache results from condylar posterior compression against the auditory meatus area. For this reason, patients may be referred by ear, nose, and throat specialists who have ruled out symptoms coming under their speciality.

DIAGNOSIS AND TREATMENT PLAN

TMJ pathology usually results in the condyles being raised and posteriorized within the glenoid fossa, with the disc being forced into an anteroinferior position. Consequently, the treatment plan strives to produce an opposite pattern to that caused by the pathology, hence the lowering and selective advancement of both condyle and disc (see clinical investigation commencing page 96). This principle is fundamental in wax bite registration for ARS fabrication.

EFFECT OF NEGATIVE OR POSITIVE LOADING ON THE TMJ

Abnormal loading may cause a loss of axial alignment between the condyle, disc, and fossa, probably leading to pathology ranging from dislocation with reduction through dislocation without reduction to final destruction with internal joint derangement. Where compression has contributed to alteration of the condyle and fossa bony tissues, articular distraction will aid remodeling of the eroded tissues until an acceptable functional compromise is reached.

Clearly, the outcome is more likely to be successful for patients who are younger and have less severe damage at the start of treatment.

To summarize, a posterosuperior condylar position associated with axial misalignment and excessive loading on TMJ structures plays a major role in the progression of damage. Conversely, pathology cases may benefit from distraction holding the articular components apart and thus contributing to recovery. If this is so, then it may reasonably be supposed that in nonpathologic cases, distraction of articular structures may bring about skeletal changes that can be exploited during therapy. Affixation of bone on the forward side, in the posterior fossa wall and on the posterior condylar surface, could bring about forward mandibular shift (see Pancherz' studies on Herbst appliances).

ARTICULOMUSCULAR INTRACAPSULAR PATHOLOGY: THERAPEUTIC ANTERIOR REPOSITIONING SPLINT

It rearranges and maintains correct three-dimensional (3D) articular relationships during the entire treatment procedure from phase I through phase II

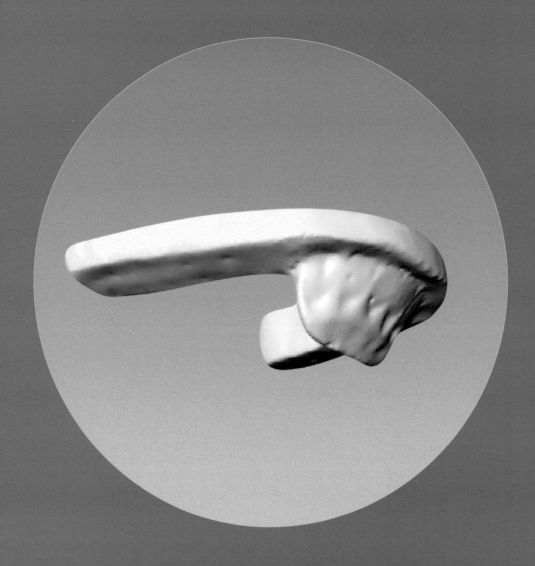

DESCRIPTION

This splint is used to reposition both the mandible and the individual condyles in the three planes of space. It consists of:

- An **intraoral acrylic resin splint** indented on the maxillary arch
- A **smooth posterolateral wedge** contacting the mandibular teeth simultaneously at a number of points
- An **anterior flange** to establish the anterior, transversal, and vertical position of the mandible and, consequently, of both condyles

The therapeutic position taken with wax bite registration is fixed and the setup mounted on the occlusor, confirming the position for the entire course of treatment. Instead of retention clasps, the splint is stabilized on the maxillary teeth by fitting fractionally higher than the equator toward the root. For this purpose, it can be useful to work with a parallelometer.

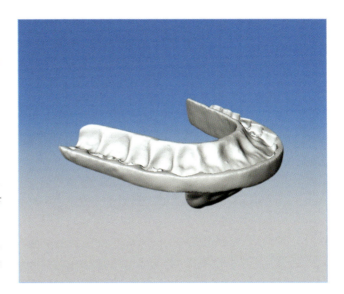

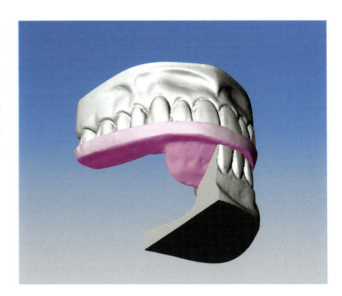

ARS: THERAPEUTIC POSITION REGISTRATION (MUSCLE-LED CLOSURE)

The manual techniques for bite registration, a key step for fabrication of all splint types, have been described on page 102.

BITE REGISTRATION FOR DISLOCATION WITH REDUCTION

Establishing the therapeutic position for bite registration prior to fabricating an ARS for patients who have dislocation with reduction can be done by following the fifth procedure (horizontal and vertical manipulation) described in the section on diagnostic manipulation (see page 78). To seek the most correct position, the mandible must be manipulated while directing the patient to perform certain movements to gain his or her active cooperation.

1. Place the index finger under the patient's chin, the thumb in the symphysis. This enables movements to be guided by the clinician.
2. Attempt to rotate the posterior mandibular area, and therefore the condyles, downward.
3. While helping the patient to protrude the mandible as far as possible, ask the patient to open and close the mouth while maintaining the protrusion. The click should disappear in the maximum protrusion position.
4. Still working together, have the patient continue to open and close the mouth while retruding the mandible fractionally, one millimeter at a time. At one point, the click will reappear. The therapeutic position judged to be correct for bite registration is the furthest retruded position of mandible opening and closure immediately prior to the click returning.
5. Determine the thickness of the wax (at least 1.5 mm) directly in the patient's mouth. The wax must not be perforated at any point.

BITE REGISTRATION FOR DISLOCATION WITHOUT REDUCTION AND DERANGEMENT

Likewise, therapeutic position bite registration should follow essentially the same steps as just described. The greater severity of tissue destruction in patients suffering from derangement and dislocation without reduction, the fewer the points of reference. Therefore, it is better to ensure greater condylar lowering and forward distraction (overcorrection) to relieve compression on the joint extremities and thus aid their rearrangement.

A further point to consider is the transversal component for lateromedial condylar position correction, in which case the position to take is that given when the muscles are relaxed.

In these cases, it is improbable that the condyle will be in a central position within the fossa since it is influenced by a number of factors including articular eminence inclination (see clinical investigation by Dr Crudo on page 96) and the position of the disc, or what remains of it.

Clinical considerations

To safeguard correct bilateral muscle tension, there can be little or no tolerance in mandibular positioning on the transversal plane. However, Class II pathologies do permit a small degree of horizontal tolerance, and indeed, it may be beneficial to bring the mandible fractionally forward during bite registration and some weeks later by adding acrylic to the anterior flange area and thus addressing both negative factors. The vertical dimension is worth separate consideration since this may be a concrete, long-term way to relieve dislocation and derangement by lowering the mandible and rearranging the damaged articular structures. A clinical research study (see pages 208 to 209) shows that the amount of mandibular lowering correlates with the amount of protrusion.

Extra care must be taken with Class III patients to prevent mandibular protrusion.

GUIDELINES ON MUSCLE-LED CLOSURE IN CLASSES I, II, and III

Bite registration often leads to changes:
- *In anteroposterior relationships*
  - Class I: edge-to-edge bite or sometimes crossbite
  - Class II: considerable reduction in overjet with skeletal improvement
  - Class II, division 2: edge-to-edge bite between maxillary and mandibular incisors
  - Class III: bite deterioration

The anterior vertical height is caused by greater opening of the anterior bite from original jaw position.
- *In transversal relationships (some possibilities):*
  - If the midlines coincide in dental closure and on protrusion, the therapeutic position should be central.
  - If the midlines do not coincide in dental closure but coincide on protrusion, the correct position is when they are centered.
  - If the patient complains of earache on one side only or there is radiologic evidence of only one condyle being posteriorized, the therapeutic position is deviated toward the opposite side—that is, toward the unaffected side, thus advancing the damaged condyle.

Where it is not possible to compare upper and lower midlines, reference should be made to the gingival frenula. Both maxillary and mandibular dental midlines are acceptable on condition that there is no major dental asymmetry in either anterior or lateral areas (which is relatively common), such as complete lack of space for a canine, or where the patient has lost a first molar with consequent hemiarch collapse. In cases such as these, the gingival frenula are to be referred to.

The clinician should make every effort to achieve the following:

- Enable the **muscles** to operate in a relaxed condition. Many of the procedures previously mentioned are based on this assumption.
- Rearrange the internal structures of the **TMJs** while maintaining axial alignment between the condyle, disc, and fossa.

In more advanced cases (with tissue destruction), it is advisable to give priority to condylar distraction (see pages 100 and 101).

PHASES OF ARS FABRICATION

Since the initial laboratory work is the same as that for an SS, refer to page 129, steps 1 through 5.

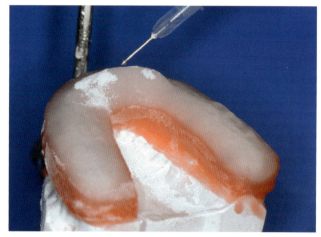

1. SALT-AND-PEPPER technique.

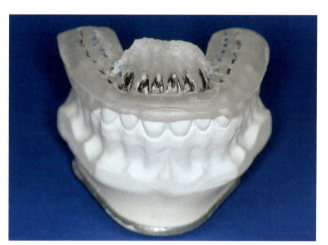

4. Marking antagonist cuspids for grinding.

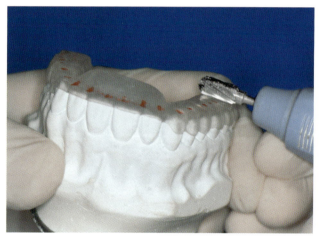

5. Resin bur rough contouring.

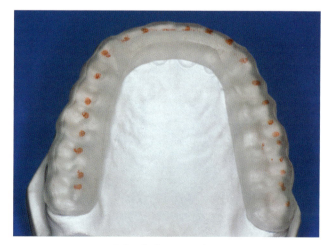

8. Detail of contact points.

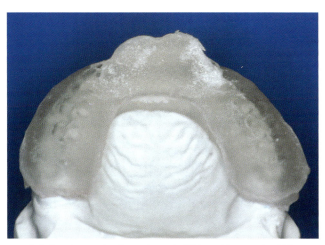

2. Splint after wax has been cleaned off (viewed from underside).

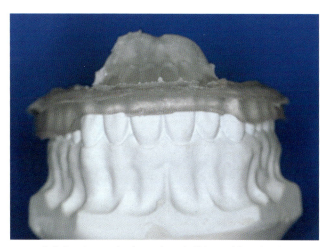

3. Splint after wax has been cleaned off (viewed from front).

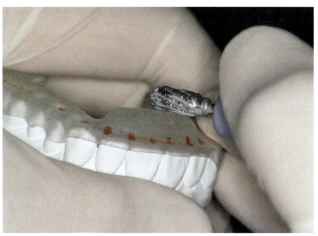

6. Flange finishing.

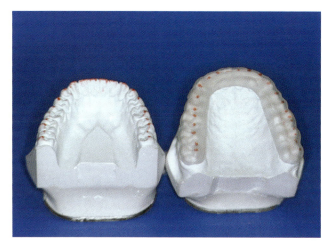

7. The splint must only touch the maxillary cast cuspids.

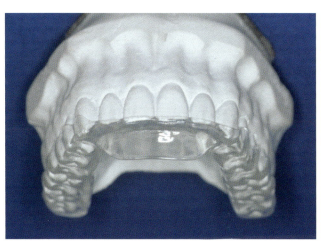

9. The ARS completed with final polishing.

TRASFORMING AN SS INTO AN ARS

Conversion can be done chairside, with the patient present for the fitting, or indirectly in the laboratory. Both procedures have their respective advantages and disadvantages.

DIRECT CHAIRSIDE TECHNIQUE

1. Using a handheld tungsten carbide bur, rough grind the occlusal surface to make it conducive to adhesion of the added acrylic.

The two alteration steps are done separately.

Flange:

2. Roll an acrylic cylinder approximately 3 cm in length with a lateral taper.

3. With the splint fitted on the patient's maxillary arch, mold the fresh acrylic cylinder to the front part, and guide the patient's mandible into the new therapeutic position.

4. Check the indentation frequently, and use scissors to trim excess resin before it hardens.

Posterior wedge:

5. If necessary, add resin over the posterior quadrants to create correct contacts with the mandibular counterparts.

6. Check the entire splint, finish, and polish.

ADVANTAGES AND DISADVANTAGES OF DIRECT CHAIRSIDE TECHNIQUE

ADVANTAGES	DISADVANTAGES
Rapidità di esecuzione	*The operator must be highly skilled in handling acrylic chairside*
Lower cost	*Shorter splint life due to infiltration of more porous resin*

ADVANTAGES AND DISADVANTAGES OF INDIRECT LABORATORY TECHNIQUE

INDIRECT LABORATORY TECHNIQUE

1. Take a mandibular impression and a maxillary impression with the splint fitted. Cast both in dental stone, and mount in an articulator using the bite registration taken in the new musculoarticular position.

2. Rough grind the splint's surfaces, and box with wax.

3. Perform progressive salt-and-pepper monomer and polymer addition and manual shaping to build up the inferior flange and bring the posterior portions into contact.

4. Build up the posterior wedges in the same manner.

5. Set the resin at a temperature of approximately 50°C and a pressure of 2 atm.

6. Finish in the normal manner.

ADVANTAGES	DISADVANTAGES
Better resin and splint quality	*Longer lab time*
Stability	*Higher cost*

ARS FABRICATION WITH COMPUTER-AIDED DESIGN/COMPUTER-ASSISTED MANUFACTURE TECHNOLOGY

*   Computerized Aided Design = progettazione assistita dal computer.

** Computerized Aided Manufacturing = costruzione assistita dal computer.

This page incorporates, for perhaps one of the first times, the application of rapid prototyping in ARS fabrication, as illustrated below. While expected to become common practice before long, this procedure is currently undergoing practical experimentation.[27] Alginate impression-based casts are scanned with a 3D scanner and processed by computer-aided design/computer-assisted manufacture (CAD/CAM) software (CADental, Structura).

The 3D splint computer model print command is sent to a rapid prototype machine for fabrication.

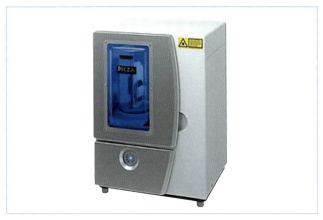

3D scanner.

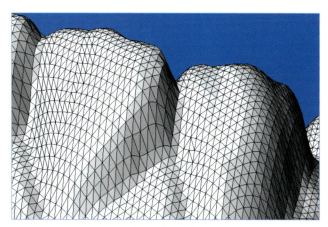

Scanned models.

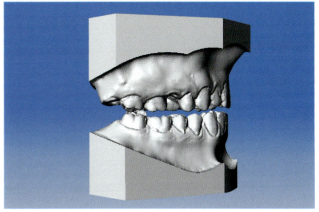

Model processing with CAD/CAM software.

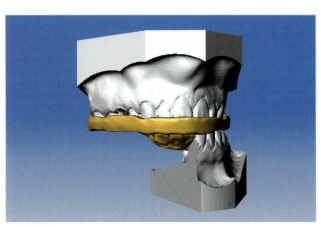

Splint computer model.

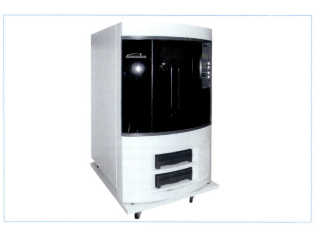

PROTOTYPE machine.

ARS: HOW IT WORKS

An ARS is used for dislocation with and without reduction and for internal derangement, even though the procedures to establish therapeutic position are separate.

The aims are similar, but the results differ:

- Where there is **dislocation with disc reduction** on opening, an ARS helps recapture the disc when possible, thus eliminating the click and obtaining functional recovery
- Where there is **dislocation without reduction** or **derangement**, the ARS helps obtain a functional adaptation by separating the osseous tissues and bringing the condyles forward and especially downward (particularly for Class III patients) to achieve the best possible rearrangement of the badly damaged structures. Some authors[28] have described the production of factors that stimulate chondro-osteogenesis and fibrogenesis in animal models consequent to anterior mandibular repositioning.

Wearing a splint is awkward for patients. The splint is cumbersome and causes speech difficulties, although these drawbacks may become less noticeable through perseverance in constant wear. However, these problems may be compensated for by the positive effect on symptoms. Where pain is the most crippling presence, the ARS may help relieve fatigue and stress by restoring normal muscle tension and more natural mandibular movements.

The patient should return for regular appointments, approximately monthly. During these appointments, the clinician makes minor adjustments, usually by eliminating acrylic over the maxillary teeth to bring them nearer to correct contacts with their antagonists. In addition, if a small click is still heard in the early opening stage, the splint may be corrected by adding acrylic to the protrusive anterior flange while the splint is worn, until the click disappears.

Note: It should be remembered that this procedure represents PHASE I of the entire musculoarticular rehabilitation. In practice, if done by an expert, it may be simultaneously combined with PHASE II orthodontic occlusal finishing.

PRACTICAL EXAMPLE: PATIENT M. G.

Without ARS

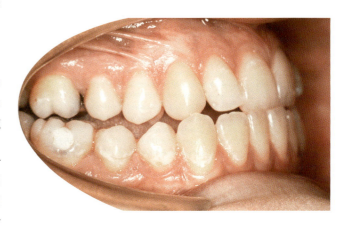

With fitted ARS

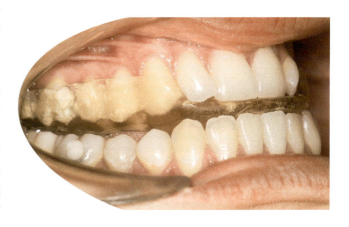

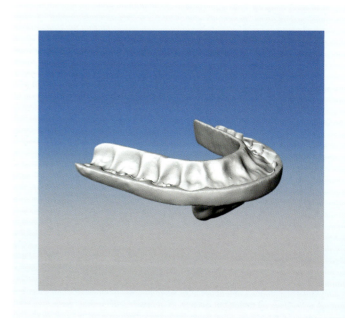

CT WITHOUT AND THEN WITH THE ARS FITTED ON THE SAME DAY

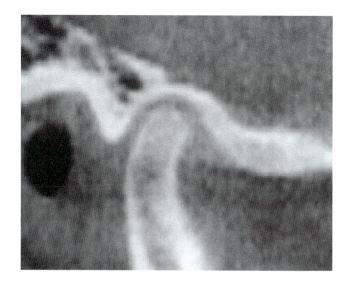

Without the splint

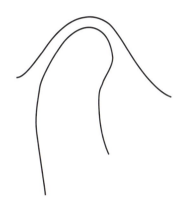

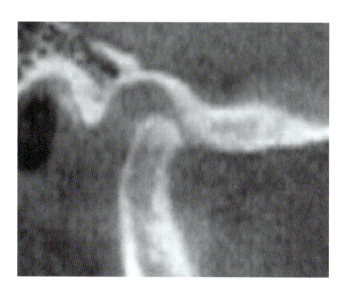

With the splint

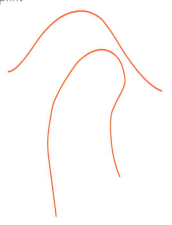

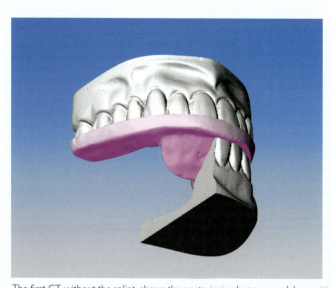

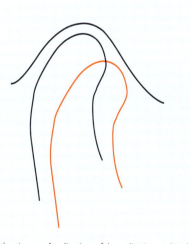

The first CT, without the splint, shows the posteriorized upper condylar position placing pressure on the tissues. Application of the splint immediately distracts the condyle downward and forward into a functionally valid position (see page 92).

MRI WITHOUT AND WITH THE ARS FITTED on the same day

In the **closed-mouth position** in pathologic maximum intercuspation, the joint components are not axially aligned, indicating a dislocation. The condyle is posteriorized, the disc is anteriorized, and the posterior articular space is reduced. In the patient's **habitual**, or **dental, closure**, note the unnatural tone of the external pterygoid muscle, in which the upper fibers inserting into the disc are contracted while the lower fibers inserting onto the condyle are stretched (see page 17).

CLINICAL EXAMPLE: PATIENT S. R.

Closed-mouth position:
dental Class I in pathologic habitual closure

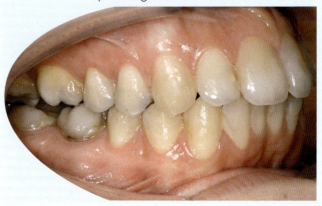

In the **open-mouth position**, the condyle, disc, and eminence are better aligned. This position creates a physiologic function with axial alignment between the joint components (see page 24). Consequently, the upper fibers of the superior bundle of the external pterygoid muscle, which insert into the disc, and the lower fibers, which insert into the condlye, have the correct length and balanced tone.

Open-mouth position:

With the **ARS fitted**, the condyle, disc, and eminence return to a correct functional recovery. They lie along the same axis with normal articular spaces and are, therefore, in correct therapeutic conditions. **Fitting the ARS** moves the condyle downward and forward. This position reduces discal dislocation and induces improved muscle balance since both upper and lower fibers of the external pterygoid muscle superior bundle present correct length and balanced tone, unlike their previous dysmetry (see page 16). This physiologic, closed-mouth position confirms the therapeutic condition established for and maintained by the splint in PHASE I, while the patient's dental relationships will be normalized during the subsequent orthodontic treatment planned for PHASE II.

Muscle-led closure:
dental Class III

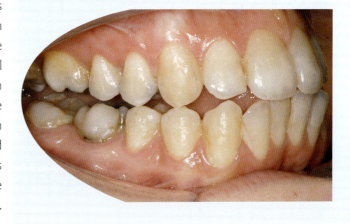

CONSIDERATIONS: The open-mouth position or fitting of the splint moves the condyle downward and forward, thus reducing the dislocation (disc recapture or reduction).

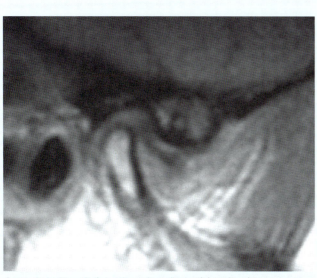

NEGATIVE PATHOLOGIC CONDITION

Mouth closed without splint

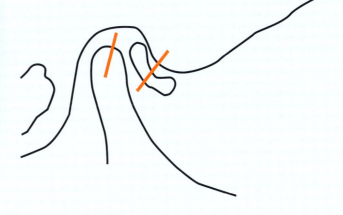

Anterior disc dislocation (unaligned loading)

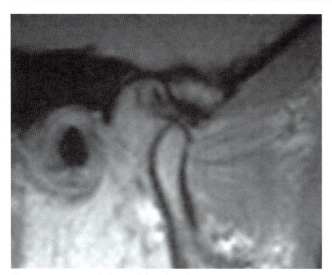

PHYSIOLOGIC CONDITION

Mouth open without splint

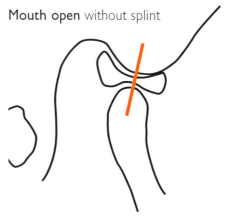

Disc recapture (aligned loading)

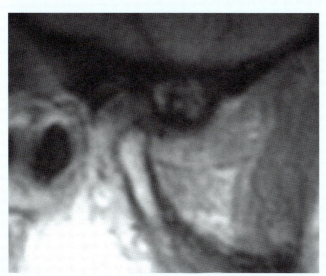

CORRECT THERAPEUTIC CONDITION

Mouth closed with ARS

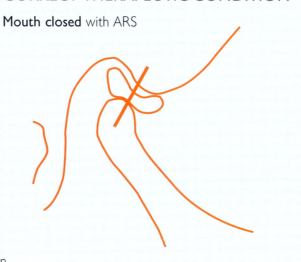

Disc recapture (aligned loading), usual therapeutic position

PHASE I: VIRTUAL ARS MUSCULOARTICULAR REHABILITATION TREATMENT

With the assistance of Dr. Fabio Ciuffolo and Structura S.a.s. for all 3D virtual treatment images

Aim: to illustrate clearly what cannot be seen when working chairside.

Some **graphic omissions** and/or limitations are present, as follows:

- The ARS often appears incomplete, especially in posterior quadrants. In fact, it is worn constantly throughout the entire treatment with ongoing alterations as necessary.

- For the sake of simplicity, fixed appliances have not been included in the 3D images but at times are illustrated separately.

- In clinical practice, acrylic is eliminated from the ARS where the bands pass and buccally where the brackets are bonded. Therefore, the splint is less voluminous than it is (intentionally) shown in these illustrations.

INITIAL SITUATION

A Class II mock-up is prepared with flaring maxillary incisors, mandibular crowding, missing maxillary first molars, and tilted and anteriorized maxillary second molars. Deep bite and midlines are off.

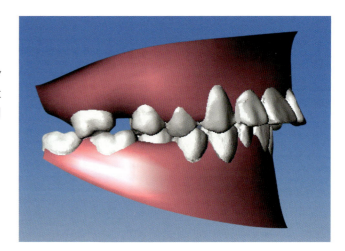

PHASE I

STEP I

MUSCULOARTICULAR THERAPY

The ARS is fitted to the maxillary arch. Wedge thickness determines vertical lift while the flange adjusts mandibular anterovertical and transversal position.

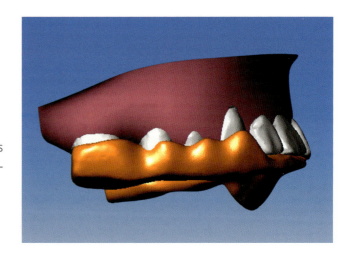

An infinite number of solutions could be applied for each patient. However, if the maxilla alone is considered, the range of options is far narrower. It cannot be stressed enough that the anterior flange anchorage area is responsible for mandibular positioning, not only posteroanteriorly but also transversally and vertically.

Posterior vertical height is determined by the thickness of the wedge.

In practical terms:
- The anterior wedge causes to a greater or lesser extent some inclination of the mandibular incisors, consequently improving any flaring present while sometimes deteriorating buccal proclination of the incisors. Where this risk is predictable, a rigid transparent guard must be applied buccally.
- Every necessary tooth movement, whether individual or in groups and in all three planes of space, can be achieved with fixed appliances with the teeth freed from the acrylic beforehand. Extrusion can be obtained by eliminating completely all acrylic from the appropriate point of the splint's occlusal surface.

INITIAL SITUATION

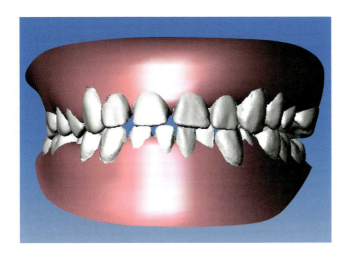
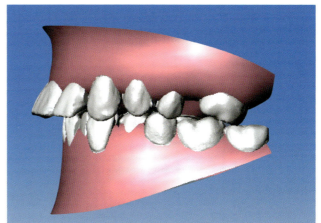

STEP I

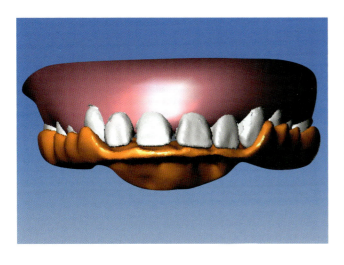
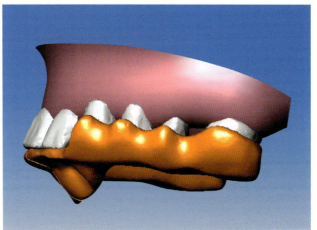

STEP I

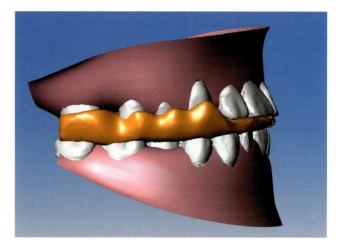

PHASE I

The splint holds the mandibular arch firmly in its therapeutic position further forward and downward.

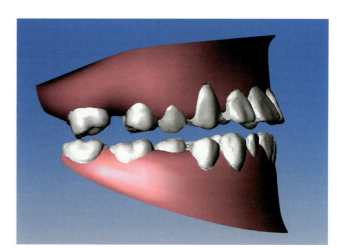

View of the jaws without the splint, showing the forward and downward therapeutic position giving greater vertical height. These changes also contribute to a functional therapeutic relationship between the condyle, disc, and articulating surface.

As a result of mandibular advance, the virtual patient's dental relationships change from a canine Class II to a Class I on the left side while on the right side the canine relationships have instead become Class III.

STEP II

PHASE I

The buccalizing effect of the splint's advancing flange has relieved anterior crowding in the anterior mandible. If necessary, the six mandibular anterior teeth can be retained with transparent buccal splinting.

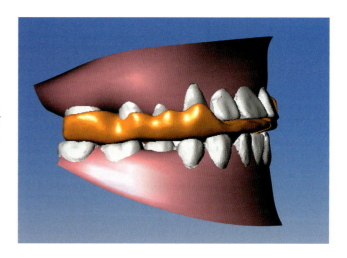

STEP I

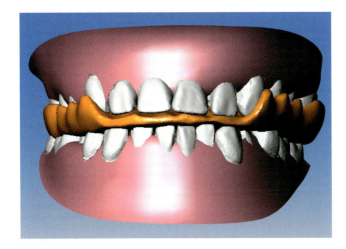
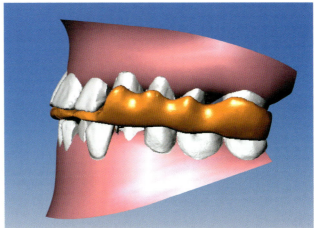

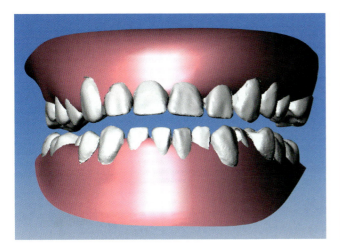
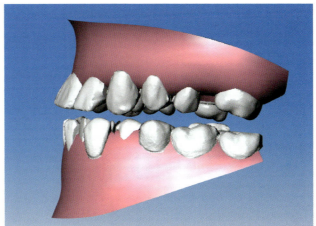

STEP II

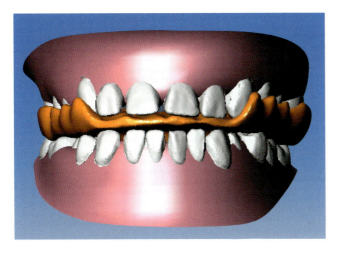
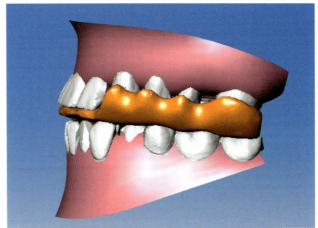

End of phase I musculoarticular rehabilitation. PHASE II orthodontic occlusal finishing is addressed on pages 214 to 219.

(See also page 205, "Considerations: Other joints versus the TMJ.")

I. OVER TIME: HOURS

22 HOURS PER DAY
(EXCEPTING MEALTIMES)

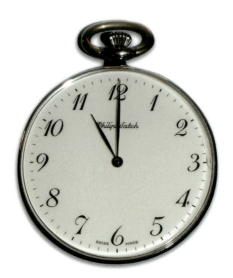

CONDITIONS

III. FIRMNESS: THE CORRECT THERAPEUTIC POSITION

VALID FUNCTION

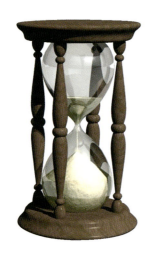

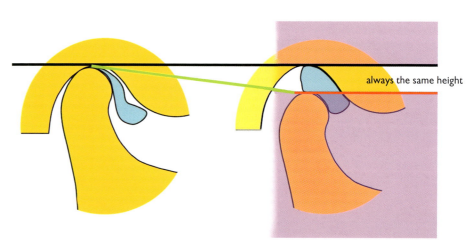

always the same height

II. OVER TIME: MONTHS

AT LEAST 10 MONTHS

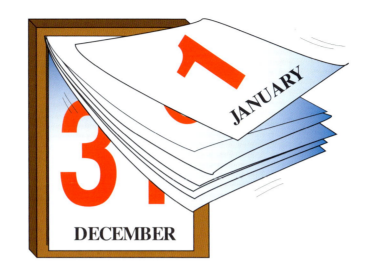

OF EFFICIENCY

MAINTAINED LONG-TERM, DURING BOTH PHASE I AND PHASE II

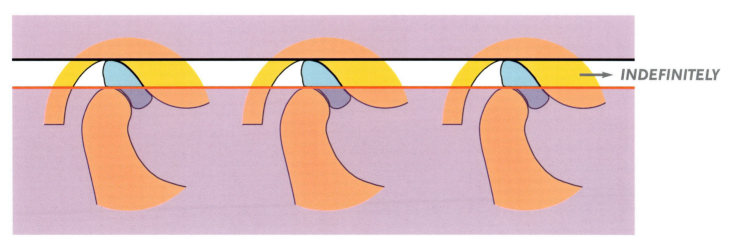

INDEFINITELY

CONSIDERATIONS: CONDITIONS OF ARS EFFICIENCY—PERMANENT STABILITY OF ARTICULAR STRUCTURES IN THERAPEUTIC POSITION

Keynote: Holding articular structures firmly in their functionally valid position, as registered with the pretreatment wax bite, must be an ongoing process throughout both musculoarticular recovery (PHASE I) and orthodontic occlusal finishing (PHASE II). This long-term stability is essential for achieving harmony between teeth, muscles, and the TMJs.

ESSENTIAL CONDITIONS FOR A POSITIVE OUTCOME

TIME
- **Hours:** The splint must be worn approximately 22 hours per day, excluding mealtimes. It may be substituted by a mandibular ARS or adaptation "A," shown on page 405, if necessary to facilitate the patient's social interaction.
- **Months:** The splint must be worn for at least 8 to 10 months in cases of dislocation with reduction to maintain the functional recovery. Where the TMJ has destruction (internal derangement) or dislocation without reduction, splint wear must be prolonged to 12 to 14 months to aid better rearrangement of the badly damaged tissues (functional adaptation).

SPATIAL FACTORS
- The splint must consistently maintain TMJ relationships in the correct orthopedic position. This "fixedness" should be interpreted more in a clinical sense than in terms of material measurement in microns. One of the most important points in the patient's interest is to ensure faithful ongoing compliance.
- The splint must permit micromovements of the joint surfaces to provide enough stimulation to cause articular rearrangement. While this is a key point in the field of general orthopedic therapy, it is less worrying in the treatment of TMD since the removable nature of a splint in itself permits some movement, both when it is removed and inserted and when the patient performs normal actions including speaking, chewing, and swallowing.

Musculoarticular rehabilitation therapy can be considered complete when the patient has a stable valid function, when the mandible opens and closes in a consistent manner, and when the opposing teeth contact in a consistent repeatable pattern despite the actual number of contacts. The teeth will subsequently be rearranged during orthodontic occlusal finishing *(PHASE II)*.

The ensuing outcome should be the best possible compromise not only in the rearrangement of the damaged anatomical parts but also in the dynamic relationships and mandibular excursions in all three spatial dimensions. From the patient's point of view, it is essential that the pain improve significantly or disappear altogether.

The objectivity of CT and MRI diagnostics is a major aid in assessing the results of treatment by showing ongoing rearrangement and restored axial alignment between condyle, disc, and fossa.

OUTCOME OF MUSCULOARTICULAR THERAPY

163

Many factors contribute to achieving an acceptable out-come. In cases of dislocation with reduction, the goal is to recapture the disc, thereby improving the articular structures and, above all, relieving the pain. In cases of dislocation without reduction and destruction, bone remodeling and rearrangement of the articular structu-res can be achieved or, at very least, the best possible anatomical compromise can be obtained, in which the posterior ligament acts as a pseudodisc. Reduction of pain and recovering of oral function are extremely gra-tifying for the patient and make the commitment of time and effort worthwhile.

(See table on pages 92 and 93.)

RESULTS OF PHASE I

Musculoarticular therapy produces rehabilitation classifiable under one or more of the four following aspects.

RELIEF OF MUSCLE
STRESS AND PAIN

ASPECT I:

CONDYLE IN
FUNCTIONAL
POSITION

ASPECT II:

AXIAL ALIGNMENT
BETWEEN TMJ
COMPONENTS

ASPECT III:

REMODELING OF
CONDYLAR HEAD

ASPECT IV:

PHASE I

MUSCULOARTICULAR THERAPY
(WITH ARS WORN CONSTANTLY)

PATHOLOGY   *FOLLOWING THERAPY*

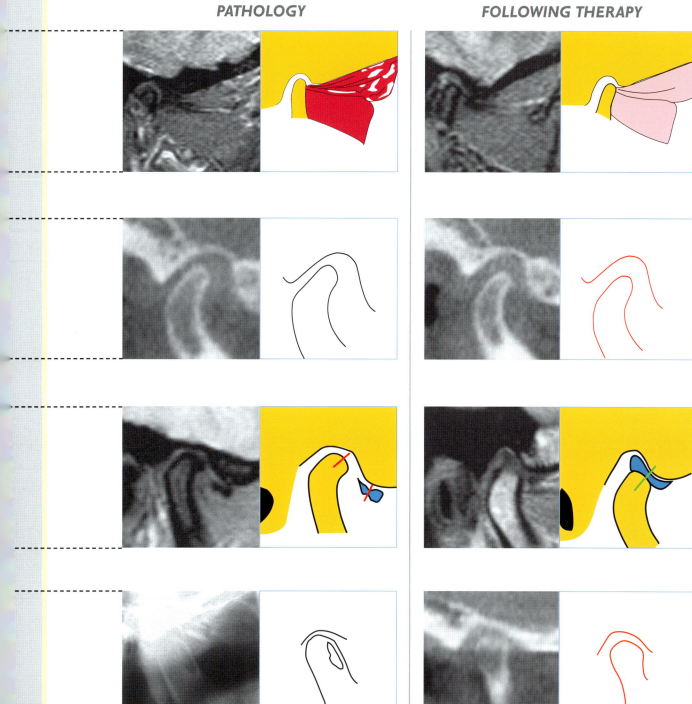

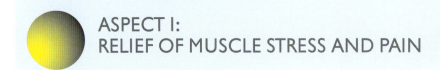

ASPECT I:
RELIEF OF MUSCLE STRESS AND PAIN

Considerations

TMDs often coexist with malocclusions, which place asymmetric loading on the TMJs with differing muscle tone, causing inflammation and edema, or fluid, on the joints. The pain is a constant, both in early stages of pathology when it is primarily of a muscular nature and in later, articular stages of TMD. The extracellular fluid formed during the phlogistic process, whether acute or chronic with flare-ups, may be localized in the muscle (especially in the lateral pterygoid, this being the most closely correlated with the TMJ) or within the joint capsule (fluid on the joint).

The advent of MRI has made it possible to evaluate not only the initial signs but also the condition throughout treatment and follow-up to observe when the symptoms disappear. The key to successful treatment lies in the ability of musculoarticular therapy to relax the muscles and consequently reduce or eliminate inflammation altogether. It is then the responsibility of the specialist dealing with orthodontic occlusal finishing to maintain this condition long-term, causing the inflammation to disappear definitively. As with all of the treatments discussed, the patient's attitude and compliance are key components of a successful outcome.

Relief of muscle stress following treatment:
Patient S. F., age 35

RIGHT SIDE

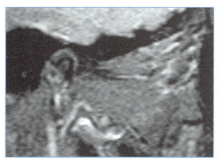 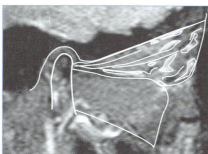 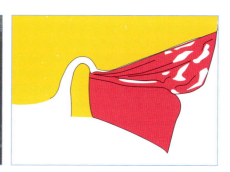

BEFORE

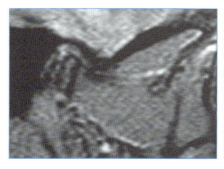 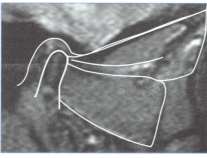 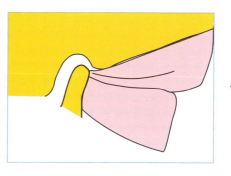

AFTER

Disappearance of fluid following treatment:
Patient A. M., age 27

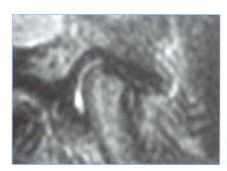 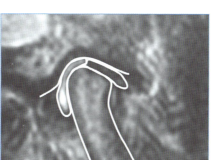 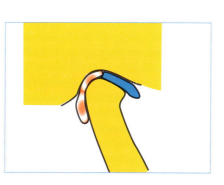

BEFORE

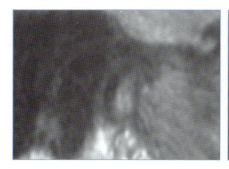 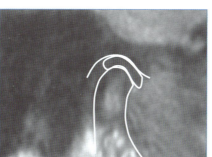 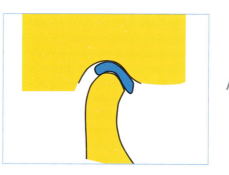

AFTER

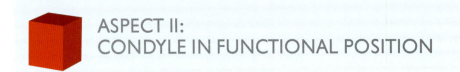

ASPECT II:
CONDYLE IN FUNCTIONAL POSITION

SPATIAL CHANGES IN THE CONDYLE-FOSSA RELATIONSHIP:

Patient: C. F., age 34

RIGHT CONDYLE ON THE SAGITTAL PLANE

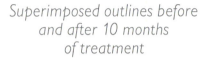

Superimposed outlines before and after 10 months of treatment

BEFORE (DECEMBER, 2001)   AFTER (OCTOBER, 2002)

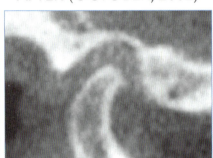
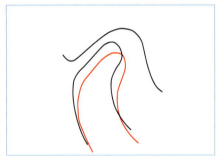

SPATIAL CHANGES IN THE CONDYLE-FOSSA RELATIONSHIP:

Patient: A. N., age 36

RIGHT CONDYLE ON THE TRANSVERSAL PLANE

Superimposed outlines before and after 14 months of treatment

BEFORE (SEPTEMBER, 2001)   AFTER (NOVEMBER, 2002)

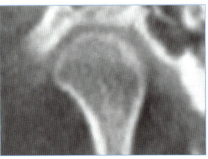
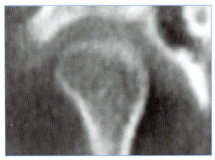
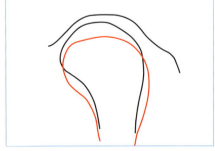

Since the condyle rarely or never lies in an anatomically correct, centered position, it is to be expected that lowering and protruding the condyle through therapy (see clinical investigation from page 96 onward) will produce varying results for a number of reasons:

- A steeper or shallower slope angle of the articular eminence
- A greater or lesser amount of damaged anatomical structures remaining
- Different conditions of the retrodiscal zone and especially of the posterior ligament, possibly being used as substitute for a ruined disc.

LEFT CONDYLE

Superimposed outlines before and after 10 months of treatment

BEFORE (DECEMBER, 2001)   AFTER (OCTOBER, 2002)

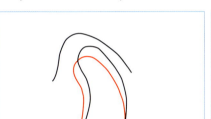 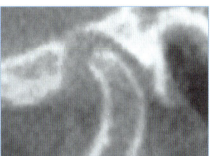 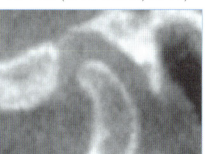

LEFT CONDYLE

Superimposed outlines before and after 14 months of treatment

BEFORE (SEPTEMBER, 2001)   AFTER (NOVEMBER, 2002)

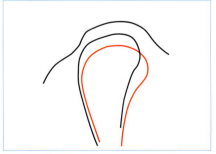 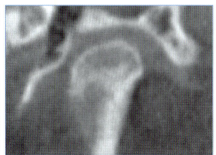 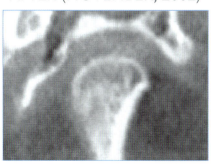

ASPECT III:
AXIAL ALIGNMENT BETWEEN ARTICULAR COMPONENTS

MRI

MRI clearly shows the alignment, or lack thereof, between the condyle, disc, and articulating surface. The static concept of geometric centering of the condyle in the fossa is superseded, in therapy, by the dynamic concept of function. Recovery is influenced by countless therapeutic possibilities and depends on the amount of damage, length of time before treatment was started, inclination of the articular eminence, and patient's age, among other factors.

Patient S. F., age 35

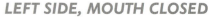

LEFT SIDE, MOUTH CLOSED

BEFORE

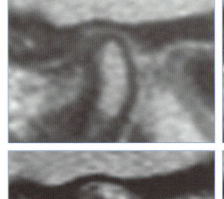
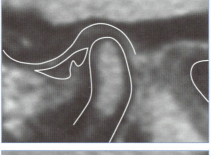
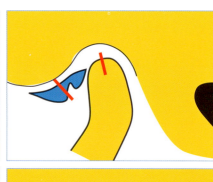

AFTER

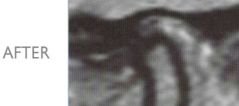
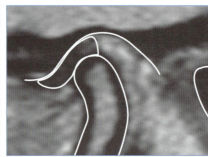
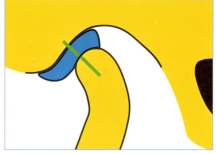

Patient: L. S., age 42

RIGHT SIDE, MOUTH CLOSED

BEFORE

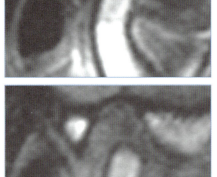
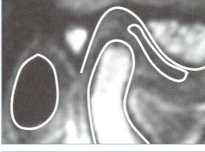

AFTER

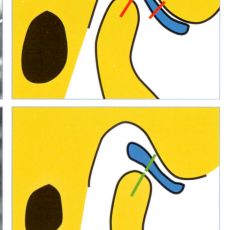

Patient: B. M. E., age 36

LEFT SIDE, MOUTH CLOSED

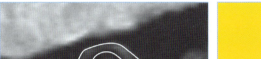

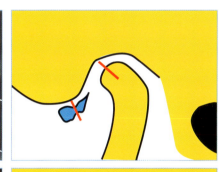

BEFORE

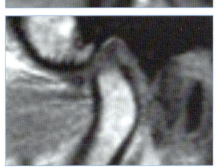

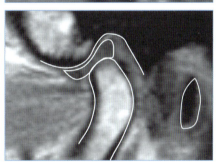

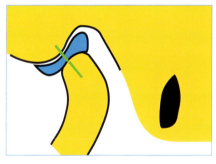

AFTER

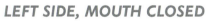

Patient: L. S., age 42

LEFT SIDE, MOUTH CLOSED

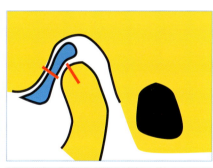

BEFORE

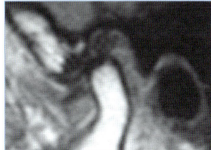

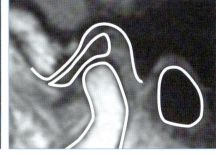

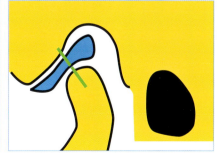

AFTER

THERAPY WITH ARS: ASSESSMENT THROUGH MRI

Patient: B. M., age 30
Case treated by Dr Fabio Ferretti

PRETREATMENT: open mouth, T2-weighted

Right side, BEFORE

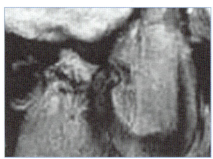 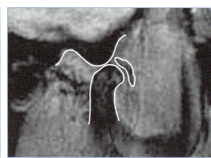 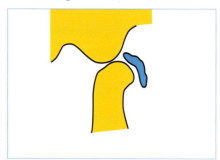

Disc dislocates anteriorly on opening.

FOLLOWING TREATMENT WITH ARS: mouth open, T2-weighted
Check-up, 1 year later

Right side, AFTER

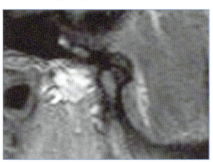 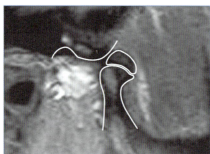 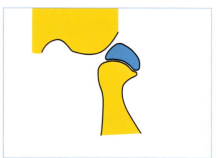

Disc partially recovered.

CHECK-UP, 5 YEARS LATER

Right side CHECK-UP

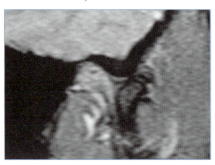 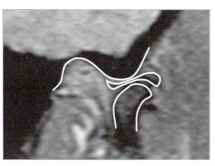 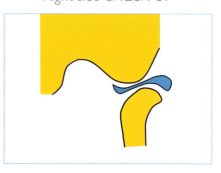

Left side, BEFORE

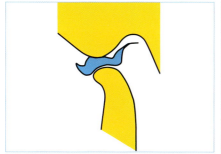 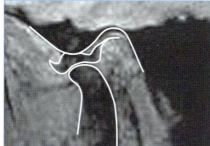 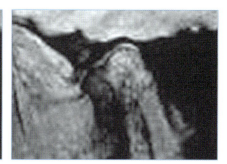

Dysmorphic disc recaptured on opening.

Left side, AFTER

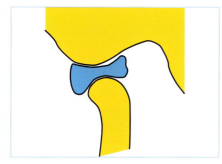 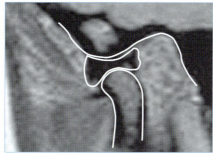 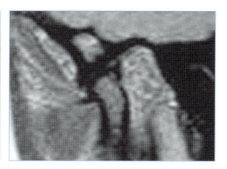

Regular disc shape recovered.

Left side CHECK-UP

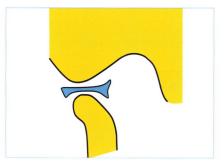 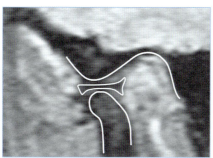 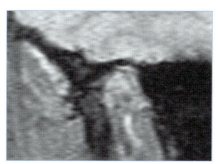

DISLOCATION WITHOUT REDUCTION: OUTCOME
Patient: L. M., age 33

Pretreatment MRI:
Click (anterior dislocation of disc without reduction)

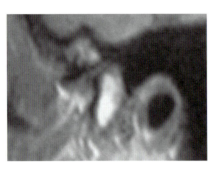 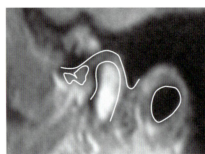 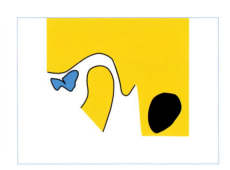

MRI following ARS therapy:
In this case, disc recovery (or recovery of what little remains) is not possible because of the potential for total destruction. Most likely, the posterosuperior ligament will be interposed between the condyle and fossa as a substitute providing disc function.

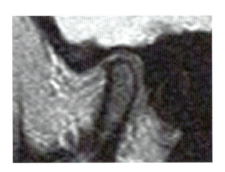 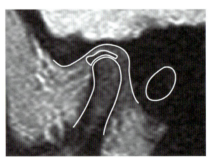 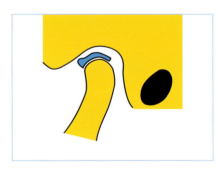

DESTRUCTION: OUTCOME

Bone remodeling and connective tissue rearrangement (theoretical example). The deranged structures can be rearranged if subjected to stable (in spatial terms) and permanent (in terms of time) action. The case is finished while maintaining the same therapeutic position established at the onset when taking the bite registration for splint fabrication.

Many references have been made to osseous structure remodeling and articular structure rearrangement, albeit using varying definitions but all with the same meaning. This confirms that anatomical remodeling is possible because of the changes brought about by the stable spatial position obtained with an ARS and, hence, the consequent distraction of the damaged articular structures. Remodeling is seen as positive changes in the bony structures' profiles and rearrangement of the other TMJ parts, even though it may not be possible to achieve a total "restitution of health." Despite some remaining damage, the best possible compromise consists of a **functional adaptation** (see pages 92 and 93).

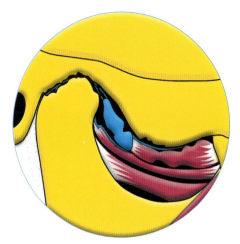

Condylar head and fossa destruction.

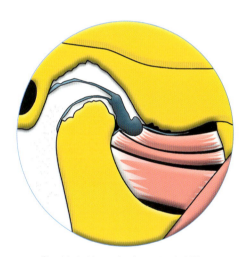

Condyle held away by the patient's ARS.

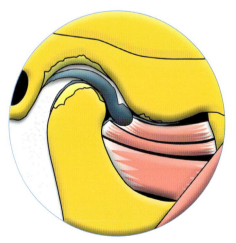

Remodeling of anatomical structures with the posterior ligament acting as pseudodisc.

ASPECT IV:
REMODELING THE CONDYLAR HEAD

Adequate ARS articular therapy can significantly benefit the condylar head and the disc (or what remains of it). In addition to restoring reciprocal axial alignment, it can produce interesting anatomical results ranging from a restitution of health in the most fortunate cases (especially where the patient is young) to bone regrowth in the condylar head and fossa profiles and the creation of a pseudodisc. Even in the most badly damaged cases, a healthy anatomical form can be achieved, giving the patient an acceptable functional activity and reduction or elimination of pain. Clearly, this can only be achieved through conditions of efficiency under which the splint provides long-term constant distraction of the damaged articular structures, a key factor in healing.

Patient I. R., age 13

RIGHT SIDE, MOUTH CLOSED

BEFORE

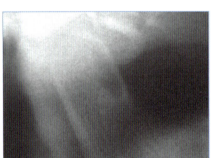
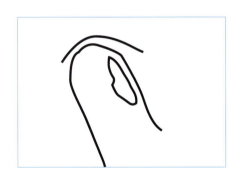

AFTER

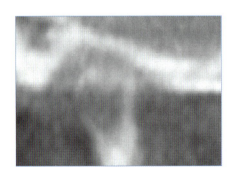
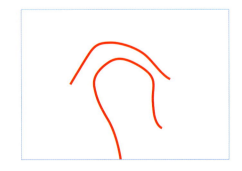

Patient D., age 11

LEFT SIDE, MOUTH CLOSED

BEFORE

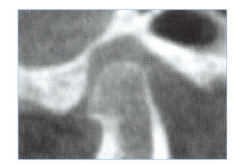 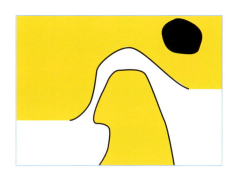

AFTER

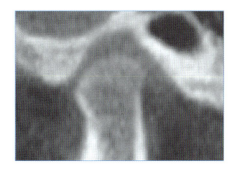 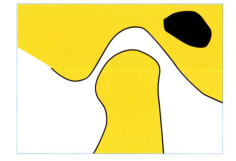

Patient A. M. P., age 43

RIGHT SIDE, MOUTH CLOSED

BEFORE

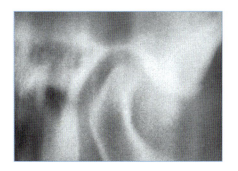 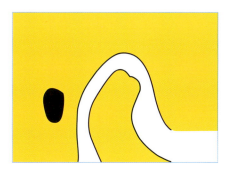

AFTER

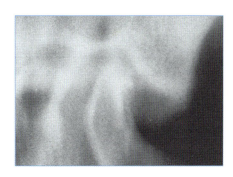 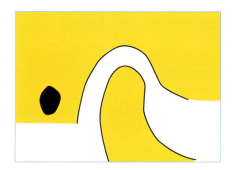

CHANGES IN ADULT PATIENT'S MANDIBULAR SPATIAL POSITION FOLLOWING ARS THERAPY

Patient: S. F., age 35

Case treated by Dr Pietro Petroni

Before ARS therapy

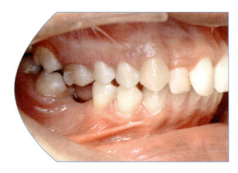
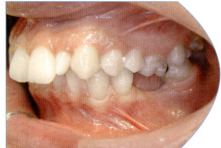
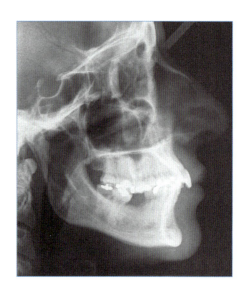

After ARS therapy

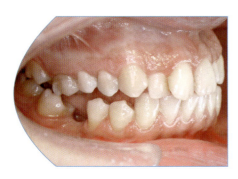
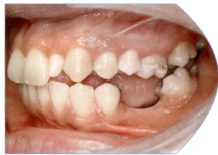
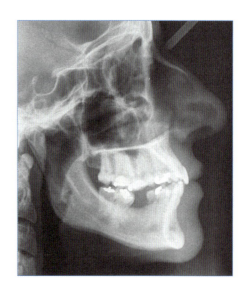

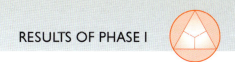

Evident changes in stable mandibular spatial position (in addition to musculoarticular therapy).

A significant procedure for correction of Class II skeletal relations.

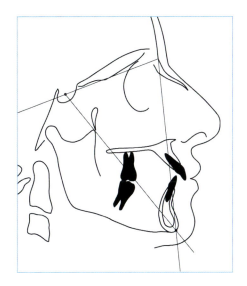

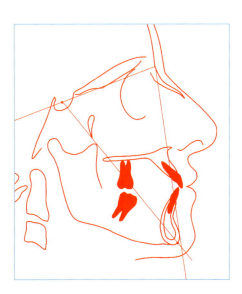

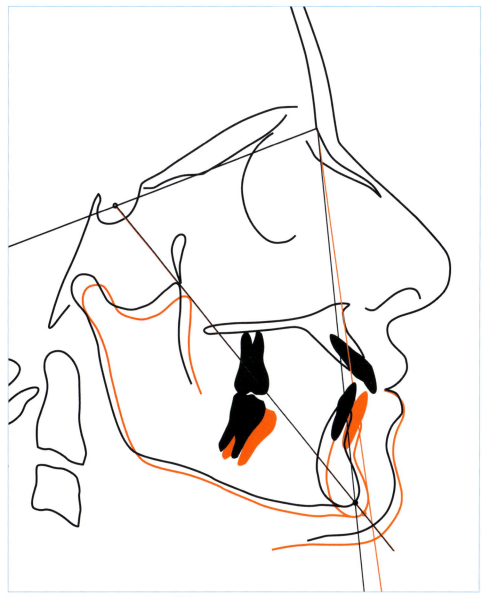

Superimposed outlines of pre- and post-ARS treatment.
Note that this outcome has been achieved as a result of the stable mandibular position sought from the onset of treatment with bite registration.

INTRACAPSULAR PATHOLOGY:
MANDIBULAR ARS FOR MAINTENANCE

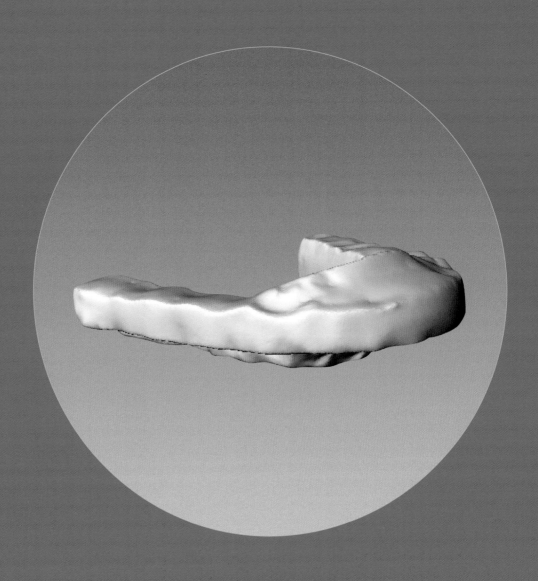

DESCRIPTION

Adult patients undergoing treatment with a traditional ARS are almost always given an additional **mandibular ARS.** This appliance indents onto all the mandibular teeth and has a smooth surface that contacts all the maxillary teeth as well as an acrylic wedge for anterosuperior incisor engagement.

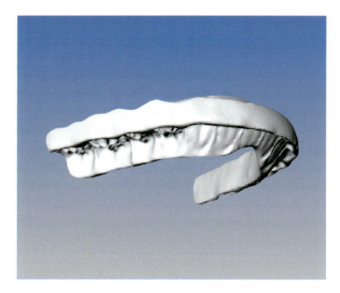

Fabrication

1. Fabrication of the mandibular ARS requires impressions. Use the maxillary ARS as a "fabrication bite" to reproduce the same spatial position in the mandible.
2. Pour and trim the casts.
3. Mount the casts in an occlusor, and block out the undercuts with thermal wax.
4. Box the model, and spread the separator.
5. Commence the progressive addition of the salt-and-pepper polymer-monomer mix.
6. Cure at a temperature of approximately 50 °C and 2 atm of pressure for about 10 minutes. 7. Finish the splint in the normal manner.

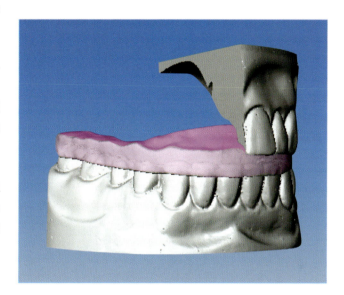

To simplify matters, the lower splint may be fabricated at the same time as the upper splint, but it should not be given to the patient until he or she has become accustomed to wearing the traditional ARS.

HOW IT WORKS

Advantages

A lower splint does not encroach on the palate, therefore it permits freer tongue movement and considerably better diction than its maxillary counterpart. This eases social interaction, an important consideration given the variety of personal and professional relationships that adult patients engage in.

Limitations

Since a lower splint provides maintenance rather than therapeutic function, it should be worn as little as possible.

Note: The new ARS adaptation "A" described on page 405 may be considered.

INTRACAPSULAR PATHOLOGY
ARS AS DISTRACTOR TO TREAT JOINT LOCKING

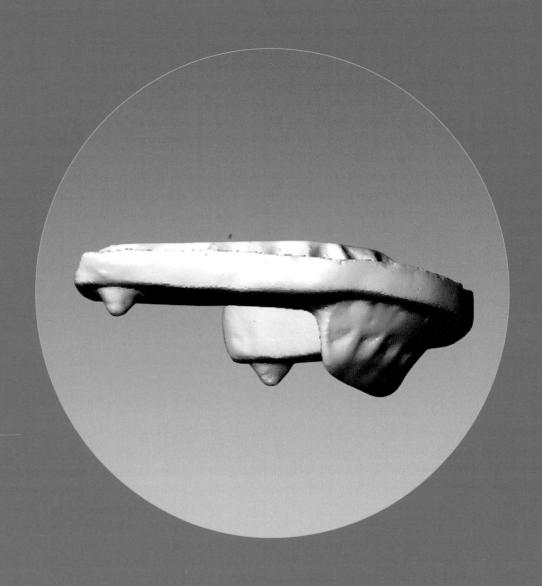

DESCRIPTION

This is a traditional ARS with the addition of two vertical acrylic cusps, approximately 3 mm high, in the posterior quadrants that indent precisely into the grooves of the opposing mandibular molars. It is used when the unlocking movement described on page 82 fails to have the desired effect, thus necessitating an integration.

FUNCTION

The patient must wear the splint for a number of days while chin pressure movements are also carried out. Immediate improvement is often noted. This is not always the case, however, especially with older patients whose pathology has developed over a consistent period of time. Where the outcome is successful, the condyle acquires a better position, and the mandible increases its range of excursions. Alternatively, it may be necessary to further increase vertical height by applying acrylic wedges directly onto the splint to separate the condyles from the fossa. On rare occasions, even the best procedures—although properly executed and repeated more than once—may fail to achieve a significant improvement. In such cases, surgery may be called for.

DESTRUCTION: CHRONIC LOCKING OVERVIEW

Locking is the phenomenon by which the patient is unable to achieve functional movements in one or both TMJs. It may be classified as:

- **Acute or chronic**, according to the length of time since onset of pathology. An acute pathology persists for a few minutes or a few days. A chronic pathology persists for years.
- **Muscle- or TMJ-related**, according to the part most affected and/or damaged.

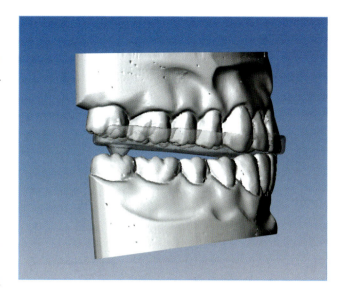

When anything that induces muscle relaxation leads to increased movement, locking is **muscle-related**, the differentiating pathognomic element being the ability to protrude the mandible and perform lateral excursions. In contrast, TMJ-related locking occurs when the disc is unable to reduce and is usually accompanied by severe tissue damage within the joint. If both TMJs are affected, the patient cannot protrude the mandible whereas homolateral deviation toward the affected side in opening and protrusive movements and limited controlateral movement during lateral excursions are characteristic of a single TMJ being affected.

In these conditions, the condyle is no longer able to recapture the disc, which ends up torn, compressed, or flattened with its ligamentous parts destroyed and largely substituted by the posterior ligament. Severe progressive damage also extends to the bony parts, both the condylar head and the fossa, and takes the form of areas of missing bone, spurs, flattening, and craters, as described in the introduction to TMD on page 140.

INTRACAPSULAR PATHOLOGY: CONDYLAR HYPERMOBILITY AND LIGAMENTOUS LAXITY
(Altered position)

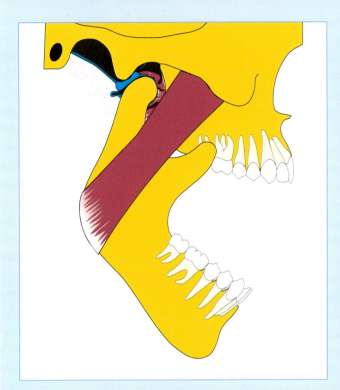

VIRTUAL THERAPEUTIC PROCEDURE

DIAGNOSIS

Greater-than-usual ligamentous elasticity can be summarized as "loose ligaments." A simple test that should be systematically included when examining a new patient consists of lifting one of the patient's hands and flexing one or more fingers backward to ascertain the range of movement. A person with ligamentous laxity is more prone to TMJ dysfunctional pathology.

Under normal conditions, the body's ligaments control and limit joint excursion. When ligaments are loose, the joints perform increased excursions, and the tone of the peri-articular muscles is always altered. This condition is more common in females, and their greater tendency to TMJ hypermobility makes them more likely candidates for joint pathology.

The most common symptom of hypermobility is an increase in excursions (maximum mouth opening greater than 50 mm versus a mean value of 45 mm), often accompanied by a click associated with pain of muscular origin.[29–31] Diagnostic imaging confirms that as the condyle advances well beyond the articular eminence on maximal mouth opening, there is a distinct incongruence in excursions between the condyle and its disc. The condyle often advances ahead of the disc as a result of its greater range of excursion while the more stable disc remains behind. The patient has difficulty in jaw closure and suffers widespread pain not only in the muscles of mastication and posture but frequently throughout the entire head and neck. Fortunately, only a few cases reach the extreme stage of acute open jaw lock.

TREATMENT PLAN AND THERAPY OF JOINT LOCK DUE TO LIGAMENTOUS LAXITY: UNLOCKING MOVEMENT

If the patient's jaw remains locked open, face the patient, and place the thumbs lateral to the mandibular third molars on the buccal shelf of bone. Place the remaining fingers and palms so as to grip the teeth and lower mandible. Lower the mandible by rocking the jaw downward and then backward.

Once the emergency has subsided, the patient must be advised to systematically limit jaw opening to not more than 20 to 22 mm to prevent dislocation of the condyle. Patients are advised to be especially careful when eating and performing oral hygiene and even more so when yawning, which should be limited as far as possible.

The new ARS adaptation "B" described on page 406 can be a potentially useful aid.

PROGNOSIS

The prognosis is positive in cases of luxation followed by recovery, especially if the patient cooperates consistently. Because this condition is based on a predisposition affecting all the joints in the body, it has no definitive cure.

HYPERMOBILITY VIEWED BY CT SCAN

PATIENT D. L., AGE 38

Noticeable condylar advance beyond the eminence.

Maximal mouth opening greater than 55 mm.

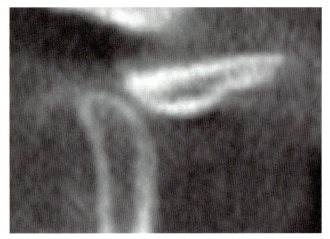

Open mouth tomogram.

HYPERMOBILITY VIEWED BY MRI

PATIENT G. I., AGE 34

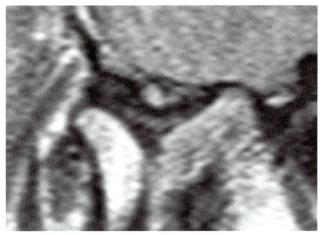

Open mouth.

HYPERMOBILITY VIEW BY MRI

PATIENT A. C., age 36

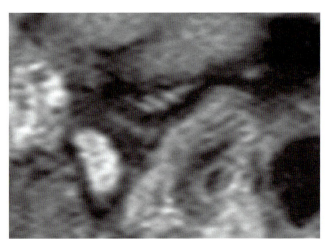

Open mouth.

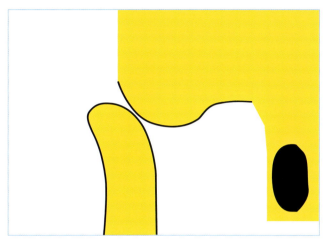

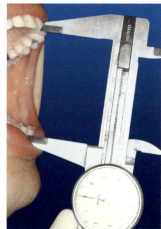

Range of opening measured with calipers.

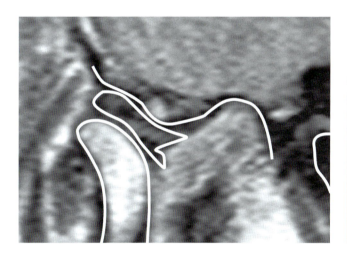

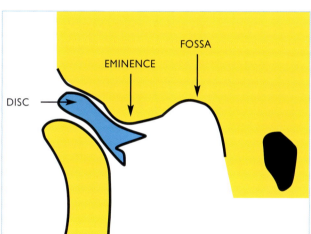

FOSSA

EMINENCE

DISC

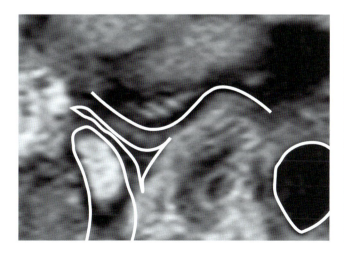

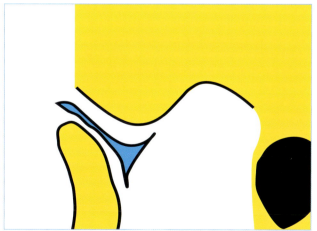

INTRACAPSULAR PATHOLOGY
MAINTENANCE SPLINT

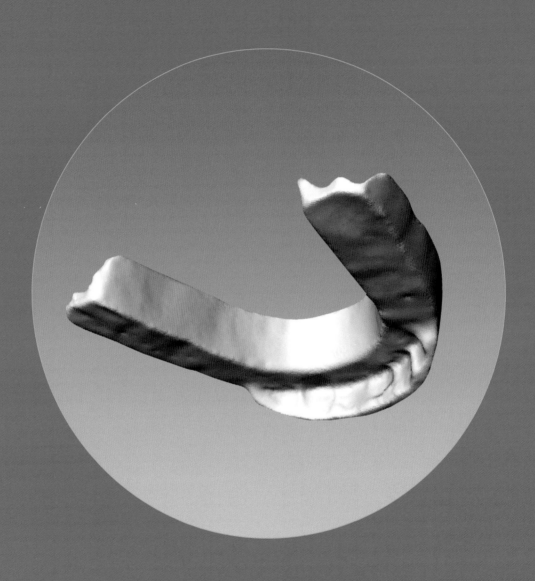

DESCRIPTION

This splint reproduces the basic features of an SS, with the addition of an acrylic band in the anterior part covering the mandibular incisors and canine buccally.

FUNCTION

The maintenance splint is used in those few cases where mandibular retrusion is required instead of protrusion. As a result, it should perhaps be defined as a posterior repositioning splint. As always, the wax bite is crucial. In this case, the clinician must exert a slight pressure on the patient's chin to retrude it a few fractions of a millimeter so that this position will be maintained when the splint is worn.

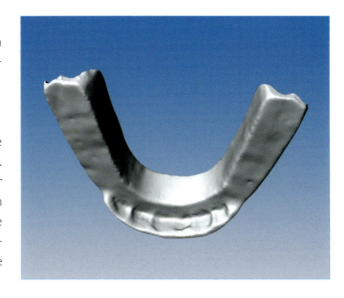

SPLINT USE WITH JOINT HYPERMOBILITY

Fabrication of this type of appliance requires that the bite registration be taken using nonstandard methods. The appliance can be indicated for patients suffering from condylar hypermobility due to ligamentous laxity resulting in mandibular excursions that exceed—often significantly—the mean maximum mouth opening value of 45 mm.

Two procedures underlie the basis for treatment:
- Advise the patient to limit mouth opening movements at all times to not more than 20 mm, even when eating.
- In more complex cases, advise nighttime splint wear.

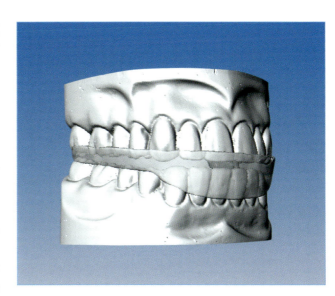

For a good number of patients, mainly female, care not to open the jaws too far (which prevents the condyle from passing the articular eminence) may suffice to eliminate the click and the pain. Although simple advice, if acted upon it may produce surprisingly positive results with patient compliance kept to a minimum.

(See new ARS adaptation "B" described on page 406).

RARE POSTERIOR DISLOCATION OF THE DISC

Patient: F. C., age 30

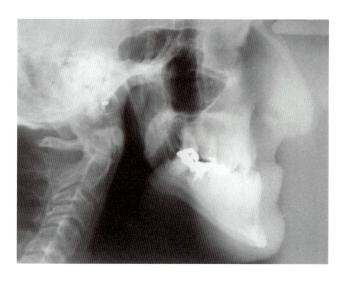

CONDITIONS HIGHLIGHTED BY IMAGING

Bilateral TMJ MRI. Condylar-centering axial T1-weighted sequences were taken, along with closed-mouth proton-density-weighted and T2-weighted oblique sagittal sequences, closed-mouth proton-density-weighted oblique coronal sequences, and open-mouth proton-density-weighted oblique sagittal sequences.

CT of facial bones. Thin-layer axial scans were taken with an osseous-dental algorithm creating oblique sagittal closed-mouth and open-mouth images and closed-mouth oblique coronal images of both TMJs.

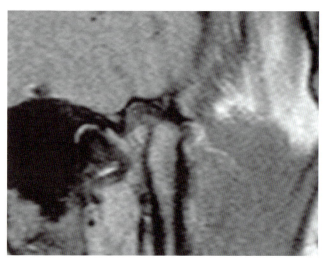

THE DYSMORPHIC CONDYLE IS CAUSED BY CURRENT ARTHROPATHY. BOTH TMJS HAVE EXTREMELY LIMITED FUNCTION, AND THERE IS A RARE POSTERIOR DISLOCATION OF DISC (see also page 274).

RADIOLOGIC DEDUCTIONS

The extremely rare (1.5%) posterior dislocation of the disc32 appears to be associated with posterior open bite and may be caused by one of two factors:

- Trauma
- Perforation of the disc with the anterior band dislocated forward due to traction from the pterygoid and the posterior band dislocated backward as a result of traction from the posterior ligament elastic upper lamina

Right side, mouth open.

CLINICAL CONSIDERATIONS

The clinician may wonder whether the considerable difference between skeletal and dental relationships may have caused paradoxical functional alterations to the extent of causing an inversion between condyle and disc.

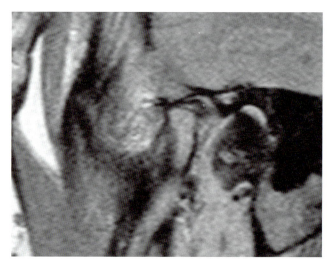

Left side, mouth open.

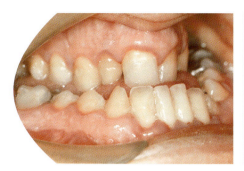
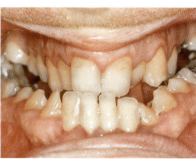
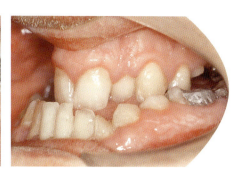

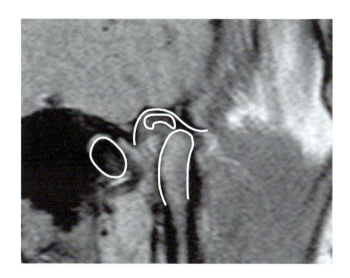
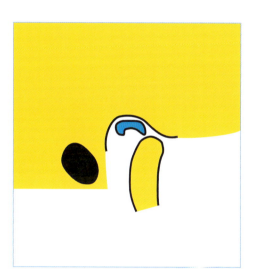

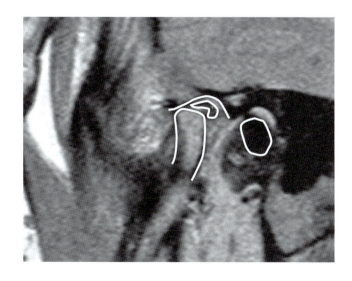
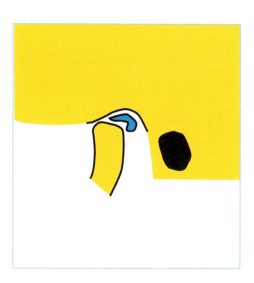

RANGE OF SPLINTS

SIX-POINT SPLINT

STABILIZATION SPLINT

MICHIGAN PLATE

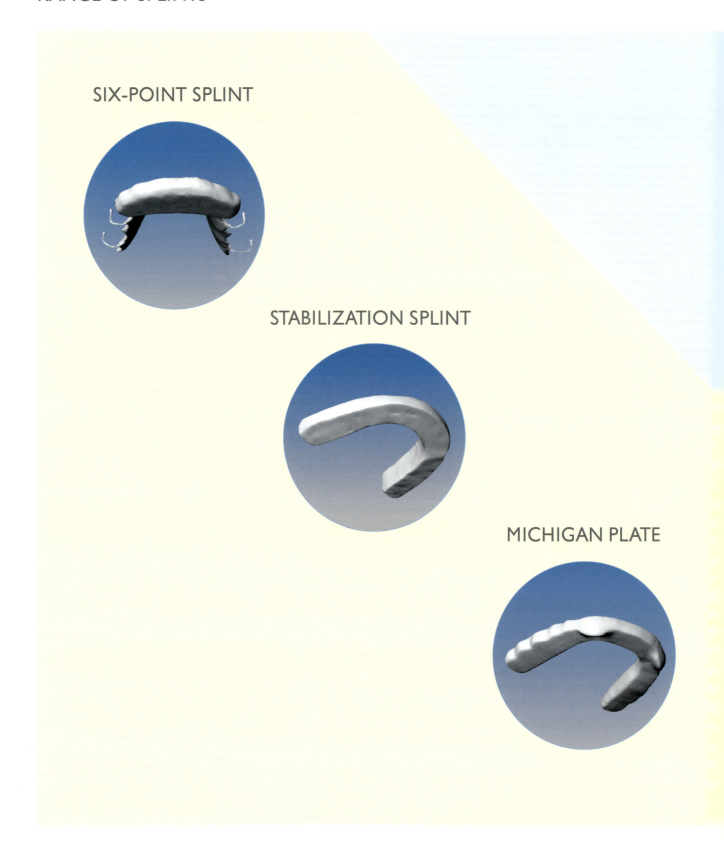

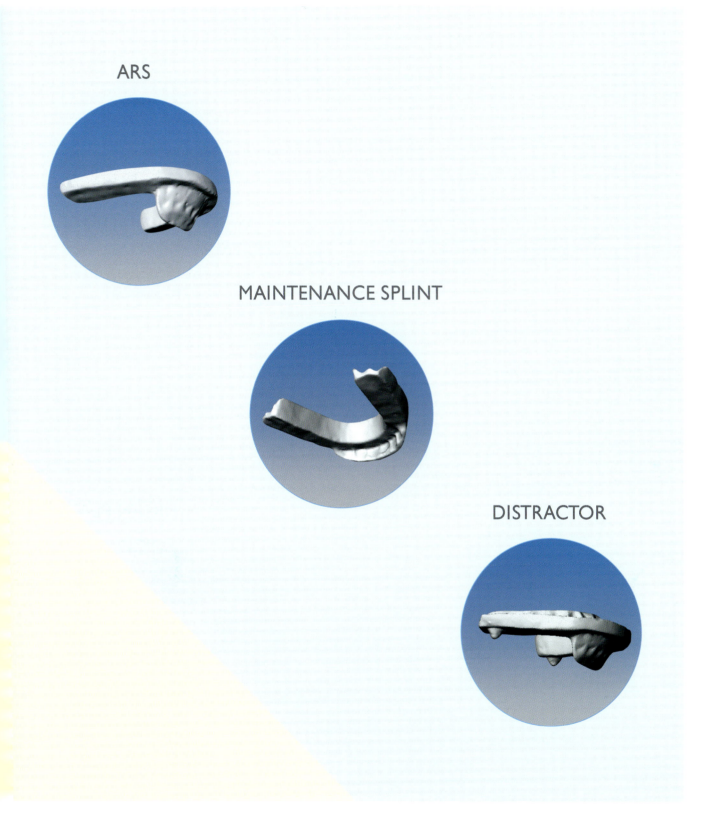

ARS

MAINTENANCE SPLINT

DISTRACTOR

To complete the range, reference should be made to the new:

ARS adaptation "A," page 405

ARS adaptation "B," page 406

CONSIDERATIONS: PHARMACOLOGY VERSUS SPLINT TREATMENT

Much has been written concerning the choice of splint versus pharmacologic treatment.[33,34] The latter is aimed mainly at relieving muscle tension and pain. Pharmacologic treatment may also benefit the patient's attitude since the pain is usually genuine and is often not treated with the proper consideration. Splints, on the other hand, are used to restore a correct relationship among damaged articular structures. Muscle tone must be normalized and the condyle-disc-articulating surface placed in axial alignment to relieve the underlying cause of the pain.

As previously described on page 20, despite some unique features, the TMJ is comparable to any other joint of the human body. This similarity suggests that treatments effective with other joints may also be successful with the TMJ. Treatment with an ARS brings about orthopedic joint repositioning and rearrangement by giving the component parts temporal and spatial stability, enabling them to heal as best they can.

Both pharmacology and splints can contribute to joint healing, and indeed, they often complement one another. What matters most is that the cause of the pathology, not just the symptoms, be resolved.

SPLINTS: A SUMMARY

TYPE	INDICATION
DIAGNOSTIC: - Six-point	- Extracapsular or musculodental pathology
DIAGNOSTIC-THERAPEUTIC: - Stabilization Splint (SS)	- Intermediate pathology. Nonspecific muscle and TMJ relaxation
Integration: - Michigan Plate	- Of particular interest for prosthodontists

THERAPEUTIC:
 	
- Anterior Repositioning Splint (ARS)
 	
- Modified version "A"
	- Intracapsular pathology:
	    - Dislocation with and without reduction
	    - Destruction of the anatomical structures

Integrations: - ARS for Class III (not presented elsewhere in this book)	- Same indications as traditional ARS, but selective for this type of pathology
- Lower ARS (not shown in previous graph)	- Principal effect of maintaining therapeutic position obtained with a traditional ARS and to facilitate social interaction
- Distractor with posterior wedges	- To treat monolateral or bilateral TMJ lock
- Maintenance splint - Modified version "B"	- In cases of articular hypermobility

SURGICAL TREATMENT OF TMJ INTERNAL DERANGEMENT

Indication and techniques proposed[35–39]

Dr Franco Carlino, Specialist in maxillofacial surgery, Maxillofacial Surgery Unit, "S. Camillo" Hospital, Forte dei Marmi (LU), Italy

Surgical techniques for correction of TMJ internal derangement have become common in many countries—especially in the English-speaking world where many varieties are available and they generally have a favorable success rate. Their current lack of popularity in other countries results from lack of information and, consequently, the fear that they are better avoided.

A thorough examination of the relevant literature reveals that surgery of the TMJ, when performed in accordance with properly established indications and techniques, deserves its rightful position as a remedy for dysfunctional pathology. Nevertheless, full-blown TMJ surgery is a last resort in treating TMD. Its use should be limited to those patients (approximately 10%) who fail to respond to the more conservative treatments described in this text. The vast majority of these patients (roughly 90%) can be treated with minimally invasive surgical techniques (arthrocentesis); thus only the remaining 10% of these patients—a mere 1% of all patients with TMJ dysfunction—are candidates for genuine surgery.

To understand the principles underlying TMJ surgery, it must be remembered that joint pain can arise from a "mechanical" fault, such as compression of the highly innervated bilaminar zone of the articular disc or posterior ligament, or from a chemical cause, such as the intra-articular buildup of substances mediating pain and inflammation or alteration of the viscosity and/or chemical composition of the joint's synovial fluid.

It should also be clarified that TMJ pathology exists in myriad forms and symptoms, the intensity and manifestation of which vary enormously from one patient to another, partly due to the considerable effect of each individual's psychoemotive contribution. In any case, the clinician should be fully aware that it is unrealistic to hope to completely and definitively solve all facets of every patient's symptomatology.

More realistically, the clinician can use all possible means, including surgery, to establish a clinically acceptable condition that will not interfere with patients' daily life (eg, rest, nutrition, work, family life), especially with their normal interpersonal relations. This does not exclude the hope that in some fortunate cases, the patient may achieve a total rehabilitation. Unfortunately, however, symptoms sometimes seem to resist even the best therapeutic solution.

According to the guidelines of the American Society of Temporomandibular Joint Surgeons, the techniques currently available in TMJ surgery are:
- Arthrocentesis
- Arthroscopy
- Arthrotomy
- Osteotomy of the mandibular ramus (condylotomy, vertical osteotomy, sagittal osteotomy) or indirect arthroplasty
- Joint reconstruction.

TYPE OF PROCEDURE	
1. ARTHROCENTESIS A straightforward, frequently used, minimally invasive procedure (described on pages 198 and 199)	
2. ARTHROTOMY	
3. ARTHROSCOPY	
4A. CONDYLOTOMY/OSTEOTOMY OF THE RAMUS (indirect arthroplasty)	
4B. VERTICAL OSTEOTOMY (Partial elevation of the medial pterygoid insertion points is important) With reference to condylar repositioning within the fossa, this procedure gives a very similar result to that of ARS therapy, with the condyle remaining seated further downward and forward. The procedure is described in detail on pages 200 and 201.	
5. TMJ RECONSTRUCTION	

INDICATION AND RESULTS

Indicated for cases of acute sudden limited opening not associated with trauma (acute closed-lock).

Commonly known as open surgery, this technique is still very common in the English-speaking world. It often results in restricted jaw movement as a result of scarring

This is the same technique performed on other joints by orthopedic surgeons, consisting of inserting a fiberoptic telescope (videoarthroscope) into the upper joint compartment. There is often insufficient correlation between **preoperative clinical data, intraoperative arthroscopic monitoring, and postoperative clinical results**. For instance, patients whose MRIs showed disc luxation without reduction can give an **arthroscopic image** of severe chondromalacy. Likewise, objective symptoms such as **functional limitation** and the severity of TMJ **noise** cannot predict postarthroscopy clinical results.

Rationale for treatment: to obtain spontaneous **displacement** of the condylar fragment in a caudal and forward direction to increase the intra-articular space (indirect arthroplasty) in practice.

Indication: initially only in cases of joint pain with discal dislocation with reduction. It may then be extended to cases of nonreducible dislocation or disc perforation.

Results: according to current literature, 92% clinical healing rate referred to the pain syndrome.

Possible complications of condylar/vertical osteotomy: include infection, nerve injury and occlusal changes, and **condylar luxation** following condylotomy or vertical osteotomy as a result of excessive detachment of the internal pterygoid insertion. **Securing the osteotomy segments** helps prevent spontaneous luxation of the condyle.

Reconstruction of the TMJ yields predictable and achievable results.
Cases which do not respond to the above surgical techniques must undergo joint reconstruction either with autologous bone graft (rib, clavicle) or with total prosthetic replacement (both condyle and glenoid fossa).

The following pages contain a description of perhaps lesser-known yet clinically useful techniques.

ARTHROCENTESIS

This practice is the simplest and least invasive form of surgery available to treat TMJ dysfunction. Arthrocentesis involves lavage, or flushing, of the upper TMJ compartment with a sterile solution. The area is anesthetized, and two needles are inserted. The needles are attached to catheters that regulate the input and outflow of the solution, creating a continuous flush cycle.

The purpose of the procedure is to restore normal disc mobility. Adhesions are lysed as the solution is injected between the roof of the articular cavity and the disc itself. Flushing with a copious quantity of saline solution (500 ml) dilutes the joint's own fluid, which reduces the concentration of substances causing pain and inflammation. Important mechanical and chemical benefits are achieved, including removal of pain-inducing intra-articular substances, freer rotation of the disc, and reduction in discal interference-related noise.

As it is currently performed, arthrocentesis was developed and perfected by Dr D. W. Nitzan[38] as a method of addressing acute closed-lock. This definition is restricted to the jaw lock arising within 3 months of treatment. The author extended this indication by applying the procedure to the treatment of other dysfunctional conditions. As a result, it is frequently used as a first step in managing almost all patients who fail to respond to conservative methods.

The author believed that TMJ lock arose primarily from an increase of intra-articular pressure caused by parafunction (clenching and grinding). This pressure, in turn, compresses the articular disc against the glenoid cavity roof, expelling synovial fluid and creating a vacuum between disc and cavity roof (the so-called stuck disc phenomenon). When attempting to open the mouth, the patient provokes traction on the disc, which is unable to move as a result of vacuum suction. Tension on the posterior ligament and compression of the bilaminar zone generate pain. The result is a self-maintaining vicious cycle of pain with defensive muscle contraction and limited opening. Simply inserting a hollow needle into the superior compartment lets in air, eliminates the vacuum, and restores partial disc mobility.

Subsequent flushing of the superior compartment with saline solution restores normal discal dynamics; dilutes the synovial fluid, which in these patients always shows increased viscosity; overcomes the fibrous adhesions formed within the joint; and lowers the concentration of pain- and inflammation-mediating molecules (eg, bradykinins and interleukin-9).

In practical terms, arthrocentesis consists of inserting a first needle along the tragus-ocular line 1 cm anterior to the tragus while palpating the zygomatic arch manually until the needle tip is felt to have reached a point corresponding to the superior margin of the glenoid cavity. The needle is then pointed downward around the bony zygomatic profile until it comes into contact with the articular capsule. Next, the needle is sunk into the articular cavity by approximately 1 cm, and local anesthetic is injected, followed by saline solution, until the cavity is completely distended (usually 2 to 3 mL). The saline solution irrigator is connected to the needle, and a second needle is inserted approximately 1 cm anterior to the first and slightly lower (Fig 1) as an outflow catheter, at which point lavage commences (Fig 2).

The cavity is flushed with approximately 500 mL of solution while the patient is asked to perform opening, lateral, and protrusive movements during the entire procedure, which continues until the patient is able to reach acceptable interincisal opening (40 mm).

For the next few days, it is important that the patient wear the occusal plate (bite) to help rest the joint, eat soft foods, and do the resistance exercises/physiotherapy recommended by the clinician.

This rapid outpatient procedure has no drug-associated collateral risks, the only substances used being sterile solution and a common local anesthetic. Despite its simplicity, it has a good success rate, especially in terms of improved mouth opening and joint noise. The results are especially good when the pathology is relatively recent. A further advantage is that arthrocentesis may be repeated more than once with the same patient. It is not uncommonly the treatment of choice for many people who return—usually every 2 to 3 years—when their TMJ pathology flares up again. The cost-benefit ratio of arthrocentesis is extremely favorable since it relieves pain symptoms in 90% (see page 195) of patients referred to the maxillofacial specialist.

One short-term after-effect of the procedure is swelling at the injection site due to an accumulation of fluid below the skin. The swelling disappears in a matter of hours or days at the most. Any pain, although uncommon, can be controlled with over-the-counter painkillers. More likely, the patient will experience a feeling of numbness accompanied by fluid in the auditory meatus, which is reabsorbed within a few days.

Other after-effects are caused by permeation of the local anesthetic into the surrounding area, occasionally extending to the facial nerve with resulting difficulty in moving the eyelids, forehead, and/or mouth. These effects are temporary and wear off after a few hours. Very rare cases have been reported of permanent anesthesia of the skin in the temporal region due to accidental puncture of the auriculotemporal nerve.

Another common occurrence is the inability to close the jaws fully on the side where the procedure was done because accumulated liquid in the TMJ forces the mandible downward and prevents the homolateral opposing teeth from occluding. This effect is also temporary.

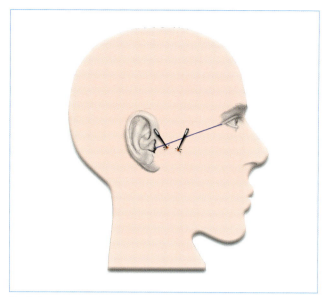

Fig. 1 Entry points of the two needles used for arthrocentesis. With the tragoocular line used as reference, the first needle is inserted 1 cm anterior to the tragus and 2 mm below the line, while the second needle is inserted 1 cm further forward and 1 cm below the first.

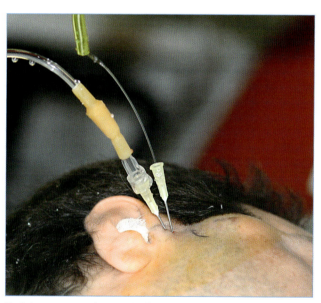

Fig. 2 Intraoperative photograph of arthrocentesis of the right TMJ. Note the two needles, one of which is connected to the irrigator by a drip tube while the other allows the sterile solution to drain out.

No known cases of TMJ infection following arthrocentesis have been reported, although this event is theoretically possible and makes it advisable to administer a preventive course of antibiotics as a matter of routine.

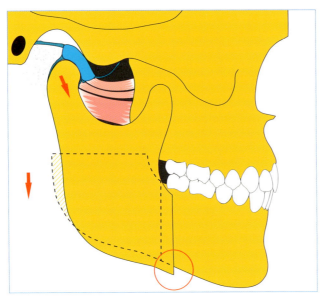

Fig. 3 Drawing of sagittal osteotomy of the mandibular ramus to provide anterocaudal condylar distraction.

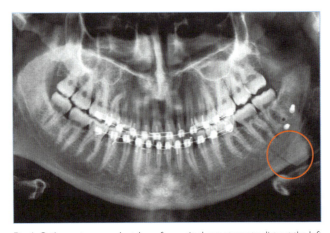

Fig. 4 Orthopantomography taken after sagittal osteotomy to distract the left condylar segment in an anterocaudal direction. Note the protruding segment showing on the lower edge of the mandibular ramus, which confirms the translatory movement.

OSTEOTOMY OF THE MANDIBULAR RAMUS (CONDYLOTOMY, VERTICAL OSTEOTOMY, SAGITTAL OSTEOTOMY) OR INDIRECT ARTHROPLASTY

The various techniques for osteotomy of the mandibular ramus aim to shift the articular condyle downward and forward to increase the intra-articular space. This change eliminates the pressure exerted by the condyle on the posterior portion of the articular disc and its posterior ligament and, as a result, removes the chief cause of TMJ pain. As with an arthrotomy, this technique increases intra-articular space without removing the disc or filing down the condylar head. Furthermore, by moving the mandibular ramus, the result is achieved indirectly and from a distance. Therefore, this method is also referred to as indirect arthroplasty (or arthrotomy).

The original technique consisted of a simple cut across the lower condylar neck (condylotomy) imitating a normal lower condylar fracture and proceeding with standard treatment for condylar fractures. After short-term maxillomandibular fixation (approximately 10 days), the joint is mobilized, and rehabilitation is started with Class II anteroposterior intermaxillary traction as normally used for condylar fracture. The underlying principle is that while the jaws are held locked, the masticatory muscles inserting onto the condyle (external pterygoid) exert traction, pulling the condyle downward and forward since there is no osseous fixation to hold it in place. As the segment moves into this new position, pressure on the joint is relieved as described above.

Osteotomy has since been modified from a simple condylotomy to vertical osteotomy, with the cut being made along the entire vertical length of the mandibular ramus to provide greater contact surface between bone extremities. Unlike the previous form, this technique requires partial detachment of the internal pterygoid muscle insertions from the medial surface of the mandibular ramus since this muscle would otherwise exert traction in the opposite direction from the external pterygoid (ie, in a superomedial direction), therefore preventing translation of the condylar segment in the desired direction.

Yet another modification has recently been proposed involving a complete sagittal split osteotomy of the ramus (as performed to correct skeletal malformations), after which the proximal segment is manually moved downward and forward by 2 to 3 mm before being fixed in this new position with the necessary wires, screws, and/or plates to ensure it remains in the intended position. Figures 3 and 4, respectively, illustrate the operative principle and show a postoperative orthopantomography of this type of procedure.

The chief advantage of these techniques is that they are all extra-articular. Access to the surgical site through the mouth, without entering the TMJ space, prevents the potential complications previously mentioned associated with nerve damage and intra-articular scarring, which may subsequently limit joint movement.

These procedures relieve pain symptomatology by acting on the compression phenomenon at the root of the pain. They also achieve good results in reducing joint noise and improving mobility. Some complications, of course, may arise, such as interference with sensitivity of the lower lip, tongue, and cheeks as a result of injury to the inferior alveolar nerve—the same drawback associated with any mandibular osteotomy for orthognathic purposes.

A particular complication of this type of procedure is the onset of a postoperative malocclusion, generally in the form of anterior open bite, mandibular retrusion, and, in monolateral cases, mandible shift towards the side operated on. The cause of these phenomena is the traction exerted by the ligaments, which react to the downward and forward translation by trying to return the mandible backward and rotated upward into its original position. To prevent this occurrence, it is mandatory, after maxillomandibular fixation removal, that the patient follow the muscle and joint rehabilitation program set by the surgeon and involving exercise elastics exerting Class II anteroposterior traction with the aim of combating this negative pull. Failure on the part of the patient to keep to this routine may result in a malocclusion with mandibular retrusion, open bite, and possibly mandibular asymmetry. Furthermore, there is the risk of defeating the surgical outcome if the mandible is allowed to return to its original position and joint pressure resumes as before.

Postoperative malocclusion occurs more commonly in edentulous patients, in whom it affects the replacement teeth since their postoperative occlusion cannot be controlled. Another group commonly affected by malocclusion is patients who have previously undergone surgery for mandible advancement. In these patients, it may be very difficult to prevent a lapse back into Class II malocclusion.

Another potential occurrence following a condylotomy or vertical osteotomy is condylar luxation anterior to the articular eminence. This may be caused by the downward and forward translation of the condylar head resulting from the pull of the muscles without real control. If the condyle pops out of its seat and dislocates forward of the eminence, surgery will be necessary to return it to its correct position.

It was precisely to prevent this complication that a modified procedure was introduced consisting of sagittal osteotomy with the osseous segments fixed intraoperatively so that the condyle is unable to move inappropriately from the established position. It is highly unusual for this procedure to be followed by a complete return of the pain symptomatology, noise, and functional limitations. The possible exceptions are edentulous patients, for the reasons described above, or patients whose preoperative joint conditions included advanced articular degeneration, disc perforation, or macroscopic erosion of the condyle and articular fossa.

REFERENCES

1. Laskin DM, Greene CS, Hylander WL (eds). TMDs—An Evidence-Based Approach to Diagnosis and Treatment. Chicago: Quintessence, 2006.
2. Okeson JP. Orofacial Pain: Guidelines for Assessment, Diagnosis, and Management, ed 1. Chicago: Quintessence, 1996.
3. Vickers ER, Cousins MJ. Neuropathic orofacial pain. Part 2—Diagnostic procedures, treatment guidelines and case reports. Aust Endod J 2000;26:53–63.
4. Visscher CM, Lobezoo F, De Boer W, Van Der Zaag J, Naeije M. Prevalence of cervical spinal pain in craniomandibular pain patients. Eur J Oral Sci 2001;109:76–80.
5. Ciuffolo F, Manzoli L, Ferritto AL, Tecco S, D'Attilio M, Festa F. Surface electromyographic response of the neck muscles to maximal voluntary clenching of the teeth. J Oral Rehabil 2005; 32:79–84.
6. Milani RS, De Periere DD, Lapeyre L, Pourreyrone L. Relationship between dental occlusion and posture. Cranio 2000;18:127–134.
7. Fujimoto M, Hayakawa L, Hirano S, Watanabe I. Changes in gait stability induced by alteration of mandibular position. J Med Dent Sci 2001;48:131–136.
8. Gangloff P, Louis JP, Perrin PP. Dental occlusion modifies gaze and posture stabilization in human subjects. Neurosci Lett 2000; 293:203–206.
9. Monzani D, Guidetti G, Chiarini L, Setti G. Combined effect of vestibular and craniomandibular disorders on postural behaviour. Acta Otorhinolaryngol Ital 2003;23:4–9.
10. Sessle BJ. Peripheral and central mechanisms of orofacial pain and their clinical correlates. Minerva Anestesiol 2005;71:117–136.
11. Simons DG, Travel JG, Simons LS. Myofascial Pain and Dysfunction: A Trigger Point Manual. Baltimore: Lippincott Williams and Wilkins, 1998.
12. Huang GJ, LeResche L, Critchlow CW, Martin MD, Drangsholt MT. Risks factors for diagnostic subgroup of painful TMD. J Dent Res 2002;81:284–288.
13. Wänman A. The relationship between muscle tenderness and craniomandibular disorders: A study of 35 year-olds from the general population. J Orofac Pain 1995;9:235–243.
14. Peterson AL, Dixon DC, Talcott GW, Kelleher WJ. Habit reversal treatment of TMD: A pilot investigation. J Behav Ther Exp Psychiatry 1993;24:49–55.
15. Seligman DA, Pullinger AG. The prevalence of dental attrition and its association with factors of age, gender, occlusion and TMJ symptoms. J Dent Res 1988;67:1323–1333.
16. Riley JL 3rd, Benson MB, Gremillion HA, et al. Sleep disturbance in orofacial pain patients: Pain-related or emotional distress? Cranio 2001;19:106–113.
17. Kaergaard A, Andersen JH. Musculoskeletal disorders of the neck and shoulders in female sewing machine operators: Prevalence, incidence and prognosis. Occup Environ Med 2000;57:528–534.
18. Svensson P, Burgaard A, Schlosser S. Fatigue and pain in human jaw muscles during a sustained, low-intensity clenching task. Arch Oral Biol 2001;46:773–777.
19. Cram JR, Kasman GS, Holtz J. Introduction to Surface Electromyography. Gaithersburg, MD: Aspen, 1998.
20. Crider AB, Glaros AG. A meta-analysis of EMG biofeedback treatment of temporomandibular disorders. J Orofac Pain 1999;13:29–37.
21. Al-Ani MZ, Davies SJ, Gray RJ, Sloan P, Glenny AM. Stabilisation splint therapy for temporomandibular pain dysfunction syndrome. Cochrane Database Syst Rev 2004;1:CD002778.
22. Eberhard D, Bentleon HP, Steger W. The efficacy of ARS therapy studied by magnetic resonance imaging. Eur J Orthod 2002;24:343–352.
23. Tecco S, Festa F, Salini V, Epifania E, D'Attilio M. Treatment of joint pain and joint noises associated with a recent TMJ internal derangement: A comparison of an anterior repositioning splint, a full-arch maxillary stabilization splint, and an untreated control group. Cranio 2004;22:209–219.
24. Santacatterina A, Paoli M, Peretta R, Bambace A, Beltrame A. A comparison between horizontal splint and repositioning splint in the treatment of disc dislocation with reduction. J Oral Rehabil 1998;25:81–88.
25. Cozzani G. Diagnosi in occlusione abituale e in occlusione centrica, M Ortod, 4-76:1–12.
26. Pancherz H, Michailidou C. Temporomandibular joint growth changes in hyperdivergent and hypodivergent Herbst subjects. A long-term roentgenographic cephalometric study. Am J Orthod Dentofacial Orthop. 2004;126:153-61
27. Ciuffolo F, Epifania E, Duranti G, et al. Rapid prototyping: A new method of preparing trays for indirect bonding. Am J Orthod Dentofacial Orthop 2006;129:75–77.
28. Rabie AB, Xiong H, Hägg U. Forward mandibular positioning enhances condylar adaptation in adult rats. Eur J Orthod. 2004;26:353-8.
29. Katzberg RW, Keith DA, Guralnick WC, Ten Eick WR. Correlation of condylar mobility and arthrotomography in patients with internal derangements of the temporomandibular joint. Oral Surg Oral Med Oral Pathol 1982;54:622–627.
30. Dijkstra PU, de Bont LG, Stegenga B, Boering G. Temporomandibular joint osteoarthrosis and generalized joint hypermobility. Cranio 1992;10:221–227.
31. Holmlund AB, Gynther GW, Kardel R, Axelsson SE. Surgical treatment of temporomandibular joint luxation. Swed Dent J 1999;23:127–132.
32. Montagnani G, Manfredini D, Tognini F, Zampa V, Bosco M. Magnetic resonance of the temporomandibular joint: Experience at an Italian university center. Minerva Stomatol 2005;54:429–440.
33. Brazeau GA, Gremillion HA, Widmer CG, et al. The role of pharmacy in the management of patients with temporomandibular disorders and orofacial pain. J Am Pharm Assoc 1998;38:354–361.
34. List T, Axelsson S, Leijon G. Pharmacologic interventions in the treatment of temporomandibular disorders, atypical facial pain, and burning mouth syndrome. A qualitative systematic review. J Orofac Pain 2003;17:301–310.
35. Dolwick MF. Disc preservation surgery for the treatment of internal derangements of the temporomandibular joint. J Oral Maxillofac Surg 2001;59:1047–1050.
36. Hall HD, Nickerson JW, McKenna SJ. Modified condilotomy for treatment of the painful temporomandibular joint with a reducing disc. J Oral Maxillofac Surg 1993;51:133–142.
37. Hall HD, Navarro EZ, Gibbs SJ. One- and three-year prospective outcome study of modified condilotomy for treatment of reducing disc displacement. J Oral Maxillofac Surg 2000;58:7–17.
38. Nitzan DW. Arthrocentesis for management of severe closed lock of the temporomandibular joint. Oral Maxillofac Surg Clin North Am 1994;6:245–257.
39. Pruitt JW, Moenning JE, Lapp TH, Bussard DA. Treatment of painful temporomandibular joint disfunction with the sagittal splint ramus osteotomy. J Oral Maxillofac Surg 2002;60:996–1002.

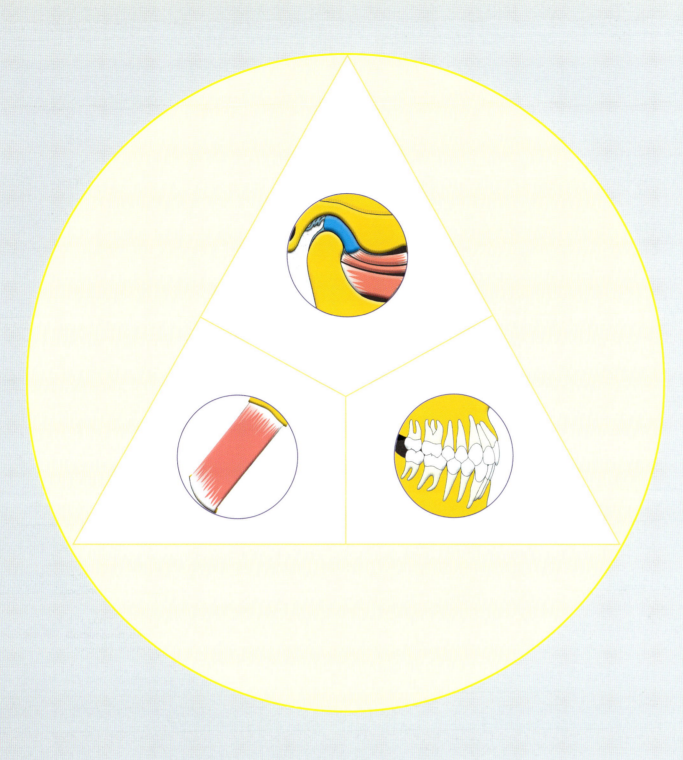

PHASE II: ORTHODONTIC OCCLUSAL FINISHING

The principal aim of occlusal finishing is to obtain correct interarch relationships in harmony with the muscles and joints. In most cases, occlusal finishing will be orthodontic. Every orthodontic treatment is a complete oral rehabilitation and as such must be treated with great care and attention, for even apparently simple cases involve the entire stomatognathic apparatus.

Treatment plan

During PHASE I, the best possible outcome in terms of muscle relaxation should have been achieved with a six-point splint, a stabilization splint (SS), or, in patients with more serious musculoarticular problems, an anterior repositioning splint (ARS). PHASE II of treatment proceeds with the occlusal finishing stage. Although this is almost always orthodontic, a range of solutions are available for each patient, and the choice will vary according to the plan established at the outset of treatment. Options include the following:

- Orthodontics is the treatment of choice. It is the means to achieve simultaneous contact between all the teeth in both arches. Orthodontics gives functional effectiveness, which is the aim of all orthodontic treatment, and ensures that the teeth are treated after the requirements of the muscles and joints are met.
- The effectiveness of occlusal adjustment[1] (selective grinding and/or adding composite) is questioned by the scientific community. Nevertheless, this procedure cannot be entirely ruled out. In certain cases it may promote long-term, stable, satisfactory occlusion and valid function.
- Where a number of teeth are missing, whether few or many, prosthetic replacement is a solution that simultaneously addresses two issues:
  - Replacement of missing teeth
  - Uniformity of occlusion with valid function, thereby completing the balance between teeth, muscles, and joints
- Maxillary surgery is another option for occlusal finishing. Before the procedure is done, it is crucial that the surgeon fix the therapeutic condyle-disc-fossa relationship by anchoring a metallic plate, or Luhr device, to a fixed cranial point such as the zygomatic bone. The device is removed postosteotomy (see page 267).
- Permanent splint wear should never be considered because of its many obvious drawbacks that include the need for frequent checkups and adjustments and a failure to actually resolve the underlying pathology. Splint wear can be useful on a temporary basis or as a last resort where the patient's finances are a key factor.
- Other forms of treatment include drugs, physiotherapy, and biofeedback training, among others. These all have their indications both as treatment of choice and as backup to splint therapy to achieve a satisfactory definitive outcome.

Particular care is required with patients scheduled to receive irreversible procedures such as prosthodontic rehabilitation, maxillary surgery, or major orthodontic treatment. In such cases, both musculoarticular recovery (PHASE I) and subsequent occlusal finishing (PHASE II) must have established, at minimum, an "acceptable" anatomical and functional condition, although the term acceptable has no clinical definition. In other words, no irreversible procedure should be attempted until the best possible compromise has been achieved for the patient's condition.

Two clinical issues must be remembered for the patient who has undergone reversible procedures[2] without musculoarticular rehabilitation or occlusal finishing:

- The patient may be satisfied and the clinician comfortable with the knowing that an improvement has been achieved.
- The clinician must never carry out procedures such as prosthodontic rehabilitation, maxillary surgery, or major orthodontic treatment unless the patient has first undergone the necessary musculoarticular therapy and occlusal finishing work. Failure to do so leads to the risk of long-term aggravation and deterioration of the underlying damage (see the warnings on page 258).

CONSIDERATIONS: OTHER JOINTS AND THE TMJ

It may be assumed that the temporomandibular joints (TMJs) are diagnosed and treated like any other joint of the human body. However, a significant difference exists between TMJ musculoarticular therapy (PHASE I) and that used to treat other joints of the human body. Most orthopedic joint treatment with casts, braces, and similar items is worn constantly (24 hours per day) and provides a fixed position for several weeks. In contrast, TMJ treatment involves nonconstant wear (20 to 22 hours per day). Patients are allowed to remove the ARS to eat and perform oral hygiene, and the length of treatment lasts much longer, from 10 to 24 months.

To reduce treatment time, it may be convenient to organize simultaneous application (see page 220) of phase I musculoarticular therapy and phase II orthodontic occlusal finishing, which often keeps overall treatment time within approximately 24 months. It cannot be stressed enough that consistent splint wear is key in achieving a successful outcome and producing significant results, even in the most challenging cases involving internal derangement or osteoarthrosis.

PHASE PLANNING

MUSCULOARTICULAR THERAPY:
WITH SPLINT WORN CONSTANTLY

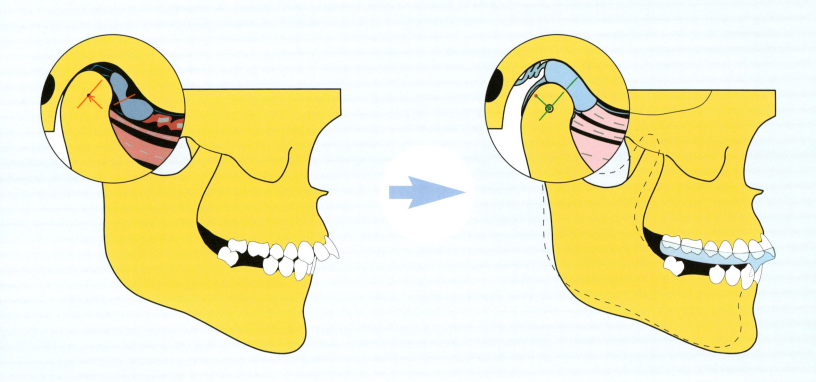

PATHOLOGY

The disc is forward and the condyle backward, with loss of axial alignment leading to muscle tension (superior bundle of the external pterygoid shortened and inferior bundle lengthened) (see page 17).

ARS causes the disc to be recaptured. Intra-articular axial alignment is restored, and muscle tension returns to the normal level.

(The illustrations are repeated as a reminder of the theoretical principles and corresponding clinical applications expressed on pages 104 and 105.)

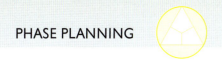

PHASE II

ORTHODONTIC OCCLUSAL FINISHING
(RESEARCH PROJECT):
WITH SPLINT WORN CONSTANTLY

VALID FUNCTION

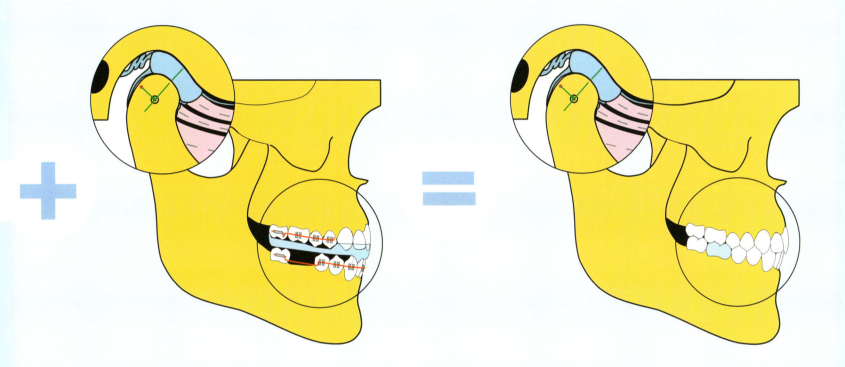

Rearrangement of the teeth through orthodontics.

A balance between teeth, muscles, and joints (completed with prosthodontics in this case).

The RESEARCH PROJECT into orthodontic occlusal finishing is based on the use of traditional fixed appliances on facial surfaces of the teeth while carefully considering the requirements for musculoarticular therapy. In combination with an ARS, these methods are usually successful.

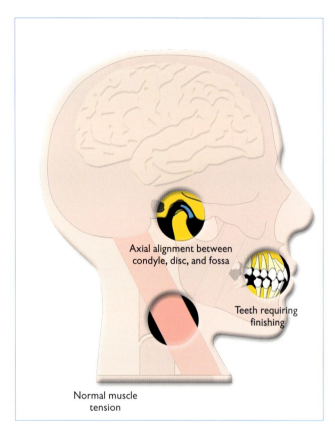

Axial alignment between
condyle, disc, and fossa

Teeth requiring
finishing

Normal muscle
tension

RESEARCH PROJECT (ORTHODONTIC)

In the treatment of disorders affecting the teeth, TMJs, and their related muscles, orthodontic occlusal finishing involves the use of any orthodontic device and fixed appliance compatible with the orthopedic splint, which the patient must wear consistently. It is essential to determine areas of anchorage (skeletal, dental, or with infraosseous screws) to alternate with areas of tooth movement, whether this be a group of teeth or a single tooth only. A section of this chapter is dedicated to explaining a dynamic process consisting of a progressive series of steps in which a single tooth at a time is shifted along the main archwire while the remaining teeth provide anchorage.

Essentially, the research project represents the implementation of PHASE II orthodontic occlusal finishing carried out subsequently to or simultaneously with PHASE I musculoarticular rehabilitation. The **teeth** must be adapted to the requirements of the **muscles** and **joints**, thus confirming the importance of these three unique yet inseparable components.

CONSIDERATIONS ON ORTHODONTIC TREATMENT

As previously stated, orthodontists must be ready to subvert traditional priorities when diagnosing and treating the unit comprising teeth, muscles, and TMJs. It is acceptable to use the **mandible** as the **guiding arch** in nondysfunctional cases, but the opposite is true in cases of dysfunction. Where there is evidence of dual bite or, worse still, signs of more significant pathology, musculoarticular rehabilitation (see PHASE I, page 86 onward) is the priority—and this must be based on the **maxillary arch, which acts as a constant therapeutic benchmark** and follows its indentation in the ARS normally used (see page 145). Iatrogenic procedures must be avoided, including forces that cause posterior compression to the condyle (Class III elastics and Delaire-like facemasks) or place the teeth outside their biologic barriers.

Before commencing phase II, the orthodontist and patient must establish whether orthodontics alone are sufficient to complete the work or whether the patient's skeletal discrepancy warrants maxillary surgery. This is especially true where the skeletal relationships—typically with Class III patients—are aggravated further by the musculoarticular therapeutic position.[3]

A key concept of the orthodontic treatment plan is for the patient to continue wearing the ARS during the tooth movement stage. This helps to maintain stable intra-articular relationships and the mandibular position established at the onset of treatment, which must remain stable until treatment is completed. For the orthodontist, this approach entails the prospect of new orthodontic procedures, such as the research project, in terms of both theoretical planning and practical applications.

THREE ANCHORAGE PROCEDURES

Depending on the patient's condition and the clinician's personal preference, orthodontic occlusal finishing may be supported by three types of anchorage: skeletal anchorage, dental anchorage, or anchorage with intraosseous screws.

I. SKELETAL ANCHORAGE

This type of anchorage stabilizes an entire jaw area or part of it. During the **first stage**, the patient continues to wear the ARS, on which the following areas are established for each dental arch:

- The **area of skeletal anchorage and musculoarticular stabilization** needed to maintain the therapeutic condyle-disc-fossa relationship and the mandibular position. This area is indicated in red in the illustrations on pages 210 and 211.
- The **area of tooth movement** required for occlusal finishing. This area in shown in green in the illustrations.

The second stage, characterized by the inversion "butterfly," occurs after the moved teeth have been properly aligned and intercuspate correctly with their mandibular counterparts (assuming that any necessary treatment of the mandibular arch has been provided). The areas are **inverted** such that:

- The **area of stabilization and skeletal anchorage**, which was shown in red, becomes the area of tooth **movement** and is therefore green.
- The area of tooth movement, which was shown in green, becomes the area of **stabilization and anchorage** and is therefore red.

II. DENTAL ANCHORAGE

(See the case study on page 294)
Currently, orthodontic occlusal finishing can be done with traditional orthodontic archwires, along which the teeth are slid by devices, the most commonly used being elastics and springs. This procedure can be defined as intra-arch and relies on the presence of space, either existing or created. It consists of tying all the teeth together into a major **anchorage** unit (red) while leaving one tooth at a time (green) free to be moved. The procedure is performed as a progressive sequence in which the tooth previously moved goes back to form part of the anchorage group. This continues until all planned movements have been completed, and the procedure may involve all the teeth in that arch or in one semiarch, as necessary.

III. ANCHORAGE WITH INTRAOSSEOUS SCREWS

This is the most effective anchorage method available today.

PHASE II:
ORTHODONTIC OCCLUSAL FINISHING
(RESEARCH PROJECT)

ARS WORN CONSTANTLY

I. BASAL, or skeletal, ANCHORAGE
Stabilizes the entire jaw or part of it and acts on both maxilla and mandible

The "butterfly"
Inversion between areas of anchorage and areas of movement

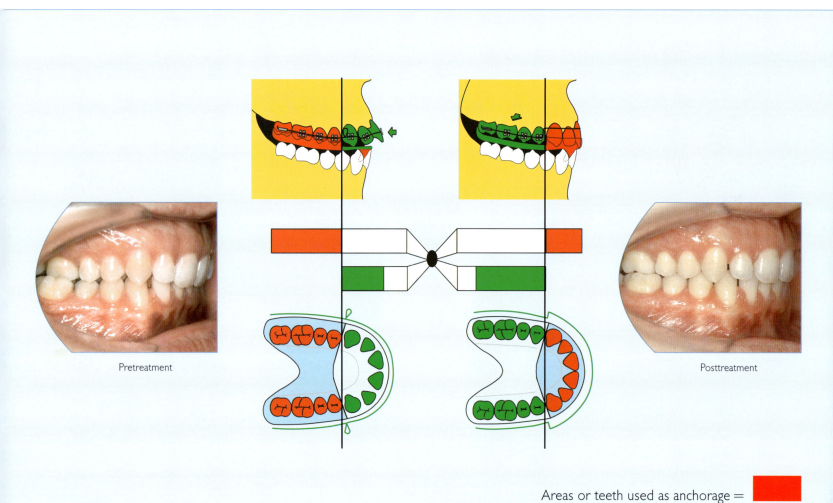

Pretreatment

Posttreatment

Areas or teeth used as anchorage =

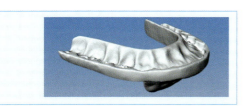

II. DENTAL ANCHORAGE

INTRA-ARCH THERAPY
All teeth are anchored except the one to be moved, which slides along the archwire
in a progressive succession that involves either the entire arch or only the right or left arch,
according to case requirements.

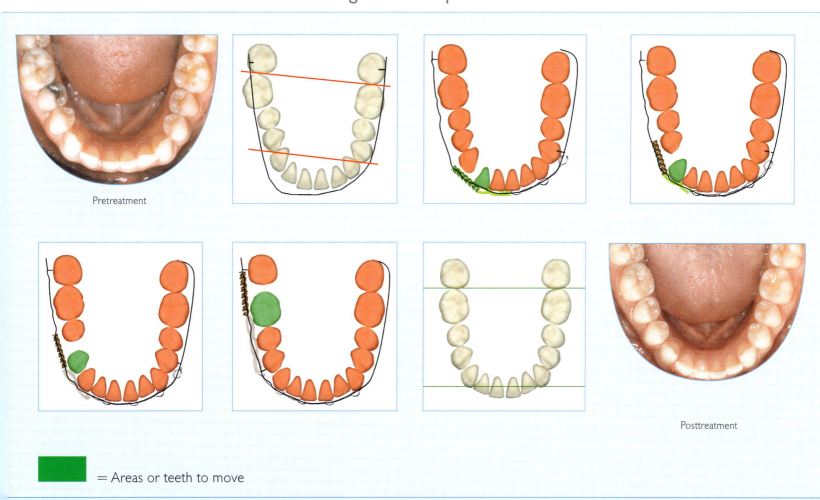

Pretreatment

Posttreatment

= Areas or teeth to move

III. ANCHORAGE WITH INTRAOSSEOUS SCREWS

Although the arches are treated individually, it is clear that they must intercuspate smoothly posttreament.
Systematic monitoring at every appointment should ensure that the correct muscle-led position is maintained.

RESEARCH PROJECT
PHASE II: ORTHODONTIC OCCLUSAL FINISHING

The therapeutic procedures of this text stem from Farrar[2]. They are consistent with the school of thought that aims to achieve rehabilitation of TMDs (referred to for simplicity as phase I) through irreversible articular and occlusal treatment (see page XII), not by following the walk-back procedure coming under the definition of reversible treatment. Because the patient must consistently wear the ARS to safeguard the renewed therapeutic position of the damaged TMJ structures corrected during PHASE I, the orthodontic appliances must be applied simultaneously. As a result, this innovative method sequentially divides individual arches into separate areas of anchorage and movement.

In an effort to illustrate the largest possible number of cases, only the orthodontic occlusal finishing procedures (PHASE II) are described.

I. VIRTUAL EXAMPLE OF PROCEDURES IN PHASE II

Three-dimensional (3D) simulation of orthodontic occlusal finishing in a Class II patient whose phase I musculoarticular rehabilitation is described in chapter 3.

II. SECTION CASE STUDIES WITH PRESENTATION OF PHASE II ALONE

Illustrated use of all orthodontic devices available, both removable and fixed, alternating between areas of anchorage and areas of movement.

I. VIRTUAL EXAMPLE OF PROCEDURES IN PHASE II

The ARS should always be worn with a fixed appliance in both the maxilla and the mandible.

ORTHODONTIC OCCLUSAL FINISHING (RESEARCH PROJECT)

In this case, spaces in the front area of the maxillary arch were closed, and the midlines were centered. On the right side, the wire was given a mesial stop on the second molar and reinforced on the left side with a bend posterior to the second molar and a loop just mesial to the left canine. This established a **multiple-anchorage unit strong enough to move the four incisors** requiring correction. The incisors were shifted left with a spring chain that made use of the space between the canine and lateral incisor. Note that anchorage was reinforced by indentation of the teeth in the resin, which surrounded all the teeth in the maxillary arch excepting those requiring movement (the four incisors). The resin was reduced as necessary to permit retrusion, and the maxillary arch was fitted with bands and brackets to provide full alignment and leveling.

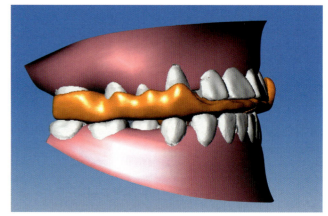

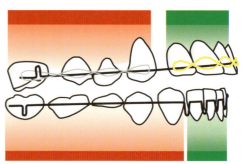

■ Areas or teeth to move
■ Areas or teeth used as anchorage

PHASE II

STEP IV

Additional resin was removed from the ARS to permit mesialization of the right canine. Anchorage was provided by placing a mesial loop on the right second molar and using extra tie wires to create a united anchorage group comprising all the teeth from the first premolar to the second molar and from the distal loop to the lateral incisor on the same side, with the archwire being bent behind the left second molar. Reduction of the splint behind the four incisors (which had previously been distalized to retrude them) left the remaining teeth firmly indented in the resin, thus reinforcing the anchorage and aiding mesialization of the actual canine. This illustrates the overall concept that **one tooth moves against all the remaining teeth, which act as anchorage.**

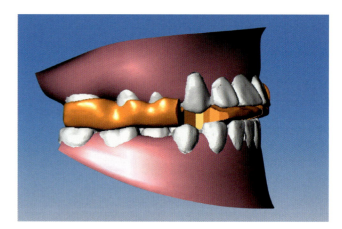

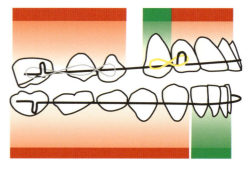

STEP III

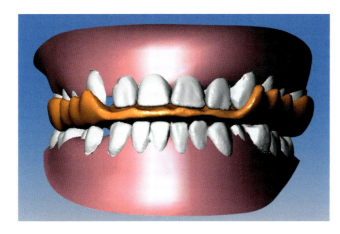
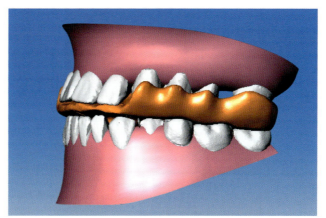

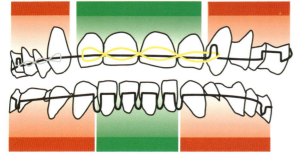
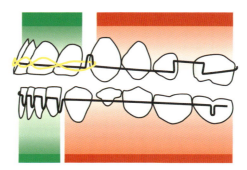

STEP IV

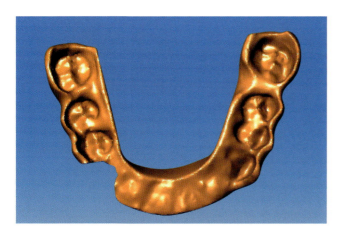
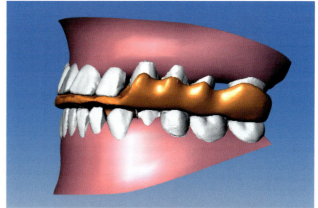

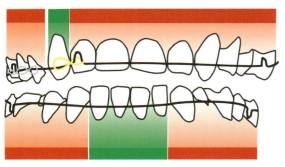
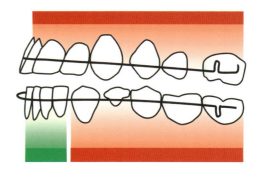

VIEWED WITHOUT SPLINT

Good intercuspation was achieved in anterior arch segments with Class I canines (both right and left) and matching interincisor midlines.

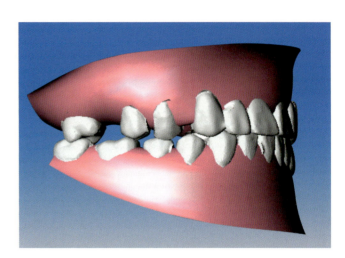

PHASE II

STEP V: INVERSION OF AREAS

With the splint in place, the patient was asked to bite into the ARS so that the **anterior maxillary sector** could act as **anchorage** to aid movement of the **lateroposterior quadrants**. Once these quadrants became **areas of movement**, enough resin in the corresponding areas was removed to permit movement of the teeth. Consequently, the ARS is deeper at the front and shallower at the back.

The increase in space between the maxillary second molars and second premolars, both left and right, produced a dual benefit: By creating space for the maxillary first molars, *(1)* it gave Class I relationships by moving the premolars forward, where previously they were in Class III, and *(2)* the posterior movement of the second molars changes their relationship from Class II to Class I.

A mandibular fixed appliance was used to flatten the curve of Spee, with an archwire prepared with loops to intrude the canines compared with the first premolars and to intrude the incisors in relation to the canines.

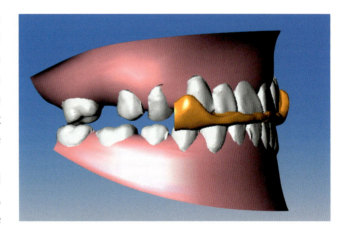

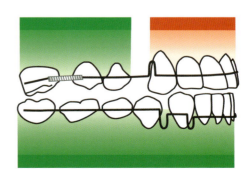

VIEWED WITHOUT SPLINT

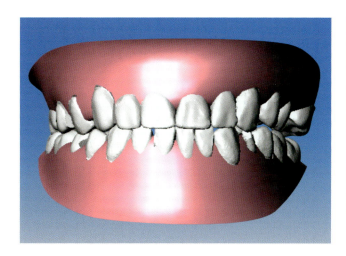
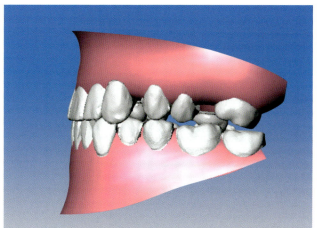

STEP V: INVERSION OF AREAS

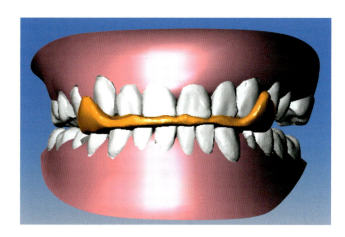
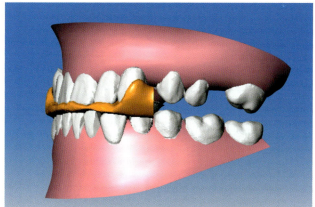

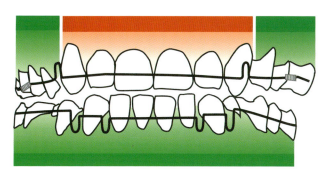
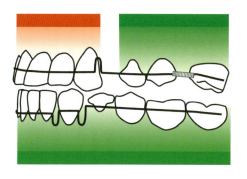

PHASE II

STEP VI

Ideal archwires were prepared to produce a coordinated effect between the maxilla and mandible to maximize intercuspation. The maxillary archwire had a utility arch between the second molar and second premolar on both the left and right sides to preserve space for the missing first molars. The ARS was monitored, resin was removed as necessary to permit minor movements of individual teeth, and the patient was asked to wear the ARS only at night.

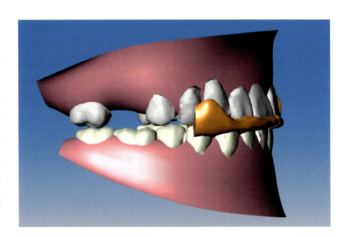

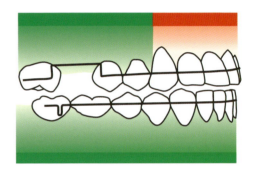

STEP VII: END OF TREATMENT

The case was completed with prosthodontics to replace the first molars, with the resin being adjusted as necessary.

The rehabilitation procedure started with TMJ therapy (PHASE I) during which a functional articular repositioning led to muscle relaxation. Completion of the rehabilitation process required that this articular position be maintained throughout treatment by means of consistent ARS wear, including during the orthodontic occlusal finishing stage (PHASE II) completed with prostheses (not shown). Although the majority of patients prefer to continue wearing their splints at night, by this point the patient has been restored to a state of wellbeing. The three key components—teeth, muscles, and TMJs—are balanced both individually and as a complete functioning anatomical unit.

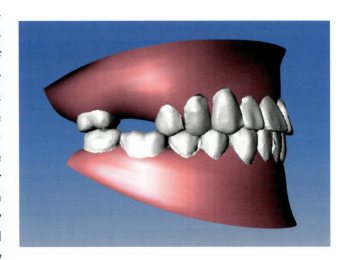

STEP VI

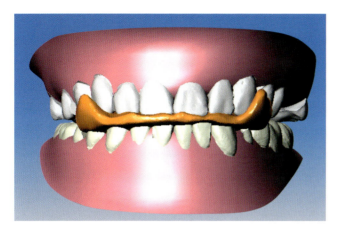
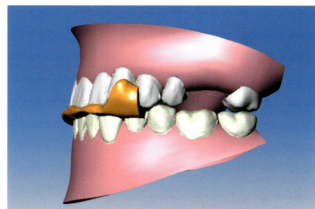

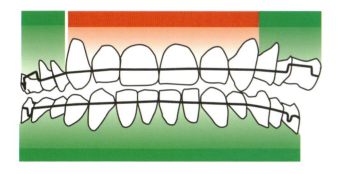
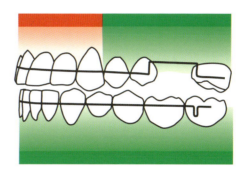

STEP VII: END OF TREATMENT
(ready for prosthetic replacement)

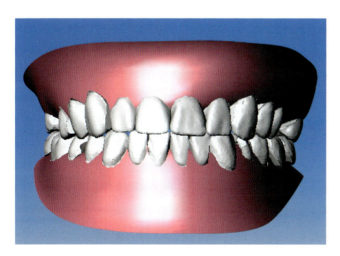
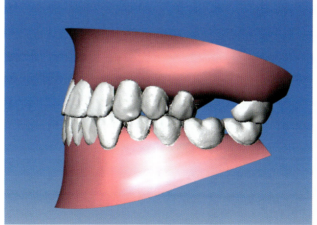

PHASE I (Musculoarticular Therapy)
PHASE II (Orthodontic Occlusal Finishing)

SEQUENCE OF TREATMENT OPTIONS

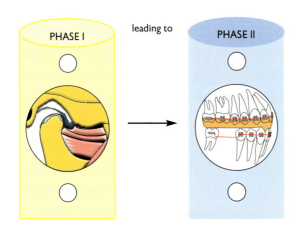

PHASE I leading to PHASE II

Musculoarticular therapy is **followed** by orthodontic occlusal finishing.

Presumed length: 28 to 36 months

Theoretical clinical implications: PHASE I could be done by a dental orthopaedic specialist.
PHASE II should be completed by an orthodontist.

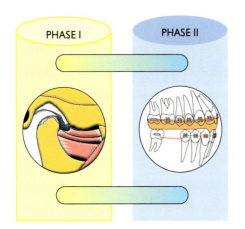

PHASE I and PHASE II performed simultaneously

Musculoarticular therapy and orthodontic occlusal finishing are performed simultaneously.

Presumed length: 22 to 24 months

Theoretical clinical implications: Both phases can be done by an orthodontist also qualified for dental orthopedics.

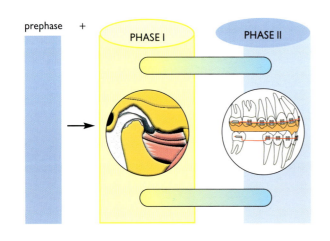

RARELY: Orthodontic prePHASE II followed by PHASE I and PHASE II performed simultaneously

An orthodontic **prephase** can be used to correct major dental discrepancies, **followed by** musculoarticular therapy and orthodontic occlusal finishing performed **simultaneously.**

Presumed length: 24 to 26 months

Theoretical clinical implications: All three phases are to be done by an orthodontist.
In conclusion: The orthodontist must also be a dental orthopedic specialist.

ADVANTAGES	DISADVANTAGES
- The clinician's effort and the patient's compliance are dedicated entirely to the first task of resolving the musculoarticular pathology. - Likewise, the same wholehearted attention is given to completing the treatment plan with orthodontic finishing to stabilize interarch occlusal relationships.	- Treatment time is longer. - Some splints are cumbersome. - With the splint removed at mealtimes, the patient may encounter difficulties due to the relatively few dental contacts.
- Major occlusal discrepancies can be corrected in a short time. - Treatment time is considerably reduced compared with the previous option since both procedures are carried out simultaneously. Furthermore, there is significant esthetic benefit due to alignment of the anterior teeth.	- It is more difficult to carry out both stages together because of overwhelming shifting of tooth anchorage and movement areas. - Some splints are cumbersome. - Each appointment will challenge the clinician to solve new issues and coordinate articular and dental problems.
- Extremely rapid improvement in intercuspation yields a vast improvement in the patient's chewing. - The splint is simpler and less cumbersome. - Overall treatment times are shorter. - Orthodontic treatment is initially done alone and only subsequently is combined with simultaneous musculoarticular therapy until completion of treatment.	- Considerable orthodontic tooth movement is during the early stages of treatment may be uncomfortable and discourage the patient, especially if there is no apparent guarantee of solving the musculoarticular pathology. - After this initial stage, the patient may give up, having obtained with the first orthodontic stage a considerable esthetic improvement and perhaps better function (only if the pathology is minor).

CHOICE OF DEVICES: REMOVABLE ORTHODONTIC DEVICES AND FIXED APPLIANCES

These are conventionally divided into two groups:

• **Removable appliances:** Expansion screws, three-dimensional (3D) (Bertoni) screws, microscrews, springs, loops, and hooks can be integrated with an ARS in the maxilla.

• **Fixed appliances:** In the maxilla, these include normal brackets bonded to the teeth's facial surfaces that do not interact directly with the splint and can be removed and adapted as required. The appliances include bonded brackets, bands, and wires, and they act on selected teeth in the areas of movement. In the mandible, the teeth are controlled with a fixed appliance. Anchorage areas are created in the mandibular incisor group, which exploits their indentation in the anterior flange and counteracts their tendency to protrude under flange pressure. The remaining teeth are free to glide against the splint's smooth lower surface. Further dental anchorage may be created in the entire mandibular arch or singly in the left or right hemi-arch (see page 211).

Note: Neither arch may be fitted with a lingual appliance while the patient wears an ARS.

Example: Splint with three-way screw

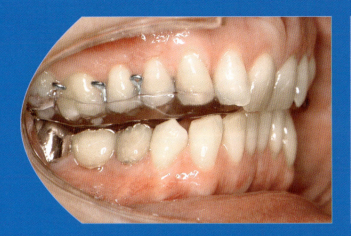
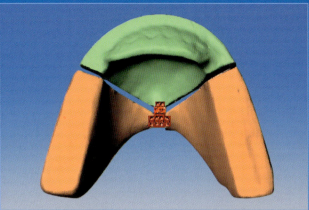

REMOVABLE ORTHODONTIC DEVICES
(eg, three-dimensional screws, microscrews)

FIXED APPLIANCES
(bands, brackets, and wires)

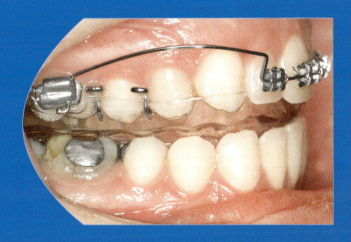
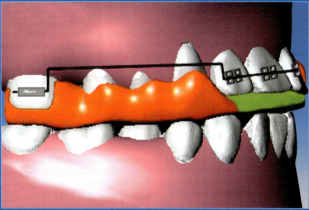

Example: Splint with maxillary fixed appliance

ADDITION OF A BERTONI 3D SCREW TO A NORMAL ARS

This procedure requires the services of a lab technician. It is done as follows:

1. Make the dental impression, and pour the cast in the same way as for a normal ARS. Trim the cast as usual.
2. Place the 3D screw in the center of the splint's palatal surface, and note its position. The corresponding surface is roughened to aid resin adherence.
3. Block out the undercuts created by the teeth's palatal surfaces. Use preshaped wax sticks to surround the areas where the acrylic will be applied.
4. Spread separator over the model, and then apply the acrylic with the salt-and-pepper technique, being careful to cover the screw extensions.
5. To polymerize the acrylic, light-cure it at approximately 50 °C and 2 atm of pressure.
6. Make the palatal surface as thin as possible to provide the least possible bulk in the patient's mouth.
7. Make three cuts in the resin to provide access to the screws that will be used for selective expansion of the oral segments.
8. Finish and polish the splint as usual.

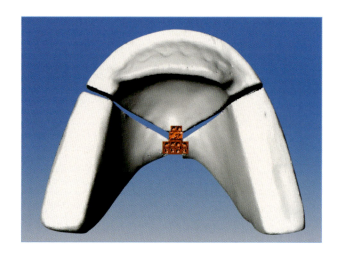

Since the most important stage in treating these patients is orthodontic occlusal finishing, the preliminary musculoarticular rehabilitation is mentioned briefly but not illustrated.

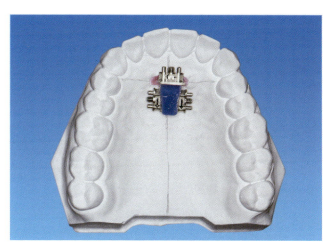

1. Place the 3D Bertoni screw on the dental stone model. The central screw area is protected with blue wax to enable easier acrylic application afterward.

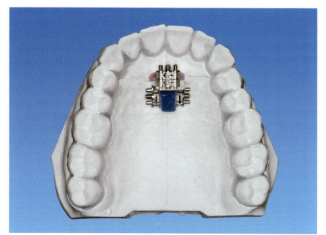

2. Block out the palatal surface undercuts with wax.

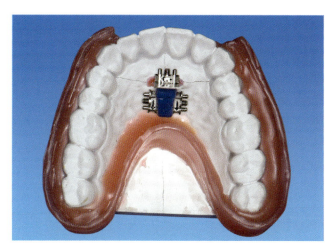

3. Mold preshaped wax sticks round the areas where acrylic is to be applied. Then spread a separator before proceeding with the salt-and-pepper technique.

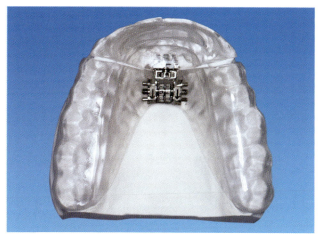

4. Finish and polish the 3D ARS. Note the cuts in the acrylic that provide access to the screws.

INTEGRATING THE ARS

A) With A 3D SCREW

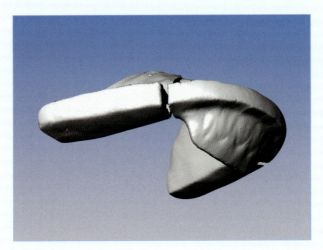
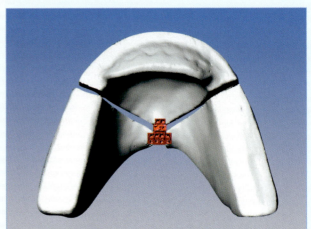

Different screw tightening options

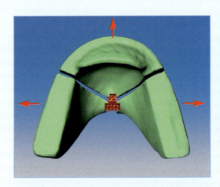
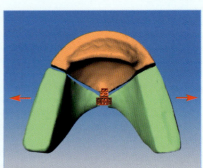

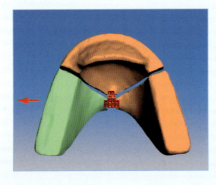
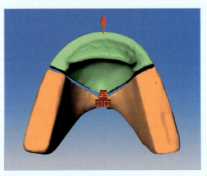
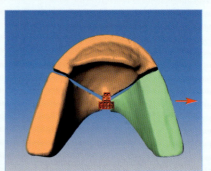

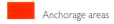 Anchorage areas   Movement areas

B) With ALTERNATIVE SOLUTIONs, for example:
– MICROSCREWS used to move single teeth

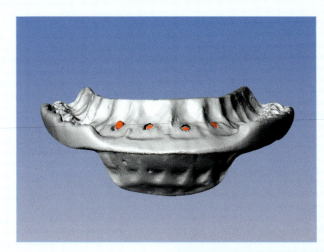
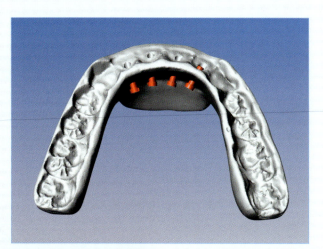

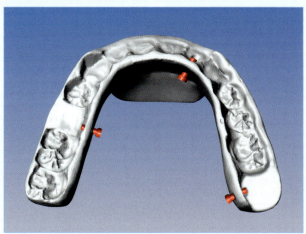

– Acrylic eliminated from SELECTED AREAS to aid spontaneous lateral or extrusive movements

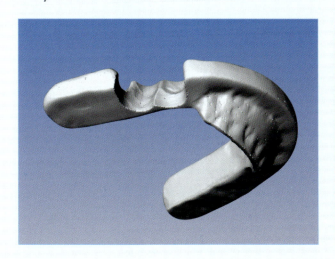
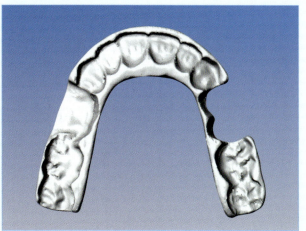

MAXILLARY ARCH: TYPE OF MOVEMENT AND DEVICES USED

TYPE OF MOVEMENT	REMOVABLE	FIXED
➤ *Protraction of maxillary incisors*	- 3D Bertoni screw, with application of anterior action only. - Single microscrews.	- Round or rectangular archwires with expansion loops, placed mesially to the first premolars or canines, plus mesial stops on the most posterior teeth for anchorage.
➤ *Retraction of maxillary incisors*	- Buccal archwire pulling inward, with loop activated with elastics (not recommended).	- Round or rectangular archwires with contraction loops placed distally to canines and activated posteriorly.
➤ *Monolateral or bilateral expansion of lateral sectors*	- 3D Bertoni screw, with application of one or both lateral screws; particularly effective when expansion is required on one side only without loss of anchorage. - One or more single microscrews, on one or both sides—to be activated on different days.	Monolateral: Round or preferably rectangular expansion archwire, selective anchorage areas with teeth tied together and other areas of individual tooth movement with resin removed as necessary. Bilateral: Expansion archwire with reciprocating areas of anchorage and movement, and resin removed as necessary.
➤ *Extrusion of anterior sector*	- Of scarce practicality. Resin can be removed from the maxillary anterior area to aid spontaneous movement.	- More efficient. Remove resin from the maxillary anterior area, and use round or rectangular archwires with extrusion loops mesial to the canines.
➤ *Intrusion of anterior sectors*	- Of scarce practicality with removable appliances.	- As above, but with intrusion loops.
➤ *Extrusion of lateral sectors*	- Remove resin from the splint vertically, where teeth require extruding, to aid spontaneous extrusion.	- Remove resin vertically from the splint where teeth require extruding. Use round or rectangular archwires with two extrusion loops.

II.   SECTORIAL CASE STUDIES ILLUSTRATING AND DESCRIBING PHASE II ALONE

The case studies presented below summarize the orthodontic procedures and appliances—both removable and fixed—most commonly used in the treatment of patients. For the sake of simplicity, details of standard fixed mandibular appliances are often omitted.

Since the most important stage concerning these patients is PHASE II - orthodontic occlusal finishing - the preliminary muscolo-articular rehabilitation PHASE I is touched on briefly but not illustrated.

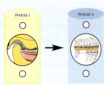

IMPROVEMENT OF INCISAL GUIDANCE WITH PROTRACTION OF MAXILLARY ANTERIORS: ARS + REMOVABLE ADDITIONS IN MAXILLARY ARCH AND FIXED APPLIANCE IN THE MANDIBLE

Patient V. S., age 41

DIAGNOSIS

This patient presented with dual bite and retroclined maxillary anterior teeth. There were problems in both TMJs. Precontacts caused deviation of approximately 4 mm during protrusive movements and a 6- to 7-mm reduction in right-side lateral movements. Deviation occurred in both opening and closing with noise and crepitus on both left and right sides. Average size indentations were present on the tongue.

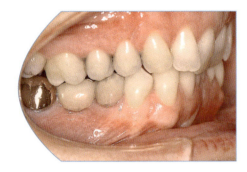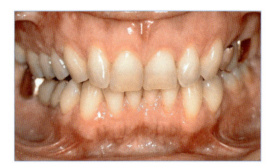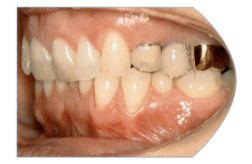

Photographs taken in centric occlusion

PHASE II	ORTHODONTIC OCCLUSAL FINISHING

Features requiring correction:
- **Retroclination of maxillary incisors with edge-to-edge bite**
- Bilateral contraction of the maxillary arch
- A slightly open bite in left and right posterior quadrants
- Accentuated mandibular curve of Spee

DEVICES USED

ARS with:

- Microscrews added to buccalize the maxillary incisors, tightened on alternate days
- 3D expansion screw activated alternately in both lateral areas
- Fixed appliance in the mandibular arch

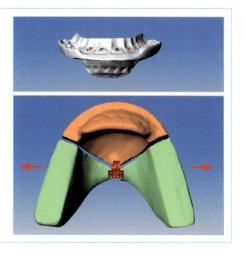

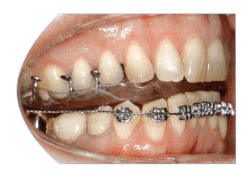

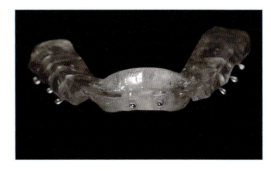

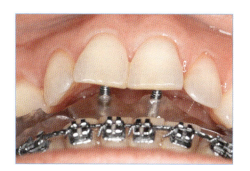

POSTTREATMENT

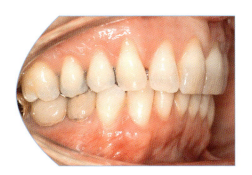

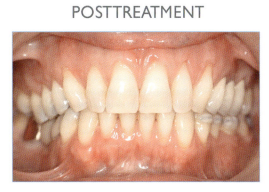

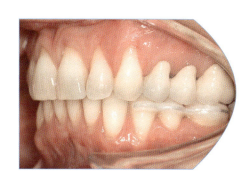

COMPARISONS

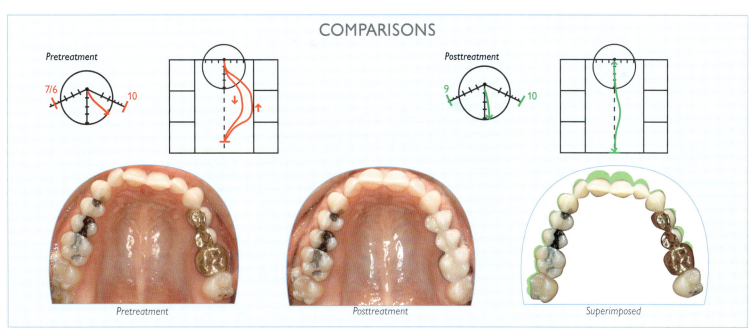

Pretreatment

7/6   10

Posttreatment

9   10

| Pretreatment | Posttreatment | Superimposed |

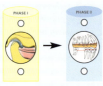

Section example 2

PROTRACTION OF MAXILLARY ANTERIORS: ARS + REMOVABLE ADDITIONS

Patient A. P., age 35

DIAGNOSIS

This patient had a Class II right side and Class I left side. The maxillary left first molar was missing, with the second molar acting as the first. Both mandibular first molars were absent, and both right and left sides exhibited severe articular pathology with reciprocating clicks.

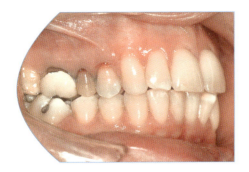
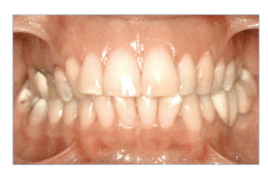
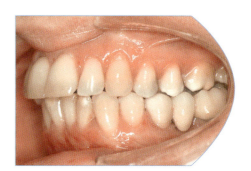

Records taken in centric occlusion

PHASE II   ## ORTHODONTIC OCCLUSAL FINISHING

Features requiring correction:
- Accentuated mandibular curve of Spee
- Considerable contraction in the maxillary arch
- Bilateral posterior open bite
- Incisal guidance

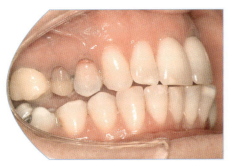
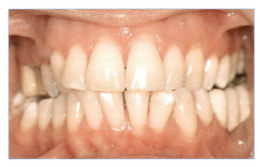
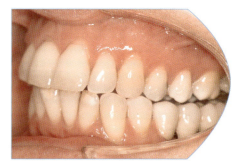

Note the few contacts between maxillary and mandibular teeth and especially anterior edge-to-edge bite.
Because the functional articular position was good and remained stable long-term, it was used as the starting point for orthodontic occlusal finishing.

DEVICES USED

Addition of 3D expansion screw to the ARS with:

- Tightening of the sole anterior screw (area of movement) to protract the incisors, while grinding resin away from the inferior flange of the ARS to prevent protracting the mandibular incisors as well

Subsequently:

- Maxillary fixed appliance with active archwire to provide bilateral expansion from first premolar to second molar, without affecting the anterior teeth
- Completion with brackets on all teeth in both jaws to provide detailed finishing of both arches

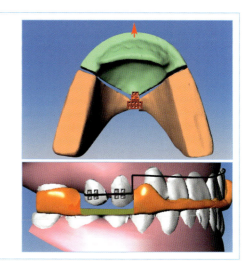

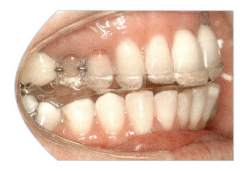
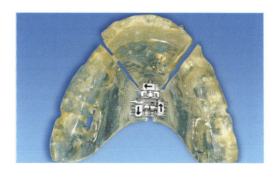
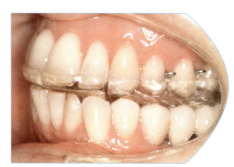

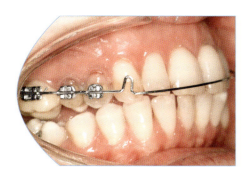
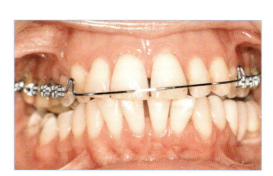
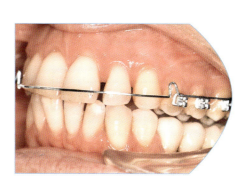

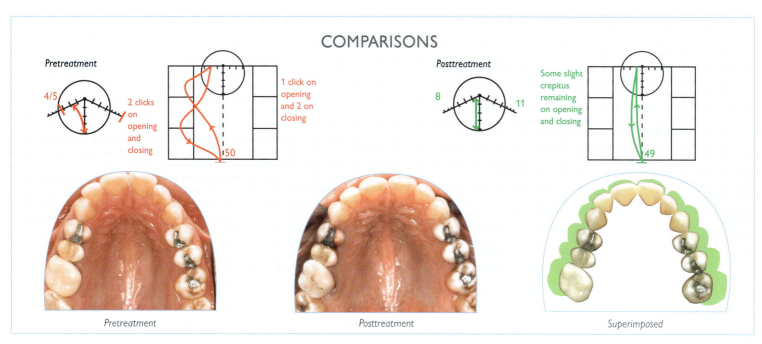

COMPARISONS

Pretreatment

4/5

2 clicks on opening and closing

1 click on opening and 2 on closing

50

Posttreatment

8

11

Some slight crepitus remaining on opening and closing

49

Pretreatment

Posttreatment

Superimposed

233

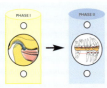

PROTRACTION AND EXTRUSION OF MAXILLARY INCISORS: ARS + FIXED APPLIANCE

Patient I. T., age 20

DIAGNOSIS

This patient presented with skeletal Class I with Class I interarch relationships on the left side but Class II on the right side. The patient experienced TMJ locking on the right side, TMJ noise, headache, facial pain, postural problems, and back pain.

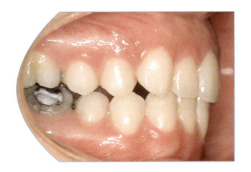 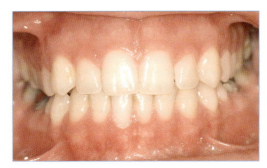 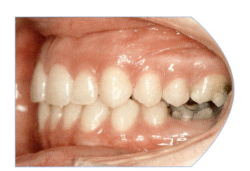

PHASE II ORTHODONTIC OCCLUSAL FINISHING

Features requiring correction:
- Retroclined maxillary incisors with edge-to-edge bite
- Transversal contraction of the maxillary arch
- ARS-induced protraction of mandibular teeth leading to Class III dental relationships on left side and Class I on right side

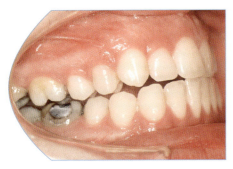 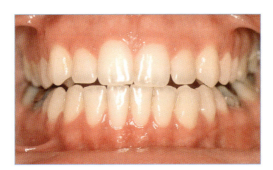 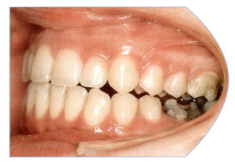

Few contacts between maxillary and mandibular teeth.
Because the functional articular position was good and remained stable long-term, it was used as the starting point for orthodontic occlusal finishing.

DEVICES USED

- Fixed appliance with utility arch to protract maxillary incisors with simultaneously use of the ARS

Details of use:

- Greater tightening of the archwire on the left side, where a dental Class III had occurred

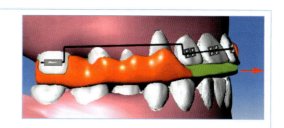

Note: The remaining minor tooth movements were "induced" with the aid of careful addition and removal of acrylic to and from the ARS, which the patient continued to wear throughout treatment. Brackets were bonded to the maxillary incisors and first molars, with the archwire shaped into a utility arch to protract and extrude the incisors, thus closing the bite. Obviously, resin was removed from the front of the splint to permit tooth movement. Instead of banding the mandibular arch, it was decided to use the forces created by the splint's posterolateral wedge. Resin was ground away from the premolar and first molar areas to allow their extrusion and, hence, to flatten the curve of Spee. In this case, a less-than-perfect outcome had to be accepted in terms of the midlines and the mandibular left canine

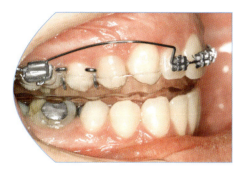
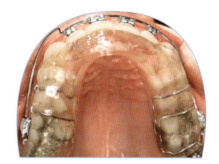
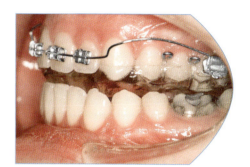

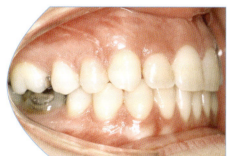
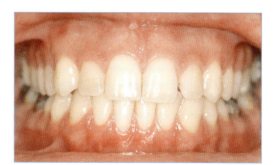
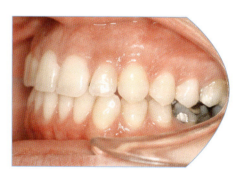

COMPARISONS

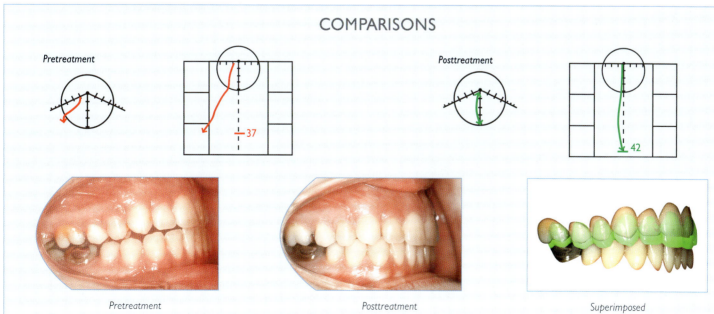

Pretreatment	Posttreatment	Superimposed

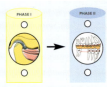

Section
example
4

RETRACTION OF MAXILLARY INCISORS: ARS + REMOVABLE ADDITIONS, WITH SUBSEQUENT FIXED APPLIANCE

Patient D. F., age 36

DIAGNOSIS

This patient was diagnosed with Class II with deep bite and a bilaterally contracted maxillary arch. The maxillary incisors were noticeably flared.

Missing teeth 6 | 8
_____
6

The periodontal condition—poor with reduced bone levels—required immediate treatment. TMJ damage was present as was widespread pain in the neck and shoulders.

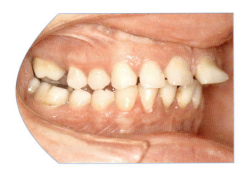
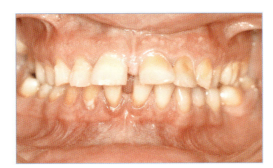
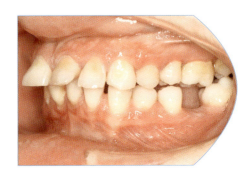

PHASE II

ORTHODONTIC OCCLUSAL FINISHING

Main features requiring correction:
- Considerable buccalization of maxillary and mandibular incisors
- Accentuated curve of Spee in both arches
- Narrow transversal dimension of maxillary arch

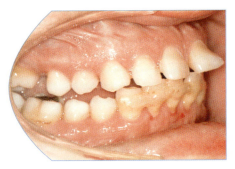
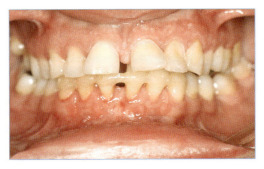
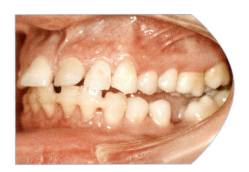

Note: During this stage, the mandibular incisors were ligated as a group from canine to canine with a transparent labial ligature to prevent further proclination.
Because the functional articular position was good and remained stable long-term, it was used as the starting point for orthodontic occlusal finishing.

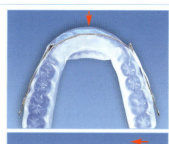
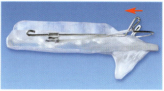

DEVICES USED

- Addition to the ARS of a labial archwire with retracting elastic (see photograph to right)
- Composite bumps applied to the center of the labial faces of the maxillary incisors and canines to act as stoppers preventing the elastic from sliding up to the gingival margin
- Complete fixed appliances in both maxillary and mandibular arches

Details of use:

- Labial arch tightened against the splint with elastics

Maxillary arch: A loop was inserted on the ARS activated by elastics to achieve retraction of maxillary anterior teeth. The unique feature of this case is that when the patient removed and replaced her splint, she also had to remove and replace the elastics!

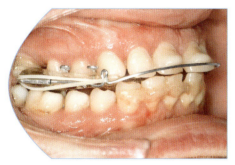
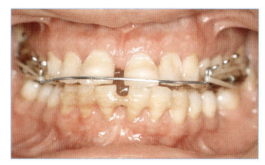
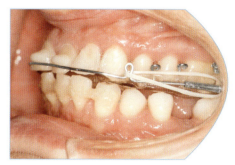

Treatment continued with complete fixed appliances in both arches and with the splint worn continuously.

POSTTREATMENT: *A compromise in interarch relationships was accepted.*

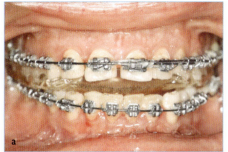
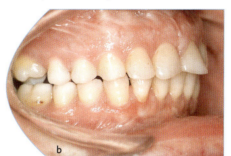
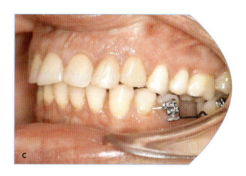

COMPARISONS

Pretreatment

Crepitus on opening and closing

Deviations on opening and closing

11   11

46

Posttreatment

11   11

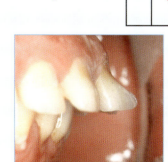

| Before ARS use | Post-splint (overcorrected) | Posttreatment (after fixed appliance) |

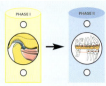

EXPANSION OF LEFT LATERAL SECTOR AND ANTERIOR SECTOR: ARS + REMOVABLE APPLIANCES

Patient L. V., age 44

DIAGNOSIS

This patient had a canine Class I relationship on dental closure on both the right and left sides (where +5 is missing). Conversely, muscle-led closure gave canine

Class II on the right side and Class III on the left side.

Teeth missing:

$$\frac{8 \mid 5\ 8}{8\ 5 \mid 6}$$

Mastication was painful, and mouth opening was limited. The left condyle was locked.

DENTAL CLOSURE

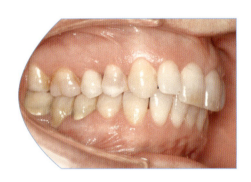 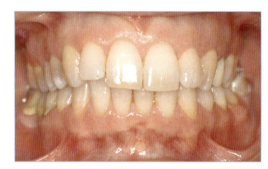 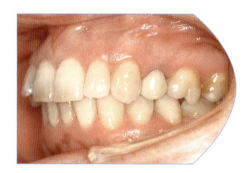

PHASE II

ORTHODONTIC OCCLUSAL FINISHING
(Initial treatment plan and only partial outcome presented in this case)

Main features requiring correction:
- Maxillary left crossbite
- Maxillary incisors slightly retroclined
- Bilateral open bite
- Narrow left hemi-arch

MUSCLE-LED CLOSURE

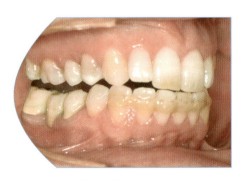 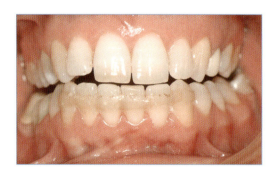 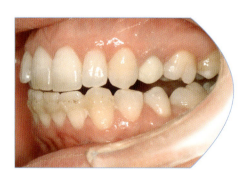

Note: The mandibular incisors were ligated as a group from canine to canine with a transparent labial ligature to prevent further proclination. Because the functional articular position was good and remained stable long-term, it was used as the starting point for orthodontic occlusal finishing.

DEVICES USED

- 3D expansion device fitted to the ARS.

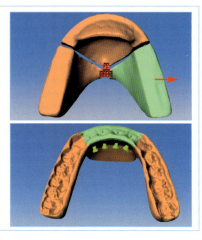

Details of use:

- Only the lateral left screw was tightened (area of tooth movement) to provoke monolateral expansion.
- Anchorage initially on the right side and front area.
- Subsequently, the left lateral area was used for anchorage, along with the right side, to allow the front teeth to move buccally aided by microscrews fitted to the ARS.

Maxillary and mandibular fixed appliances (not shown) were used to complete the best possible finishing of the interarch relationships, with particular care taken in the dynamic control of incisal guidance and left and right laterality.

Monolateral left side application of 3D screw to expand this sector alone.

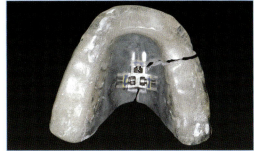

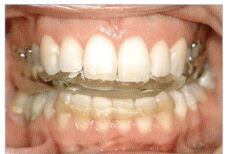

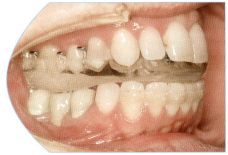

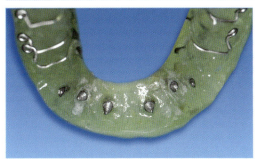

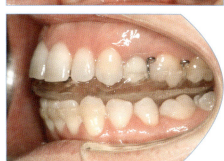

Insertion of microscrews into the anterior sector to buccalize the maxillary front teeth.

COMPARISONS

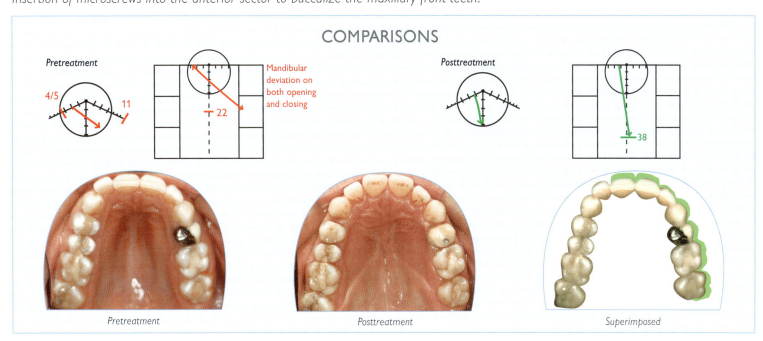

Pretreatment	Posttreatment	Superimposed

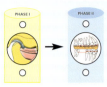

MAXILLARY ANTERIOR AND BILATERAL EXPANSION: ARS + REMOVABLE APPLIANCES FOLLOWED BY FIXED APPLIANCES

Patient P. C., age 25

DIAGNOSIS

This patient was diagnosed with a skeletal Class II and dental Class I on the right side. On the left side, there was a Class II by approximately 2 mm and accentuated curve of Spee. The maxillary arch was narrow. Also present were severe TMJ damage with clicks, deviated excursions, painful masticatory muscles, lumbar pain, and headaches. The patient reported trauma to the right side of her face.

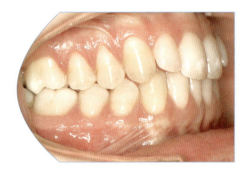 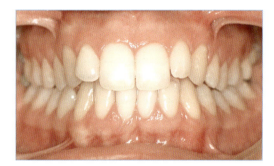 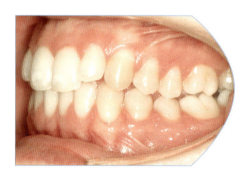

PHASE II   ORTHODONTIC OCCLUSAL FINISHING

Features requiring correction:
- Edge-to-edge incisor relationships
- Class II relationships on left side
- Narrow maxillary arch
- Bilateral open bite

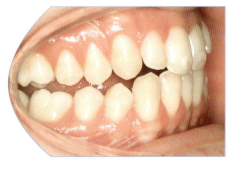 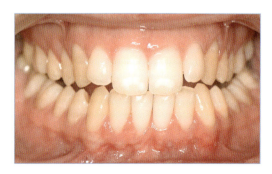 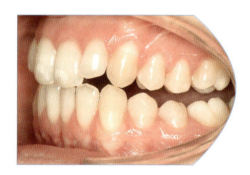

Because the functional articular position was good and remained stable long-term, it was used as the starting point for orthodontic occlusal finishing.

DEVICES USED

ARS with:

- 3D device central screw
- Microscrews on incisors and canines (in succession)

First step:

- Protraction and alignment of maxillary front teeth, using the microscrews selectively. Since this would also cause protraction of the mandibular incisors, resin must be ground away from the flange carefully and progressively to maintain the initial position.

Second step:

- Bilateral transversal expansion, alternatively tightening the lateral screws
- Maxillary and mandibular fixed appliances to provide occlusal finishing (not shown)

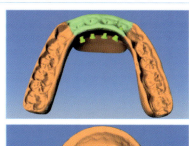
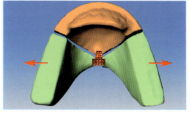

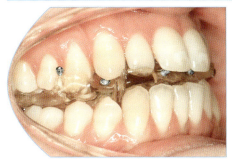
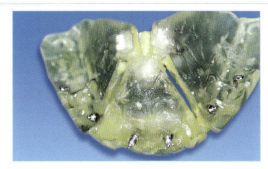
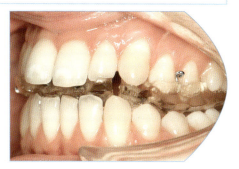

Initially, microscrews were inserted at the maxillary central incisors, followed by insertion at the canines and the lateral incisors. Subsequently, a 3D screw was inserted to provide bilateral maxillary expansion. Screw tightening must be planned carefully. In this case, it was decided to tighten the two central incisor screws, the lateral screws 2 days later, and so on.

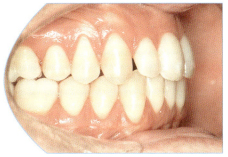
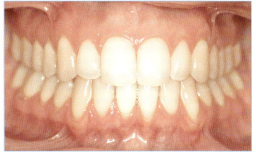
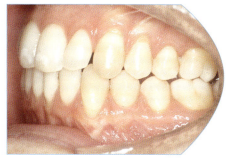

COMPARISONS

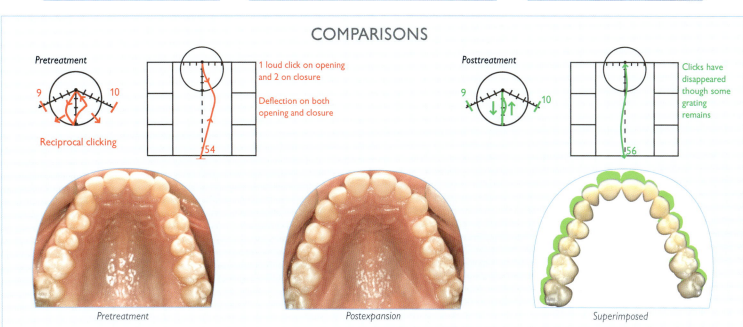

Pretreatment

9   10

Reciprocal clicking

1 loud click on opening and 2 on closure

Deflection on both opening and closure

|54

Posttreatment

9   10

Clicks have disappeared though some grating remains

|56

| Pretreatment | Postexpansion | Superimposed |

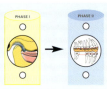

BILATERAL EXPANSION: ARS + FIXED APPLIANCE

Patient C. M., age 30

DIAGNOSIS

This patient presented with a dental Class III on the left side and a maxillary left canine crossbite. The midlines did not align. The mandible was crowded. The patient was missing the mandibular third molars, and their maxillary counterparts extruded, which was probably the main cause of the pathology. TMJ problems were present, especially on left side, with limited excursions. Cervical spine pain and lumbosacral pathology negatively affected bodily posture.

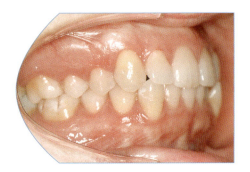 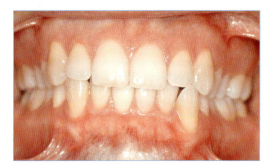 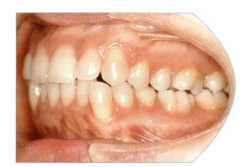

PHASE II ORTHODONTIC OCCLUSAL FINISHING

Features requiring correction:
- Bilaterally narrow maxillary arch
- Mandibular crowding
- Extraction of maxillary third molars

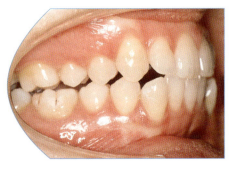 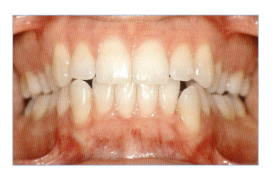 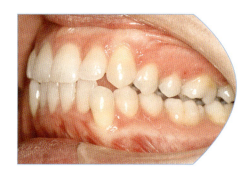

Because the functional articular position was good and remained stable long-term, it was used as the starting point for orthodontic occlusal finishing.

DEVICES USED

- Fixed appliance with brackets on right and left premolars and expanding utility arch, used simultaneously with the ARS
- Acrylic removed as needed to permit the necessary tooth movements
- Maxillary and mandibular fixed appliances for detailed occlusal finishing

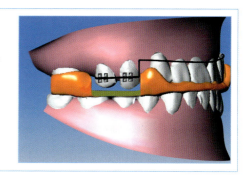

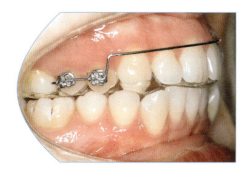
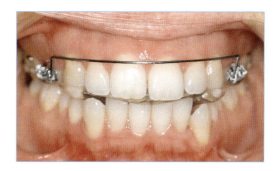
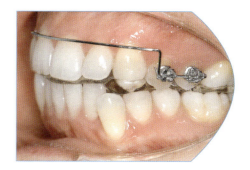

The maxillary utility arch, involving only the two premolars on both the right and left sides, provides reciprocal expansion and anchorage.

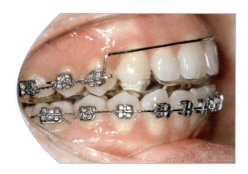
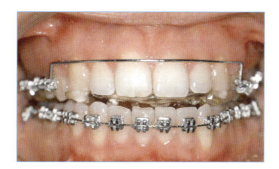
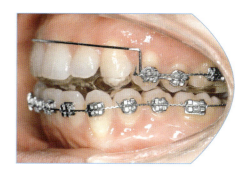

The action of the utility arch continues. After this stage was complete, full bracketing of the maxilla as well as the mandibular arch was done. It significantly improved dynamic jaw movements and interarch relationships and provided pain relief.

COMPARISONS

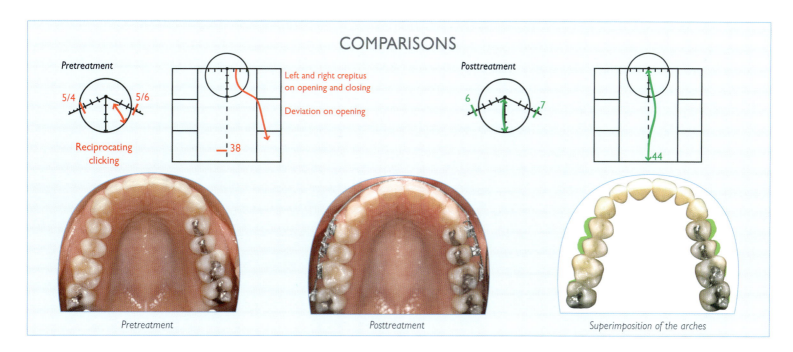

Pretreatment

5/4   5/6

Reciprocating clicking

Left and right crepitus on opening and closing

Deviation on opening

38

Posttreatment

6   7

44

Pretreatment   Posttreatment   Superimposition of the arches

243

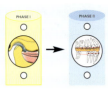

Section example 8

COMPLETE EXPANSION (ANTERIOR AND BILATERAL) OF THE MAXILLARY ARCH: USING ONLY ARS + REMOVABLE APPLIANCES, WITH A FIXED APPLIANCE IN THE MANDIBULAR ARCH

Patient P. T., age 41

DIAGNOSIS

Missing $\frac{8\ 4\ |\ 4\ 8}{6\ |\ 6}$

This patient presented with Class I skeletal and dental relationships. There was severe recession of periodontal support tissue. Limited bilateral TMJ excursions, with greater damage on left side, and joint noise were noted.

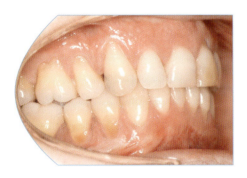
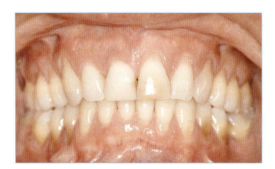
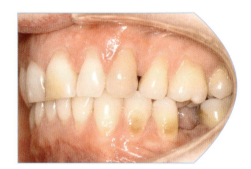

PHASE II — ORHODONTIC OCCLUSAL FINISHING

Features requiring correction:
- Thorough periodontial specialist treatment
- Bilaterally narrow maxillary arch
- Retroclined maxillary incisors with edge-to-edge bite
- Bilateral posterior open bite with accentuated mandibular curve of Spee on both sides

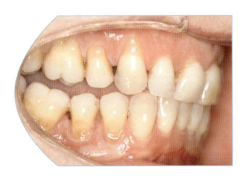
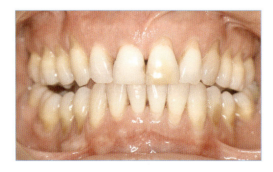
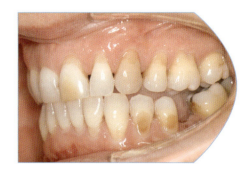

Because the functional articular position was good and remained stable long-term, it was used as the starting point for orthodontic occlusal finishing.

DEVICES USED

- 3D expansion device fitted to the ARS

Details of use:

- Each screw turned every 2 days
- Progressive removal of resin from the ARS on the mandibular contact lingual flange to prevent a contraindicated protraction
- Microscrews added on maxillary incisors to improve inclination in addition to protraction
- Complete fixed mandibular appliance, with particular care taken to achieve correct incisal guidance

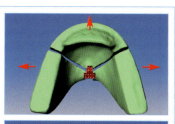
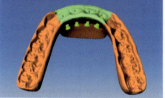

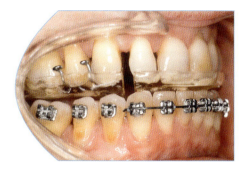
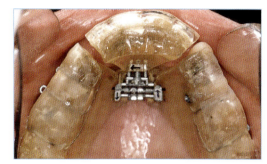
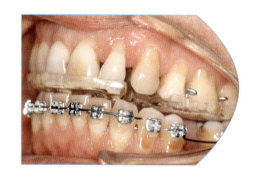

POSTTREATMENT:

Complete expansion of the maxillary arch. The final outcome (an acceptable compromise?) was achieved with the use of only removable appliances in the maxilla and only fixed appliances in the mandibular arch.

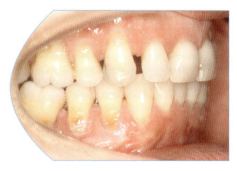
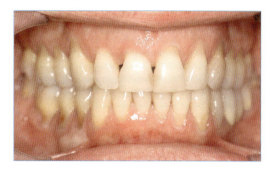
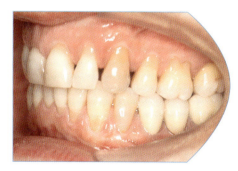

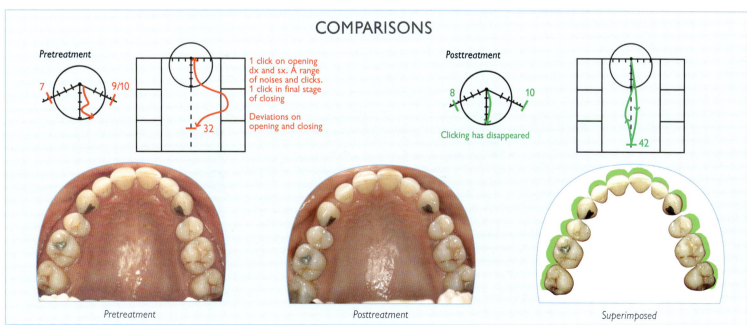

COMPARISONS

Pretreatment

7   9/10

1 click on opening dx and sx. A range of noises and clicks.
1 click in final stage of closing

Deviations on opening and closing

32

Posttreatment

8   10

Clicking has disappeared

42

Pretreatment

Posttreatment

Superimposed

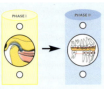

PROTRACTION AND EXTRUSION OF MAXILLARY INCISORS: ARS + REMOVABLE APPLIANCE PLUS FIXED MAXILLARY AND MANDIBULAR FIXED APPLIANCES

Patient A. D. P., age 39

DIAGNOSIS

This patient was diagnosed with an anterior edge-to-edge bite. The maxillary incisors were retroclined Class I; the mandibular incisors were crowded. Both the left and right sides exhibited clicking and lateral deviations during opening and closing excursions. The patient experienced localized headaches and widespread aching in masticatory and postural muscles.

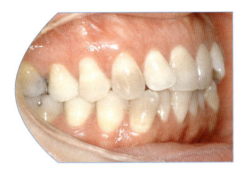
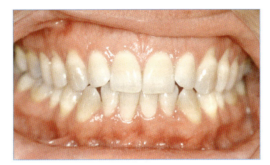
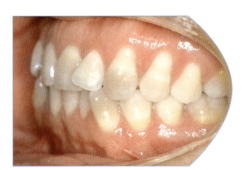

PHASE II ORTHODONTIC OCCLUSAL FINISHING

Main features requiring correction:
- Retroclined maxillary incisors with edge-to-edge bite
- Slight open bite in lateral sectors
- Incisal guidance

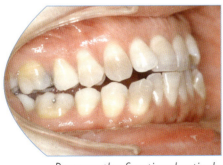
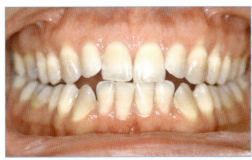
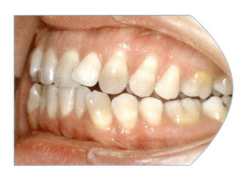

Because the functional articular position was good and remained stable long-term, it was used as the starting point for orthodontic occlusal finishing.

DEVICES USED

- Addition of maxillary incisor microscrews to the ARS.

Details of use:

- Microscrew tightening.
- No resin was removed from the ARS in correspondence with the mandibular incisors to encourage them to protract as well. The crowding was thus relieved through dental movement alone.

Following this stage, the patient had an anterior open bite, which was corrected with:

- A maxillary fixed appliance with loops in the archwire providing an extrusive effect on the incisors.

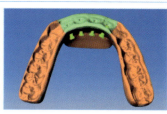

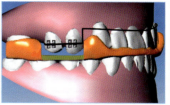

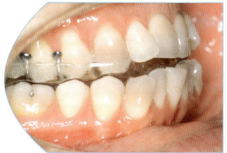

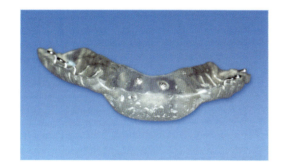

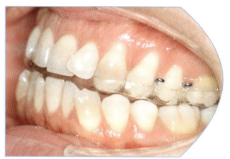

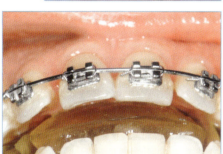

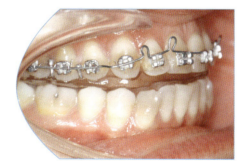

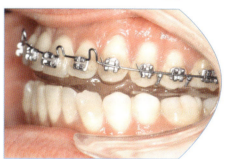

To increase the extrusive force, during a later stage the anterior archwire area was ligated to the bracket tops instead of the slots (left-hand photograph). This was done without removing the wire completely but simply by freeing it and ligating it back over the incisor bracket tops (center and right-hand photographs).

COMPARISONS

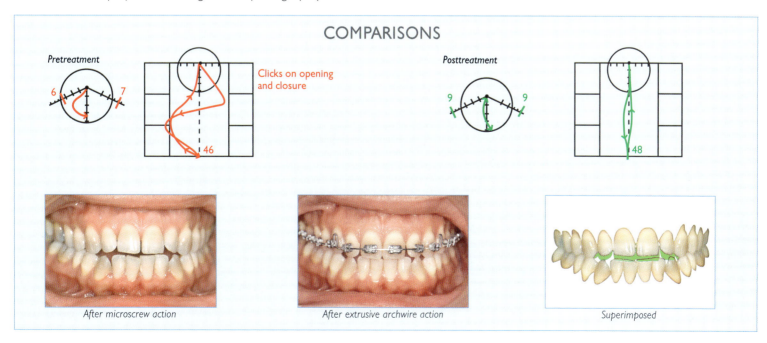

Pretreatment

Clicks on opening and closure

6 7

46

Posttreatment

9 9

48

After microscrew action

After extrusive archwire action

Superimposed

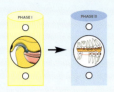

PHASE II: OCCLUSAL ORTHODONTIC FINISHING DONE WITH ONLY REMOVABLE ADDITIONS TO THE ARS
KEY FEATURE: ARS with removable additions

Patient: O. F., age 18

DIAGNOSIS

This patient presented with an asymmetric Class II on the right side only, with deep bite and dysfunctional pathology. Bilateral clicking was heard in conjunction with altered excursions at approximately 10 mm of opening and early in closing. Noises were heard during right side protrusion, lateral movements, and left side closure. The patient also complained of intermittent headaches, painful mastication, and bruxism with masticatory muscle tiredness, especially on morning awakening.

ORTHODONTIC OCCLUSAL FINISHING TREATMENT

After several months of treatment, the patient was fitted with an ARS with a 3D bilateral expansion device inserted to widen the maxilla. Microscrews were subsequently added to buccalize the maxillary incisors.

OUTCOME

Extrusion of the posterior quadrants improved the bite by opening it, and there was a slight increase in vertical height. Definite improvement in both skeletal and dental relationships was noted along with musculoarticular pathology relief.

PRETREATMENT RECORDS

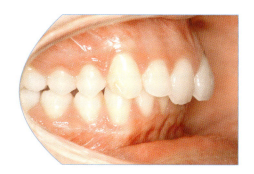 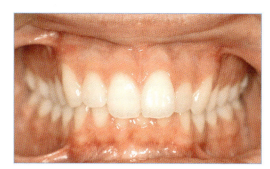 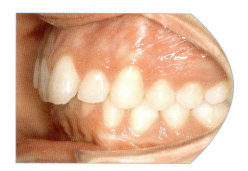

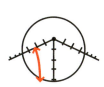

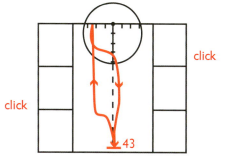

click

click

43

PHASE II   ORTHODONTIC OCCLUSAL FINISHING

Stable consistent relationships in dynamic movements and on final stage of closure were achieved with few contacts between maxillary and mandibular incisors.

This position was the starting point for the occlusal orthodontic finishing stage.

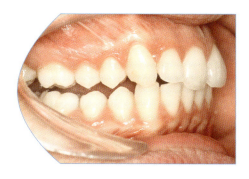 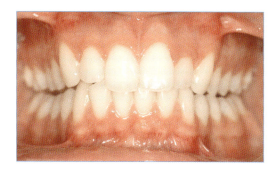 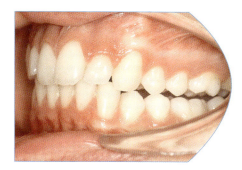

PHASE II ORTHODONTIC OCCLUSAL FINISHING

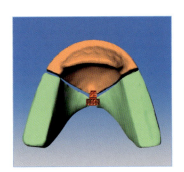
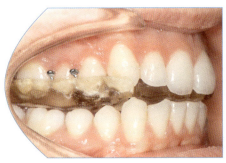
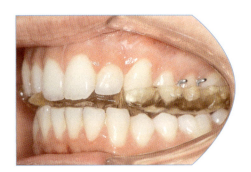

The patient was fitted with an ARS integrated with a 3D device to provide bilateral maxillary expansion, predominantly on the left side. The curve of Spee was flattened by leaving only the canines and second molars indented in the resin and by removing resin vertically from the splint over the premolars and first molars on both sides of the mandibular arch, thus aiding their extrusion. The maxillary left lateral incisor and canine were buccalized by the insertion of microscrews into the ARS, which transformed the edge-to-edge bite into an acceptable occlusion.

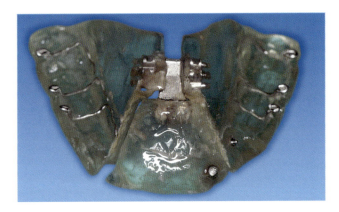
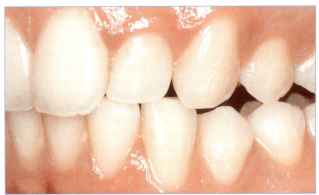

As with all patients treated with an ARS, those teeth requiring correction were determined by having the patient remove the splint and position her jaws as if she were still wearing it. This allows the practitioner to identify the teeth that need to be moved and to what extent and in what direction. A successful musculoarticular outcome is confirmed by the stability of axial TMJ anatomical component relationships as ascertained by MRI investigation or, more approximately, by the consistency of dynamic mandible movements in all three spatial dimensions (a procedure applied systematically).

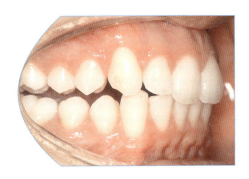
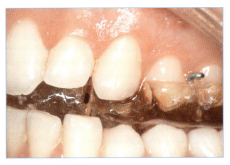
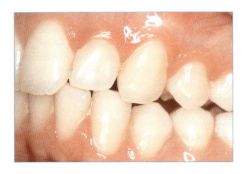

As required, resin was also removed over a number of teeth to achieve the best possible results. The amount of tooth movement was gradually reduced until this was no longer necessary since the teeth had been adapted to the patient's musculoarticular requirements and correct muscle-led occlusion had been obtained.

POSTTREATMENT

In addition to the stimulating effect on the mandible, a further point of interest with this patient—once fully grown—was the improvement of her Class II molar and premolar relationships, especially on the right side, while the canine relationship remained debatable.

This result was achieved by *(1)* shifting the right side of the mandible forward, right from the start of treatment, and *(2)* on the opposite side of the maxilla, freeing the posterior surfaces of all the teeth on the right side from the resin to permit their retraction (a similar procedure is applied when treating Class II with an Andresen activator). Some months posttreatment, the patient complained of slight muscle discomfort, which was addressed with a retainer to be worn at night.

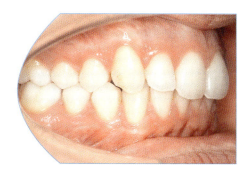
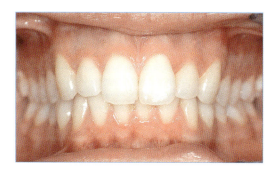
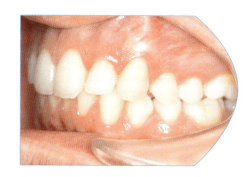

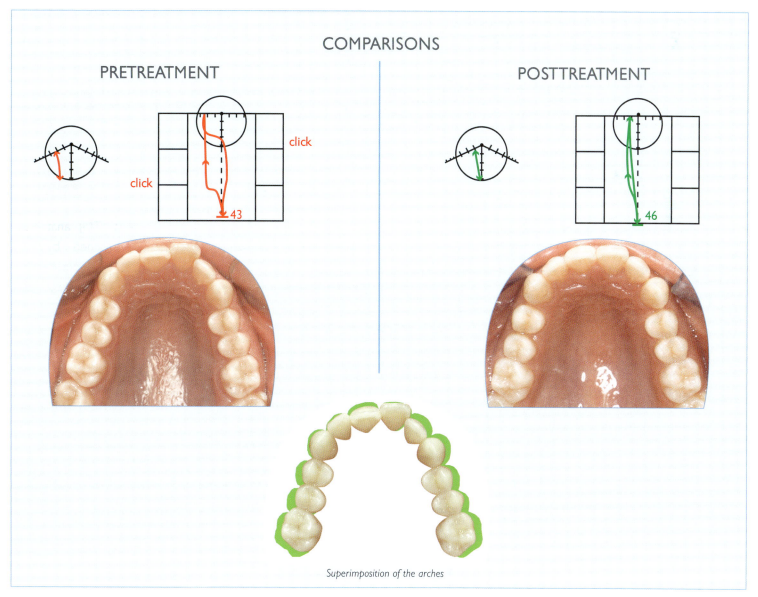

Superimposition of the arches

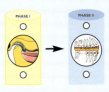

PHASE II: ORTHODONTIC OCCLUSAL FINISHING WITH FIXED APPLIANCES

KEY FEATURE: Because the patient refused maxillary surgery to correct her severe Class II, ARS musculoarticular therapy was applied for the dual purposes of *improving the TMJ pathology and the skeletal discrepancy.*

Commendable coordination was noted among the various specialists in conservative dentistry, periodontology, orthodontics, and prosthodontics.

Patient: A. M., age 40

DIAGNOSIS

The patient complained of TMJ pain, especially on the right side, involving her shoulders, neck, and head. A skeletal Class II relationship with grossly flaring maxillary incisors was evident, and the mandibular left first molar was missing. TMJ pathology due to compression, with joint noise, was more prevalent on the right side.

TREATMENT PLAN

Complete oral rehabilitation involved a number of procedures. Necessary dental treatment was taken care of, followed by musculoarticular therapy (details omitted) leading to axial relationships between the anatomical and articular components (PHASE I). Subsequently, the patient underwent orthodontic occlusal finishing (PHASE II) completed with prosthodontics. The patient continued to wear her splint to maintain the correct therapeutic position established at the outset. This position was kept stable until the treatment was completed (an irreversible procedure as classified by Farrar[2]).

At the outset, the ARS served to reposition the condyles downward and forward, which produced a significant improvement in the patient's Class II relationships, both skeletal and dental. From the very beginning, her mandibular anterior teeth were splinted labially with transparent material to limit further inclination of the incisors caused by pressure from the splint's mandibular wedge.

The first stage of orthodontic occlusal finishing involved using the maxillary posterior quadrants as anchorage to correct the incisor flare. The zones were then inverted, with the initial anchorage area being subjected to movement and the original movement area becoming the point of anchorage. Further treatment aims were to open the bite, expand the maxillary arch, retrocline the maxillary incisors, and reopen space around the missing -6 to facilitate correct dental anatomy for the planned prosthodontic replacement, all the while using the splint to maintain occlusal stability.

OUTCOME

Good maxillomandibular intercuspation was achieved with Class I relationships. The patient no longer complained of pain, and her excursions were satisfactory.

PRETREATMENT RECORDS

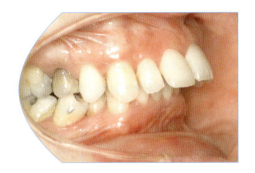 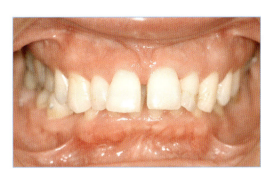 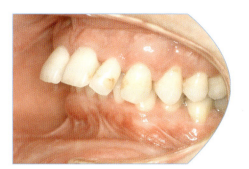

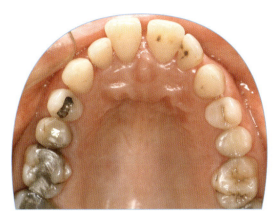 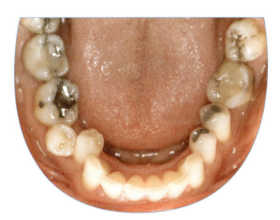

Severe deep bite and major flaring of the maxillary incisors are evident. The mandibular arch is crowded with significant dental disarray. The situation is aggravated by the missing left first molar, which enabled the neighboring teeth to crowd in and become inclined.

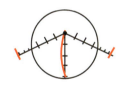

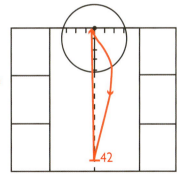

Noise

42

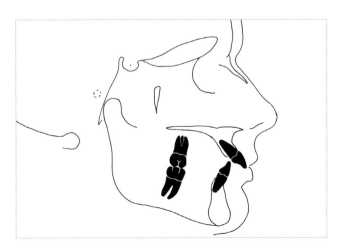

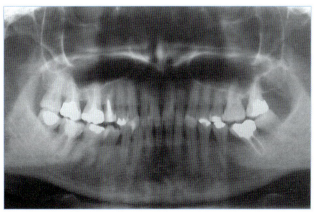

Pretreatment cephalometric tracing and OPT.

PHASE II ORTHODONTIC OCCLUSAL FINISHING

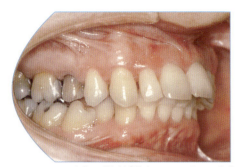
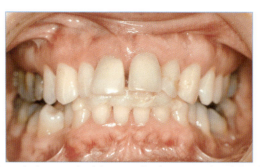
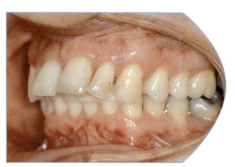

After PHASE I correction of the dental closure dual bite, orthodontic occlusal finishing commenced with the jaws in muscle-led closure alone.

Complete banding of both arches was done in several stages while the patient continued to wear her ARS. Ongoing adaptations were made to the ARS to permit gradual tooth movement and provide for the requirements of the anchorage and tooth movement areas.

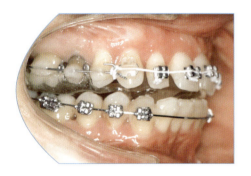
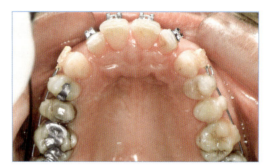
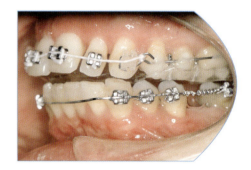

The maxillary teeth were ligated from second molar to canine with wire ties (second and first molars ligated together, first molars and second premolars ligated together, and so on) on both sides to create anchorage units. Instead of an archwire, an elastic chain was inserted into the brackets between the maxillary canines, which helped to lingualize the incisors in a short time (area of movement), primarily by causing a change in inclination as a result of the application of a single force. The two arches were treated independently due to contraindication of intramaxillary forces, and it was observed during splint-free checkups that they had come significantly closer to correct anatomical relationships and better function.

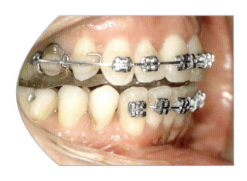
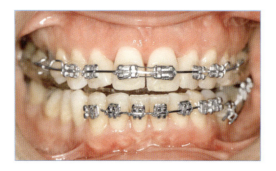
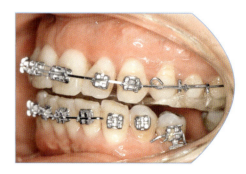

During the final stages of orthodontic treatment, the splint was progressively adapted to the changes that were taking place.

POSTTREATMENT

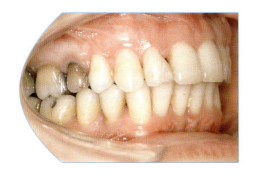
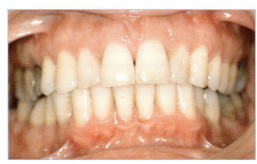
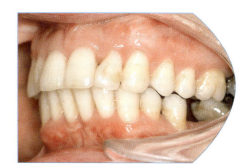

Prior to prosthodontics.

CHECKUP IN 2007: 6 YEARS POSTTREATMENT

Less-than-satisfactory outcome on follow-up: Note the left side relapse to a Class II

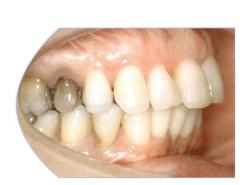
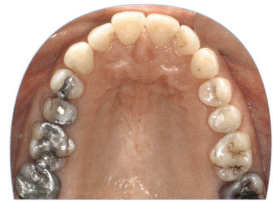
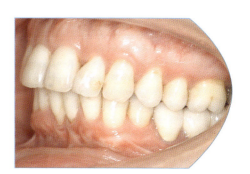

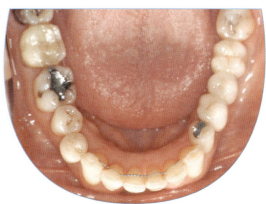

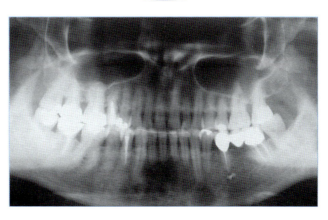

Follow-up OPT.

COMPARISONS

PRETREATMENT	START OF STAGE II ORTHODONTIC OCCLUSAL FINISHING
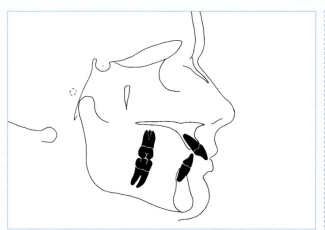	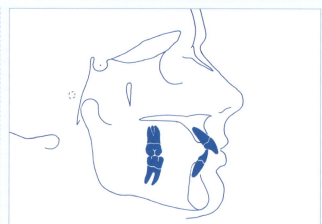
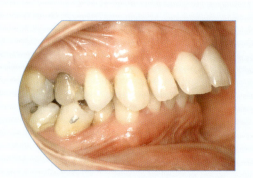	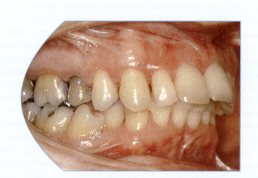

PRETREATMENT DYNAMIC EXCURSIONS

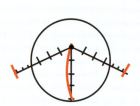

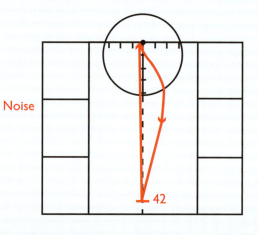

Noise

42

POSTTREATMENT

CHECKUP IN 2007 (6 years later)

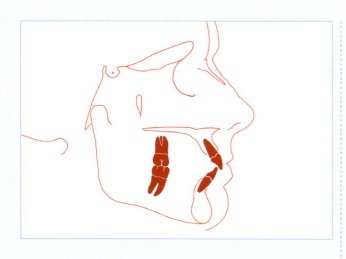

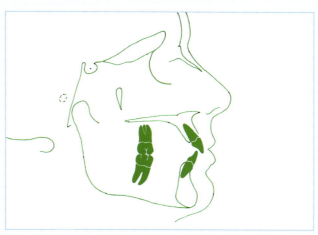

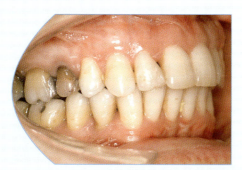

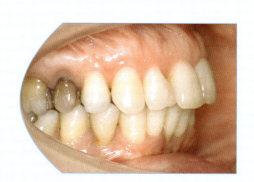

DYNAMIC EXCURSIONS IN 2007 (6 years later)

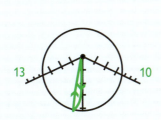

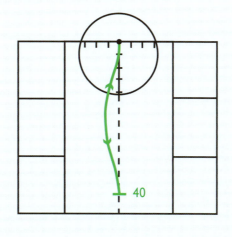

Slight grating on left side when closing. Excursions functionally acceptable.

FUNDAMENTAL WARNING

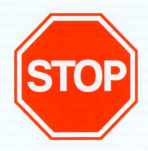

WHERE THERE IS (SEVERE) MUSCULOARTICULAR DAMAGE

Do not carry out any irreversible procedures, especially:

- Complex oral rehabilitation

- Major prosthodontic work

- Complete orthodontic treatment plans

- Maxillary surgery

Unless the underlying pathology has first been resolved (or at least the best possible compromise has been achieved) to be sure of operating in an anatomical and functional balance between teeth, muscles, and TMJs. This is the only way to ensure long-term stability of the results obtained.

Further key indicators are:

WITH ADULT PATIENTS, always carry out a comprehensive, systematic diagnosis, even if the patient does not complain of muscle or joint problems with or without pain. More often than not, these problems are there although unrecognized.
WITH CHILDREN, it is equally imperative to check the entire stomatognathic apparatus, with particular attention to the muscles of mastication and posture, to intercept a potential aggravation. It is not uncommon for head injury or trauma to lead to subsequent TMJ damage.
(See Chapter 5, Children and Temporomandibular Disorders.)

III. CLINICAL CASES DESCRIBING ONLY PHASE II INTEGRATED WITH DENTAL PROCEDURES

MAXILLARY SURGERY

PROSTHODONTIC REHABILITATION

"VIRTUAL" DIAGNOSTIC-THERAPEUTIC SETUP
for implants and prosthodontic

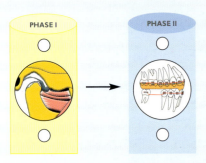

KEY FEATURE: A CASE COMPLETED WITH MAXILLARY SURGERY

PHASE II: OCCLUSAL FINISHING WITH PRESURGICAL AND POSTSURGICAL ORTHODONTICS

This case required highly complex treatment.

The clinician had to establish a stable therapeutic position for the mandible and TMJs in all three spatial dimensions, starting with extremely few interarch dental contacts. A series of impressions were taken to guide the tooth movements and prepare the jaws for the subsequent surgical stage.

The surgeon, starting from awkward skeletal relationships partly due to asymmetry, had the goal of attaining a precise intercuspation. Furthermore, the surgeon wanted to preserve the profile and smile esthetics while ensuring correct opening dynamics. During the operation, a Luhr device (or similar) was used to hold the mandible still to reproduce the exact musculoarticular position laboriously achieved during the previous orthopedic stage. The device was then removed at the end of the procedure.

The patient made a major commitment in wearing an extremely bulky splint. Much of the successful outcome of this case, in which many adverse circumstances were against her, was due to her extraordinary—or even incredible—cooperation.

Patient R. R. Z., age 44

DIAGNOSIS

The patient presented with evident severe asymmetric open bite causing an unattractive appearance and having very few posterior contacts. She had TMJ pathology with considerable damage, predominantly on the left side. The patient complained of numerous associated symptoms including headaches, preauricular pain from the right side coming on gradually and causing problems with balance, tension in the mandibular muscles, and rigid shoulder and neck muscles. Her dynamic excursions were badly deviated.

TREATMENT

PHASE I: ARS MUSCULOARTICULAR THERAPY

Although uncomfortably bulky, this splint was essential to improve the muscle and joint relationships that were causing the severe pain.

PHASE II: ORTHODONTIC OCCLUSAL FINISHING

Again an ARS was fundamental in suitably preparing the patient's jaws for the subsequent surgical procedure. This temporarily caused a major esthetic deterioration, and the patient's social life was considerably limited by her ensuing speech difficulties.

SURGERY

Complex procedures were required to bring the arches into correct alignment and intercuspation.

ORTHODONTIC FINISHING

Once normal skeletal and dental relationships had been reestablished, the patient underwent functional and postural tongue rehabilitation to fine-tune the static and dynamic dental relationships. It is suspected that the tongue may have been one of the main causes of her altered dental and skeletal relationships.

PRETREATMENT RECORDS

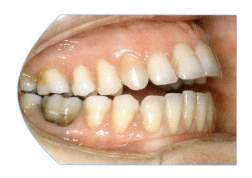
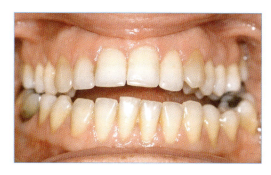
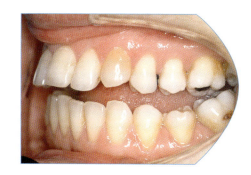

The patient exhibited marked deviation of midlines and evident asymmetric open bite, especially on the left side.

What few dental contacts remained were limited to the posterior quadrants.

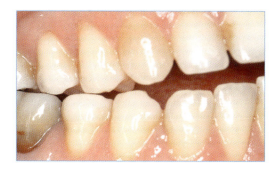
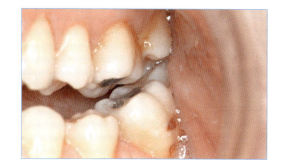

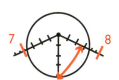
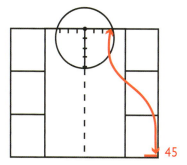

Maximum disclosure (45 mm) follows a deviating pathway several millimeters to the left. The lateral

movements (7 mm to the right and 8 mm to the left) are inferior to normal values.

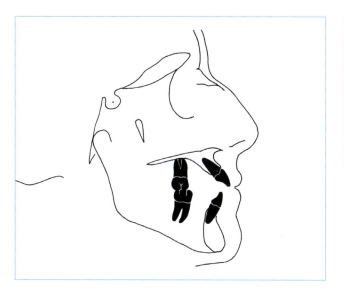

Cephalometry.

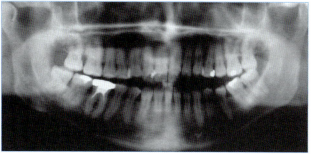

Pretreatment OPT.

PHASE II: ORTHODONTIC OCCLUSAL FINISHING

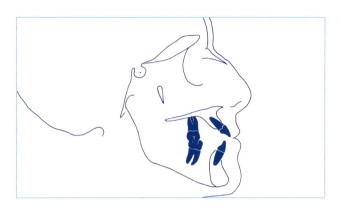

Musculoarticular therapy produced significant pain relief both subjectively and objectively with functional improvement despite aggravation of esthetics and social life caused by the cumbersome splint. Once good occlusal stability had been reached, the presurgical orthodontic stage began. An ARS was prepared for full-time wear with alterations to create anchorage and movement areas. During the first stage of this phase, anchorage on anterior and posterior teeth was used to extrude the premolars and flatten the curve of Spee, especially on the left side. Work on the mandibular teeth was then carefully planned to alternate anchorage and movement areas.

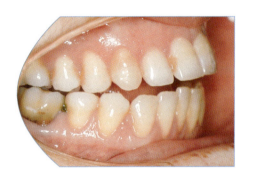
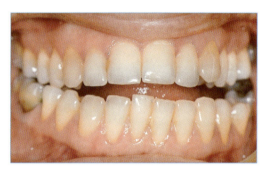
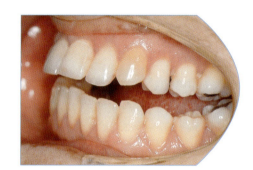

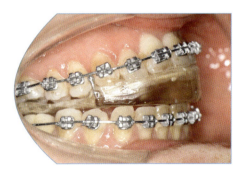
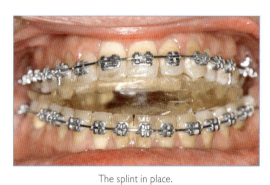
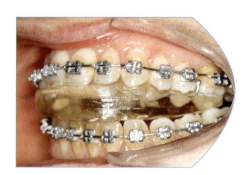

The splint in place.

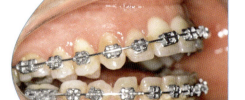
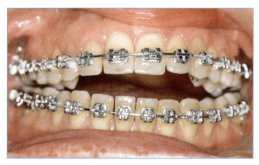
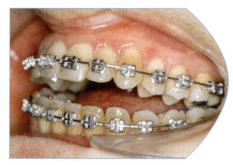

Without the splint: More impressions are taken to check intercuspation.

There are two important points in this case:

1) The patient displayed extraordinary compliance and consistency in wearing her splint for such a long time despite its awkwardness. In addition, a mandibular splint was prepared for the patient. Although it is of no therapeutic use, the mandibular splint made her social life easier and prevented the loss of functional benefit provided by the maxillary ARS.

2) Among the many procedures performed, preparation of the skeletal bases was especially important in ensuring that a correct interarch relationship was achieved. To do this, impressions were taken time and time again, and the casts used to appreciate the tooth movements were still required to enable the surgeon to plan the surgical restoration of intercuspation. The patient not only experienced diminished esthetics and comfort due to the splint's presence but also deterioration of her open bite as the curve of Spee was flattened. At this point, the clinician had serious doubts as to whether an acceptable outcome could be achieved in both skeletal and dental terms.

MAXILLARY SURGICAL PROCEDURE
(performed by Dr Paolo Ronchi)

Before starting the actual osteotomy, the surgeon fitted a plate to hold the mandible in place against the base of the cranium. This helped to secure correct condylar and disc position in relation to the articulating surface, thus ensuring that these positions will remain stable after the surgery is completed. This is described in detail on page 267.

ORTHODONTIC POSTSURGICAL FINISHING

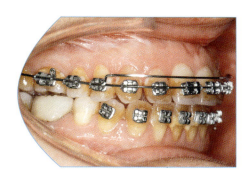
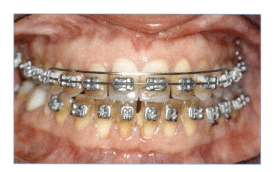
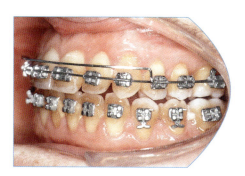
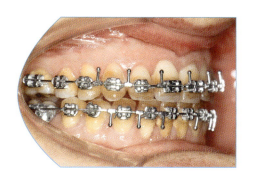
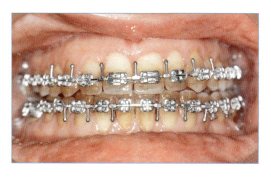
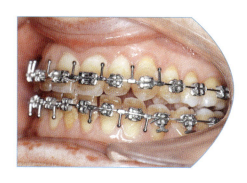

POSTTREATMENT DOCUMENTATION

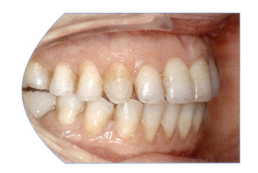 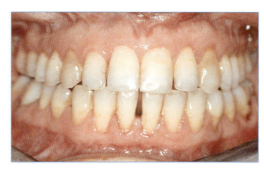 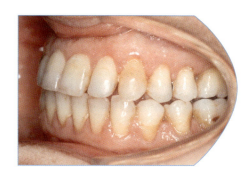

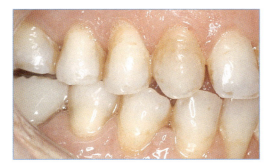 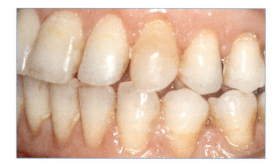

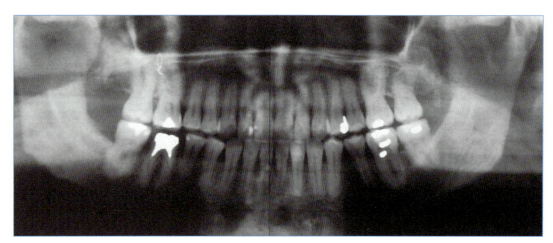

Posttreatment OPT.

COMPARISON OF CEPHALOMETRIC TRACINGS

Pretreatment

Posttreatment

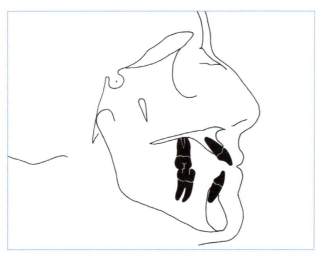 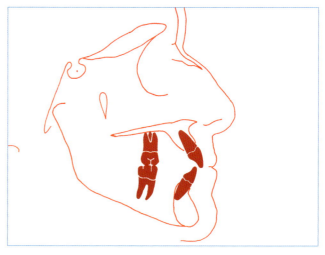

COMPARISONS

PRETREATMENT   POSTTREATMENT

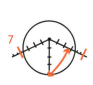 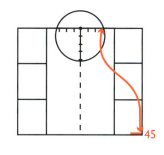   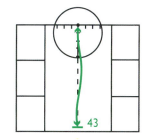

Noticeable improvement occurred in the mandibular 3D excursions, accompanied by recession of the considerable symptoms that the patient originally complained of.

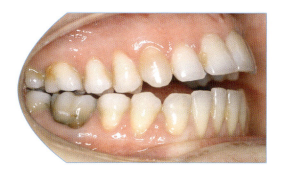 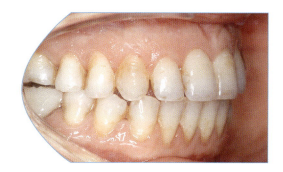

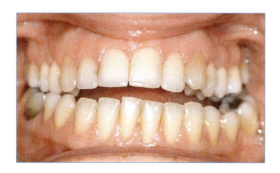 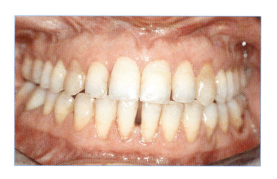

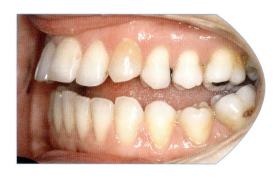 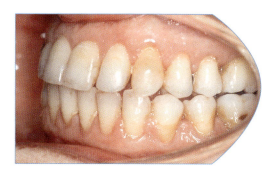

NOTE: Unfortunately, this case was completed before the advent of routine CT and MRI documentation. The mandible excursion sketches are, however, interesting to observe.

FOLLOW-UP 5 YEARS POSTTREATMENT

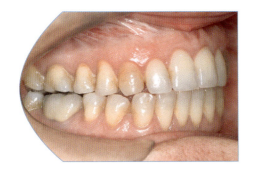
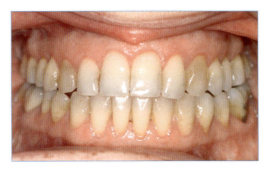
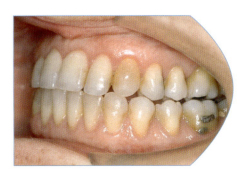

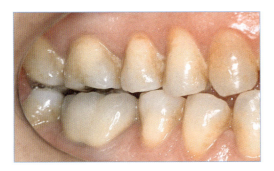
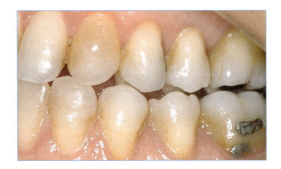

DYNAMICS

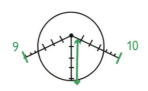

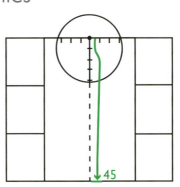

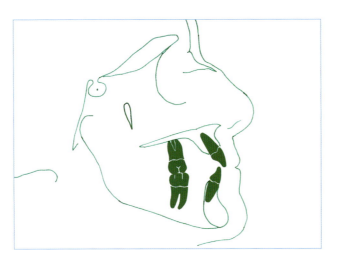

The patient's excursions and opening and closure movements are within normal ranges. Slight crepitus was observed during the final stage of opening on the right side and the final stage of closing on the left side.

Follow-up cephalometry.

ORTHOGNATHIC SURGERY ON DYSFUNCTIONAL PATIENTS
Collated by Dr Paolo Ronchi

Occlusal finishing in more serious cases of TMJ dysfunctional pathology may require surgery if there is a skeletal discrepancy between the jaws that orthodontics alone cannot correct. Condyle-disc-articular surface relations, both before and after surgery, are one of the most crucial points of orthognathic surgery and even more so when dealing with patients who have received specific musculoarticular therapy.

During orthognathic surgery, proper clinical monitoring of the TMJs and muscles of mastication, in association with correct surgical technique, ensure that satisfactory condyle-disc-articular surface relations are maintained without resorting to complicated procedures. The development of rigid internal fixation allows much swifter recovery of mandibular movements than did the former maxillomandibular fixation technique. This immediate resumption of normal functionality itself safeguards correct TMJ activity, which underlies not only a good clinical outcome but also its mid-term and long-term stability.

Achieving a satisfactory, stable outcome for patients with TMJ dysfunction treated with an ARS relies upon the following:

a) Musculoarticular rehabilitation (PHASE I)
b) Subsequent orthodontic occlusal finishing (PHASE II)
c) Maintenance of correct condylar position within the fossa throughout the entire time
d) Good muscle balance

It cannot be stressed enough that where asymmetric mandibular movements occur, as in mandibular laterodeviations or cases of dentofacial asymmetry, the risk of having altered condylar relationships are greater. In 1986, Luhr et al addressed this problem[4,5] by developing a device to hold the condyle in its presurgical tridimensional therapeutic position. In practice, the invention consisted of a T-shaped plate adapted and fixed at one end to the ramus of the mandible with the other end fixed to a cranial bone not involved in the osteotomy—to the maxilla in the case of single mandibular osteotomy or to the maxillo-malar shelf if the patient undergoes bimaxillary osteotomies (see illustration).

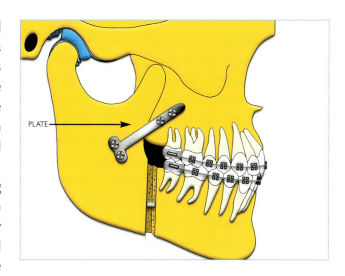

PLATE →

It is obvious that the jaws must be temporarily locked in an orthopedic repositioning hold during the procedures. The metal plate and splint are removed, and the bilateral mandibular osteotomy is performed, after which intermaxillary fixation is required to hold the jaws as established by the preoperational studies on articulator-mounted casts. The proximal fragment is therefore repositioned and the Luhr device fixed to the same screwholes as before to maintain the correct condylar-disc-fossa relationship. Only then is rigid internal fixation of the mandible done with miniplates and monocortical screws locking the segments into their new therapeutic position. Finally, following rigid fixation of the mandible, the condylar positioning device can be removed.

It seems reasonable to conclude that these devices help minimize errors in maintaining the condylar therapeutic position established from the commencement of treatment. While the use of these devices may be subject to debate in the context of "traditional" orthognathic surgery, this is not the case with dysfunctional patients. For them, every possible means **should be applied to maintain (as much as possible) the unaltered condyle-disc-fossa relationship aimed for at the start of treatment.**

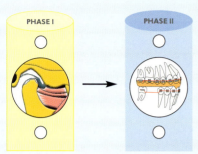

KEY POINT: CLINICAL EXAMPLE COMPLETED WITH PROSTHODONTICS

PHASE II: OCCLUSAL FINISHING: ORTHODONTICS INTEGRATED WITH PROSTHODONTICS

Procedure: At the patient's first appointment, she presented with TMJ locking and altered condylar shape and position. First, the patient was helped with unlocking manipulation, which gave immediate relief of her initial symptoms.

The orthopedic phase further reduced her negative symptomatology and improved her gait.

The orthodontic occlusal finishing (PHASE II), concluding with replacement crowns on implants, completed a program so successful that the patient did not require a retainer. Her interarch relationships were, in fact. extremely stable, both when static and during movement.

Patient A. M. P., age 43

DIAGNOSIS

At her initial examination, the patient exhibited considerable difficulty in walking due to loss of balance. She complained of frequent headaches, neck pain, reduced hearing, and painful TMJ movement, especially on maximum opening.

The following were also observed:

- Class I with several teeth lost from posterolateral areas
- Dual bite with anterolateral and vertical dislocation of approximately 3 mm
- Maximum mouth opening limited to 34 mm, deviating slightly to the right
- Joint noise, specifically crepitus

Closed-mouth lateral TMJ tomograms showed distal displacement of the left condyle while the open-mouth images showed bilateral reduced condylar excursion. The condyles, especially the right, were flattened with reduced cortical thickness.

TREATMENT PLAN

The first treatment step was joint unlocking manipulation. It was followed by orthopedic therapy and subsequently by PHASE II orthodontic treatment. Orthodontic finishing involved placement of a fixed appliance in both arches. The case was then completed with prosthodontic work.

Orthodontic treatment involved:

- Fabrication of an ARS to alternate anchorage areas with areas of tooth movement
- Rearrangement of the spaces left by missing teeth to prepare for the implants that were to be fitted 6 months before the end of orthodontic treatment

The implants and crowns were done at the office chosen by the patient.

PRETREATMENT RECORDS

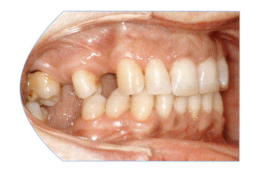 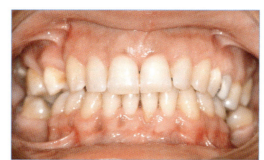 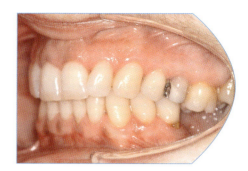

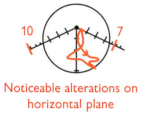

Noticeable alterations on
horizontal plane

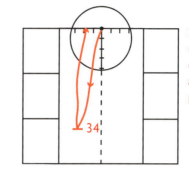

Deviation and
reduced
opening on
abnormal
pathways

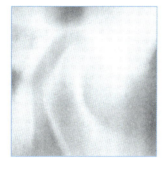 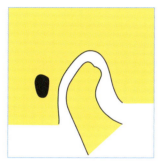 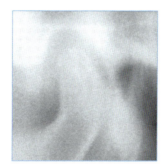 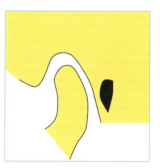

The right condyle appears flattened with reduced cortical thickness. The left condyle lies in a posterosuperior position.

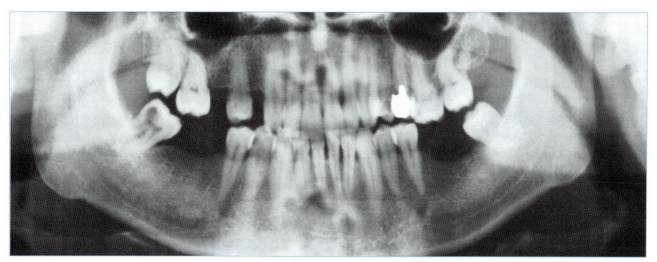

Several teeth are missing from the posterior quadrants.

PHASE II   ORTHODONTIC OCCLUSAL FINISHING

Stable, muscle-led closure resulted in significant subjective and objective improvement in symptoms with the pain being almost completely eliminated. Orthodontic occlusal finishing followed.

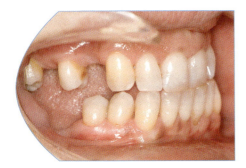 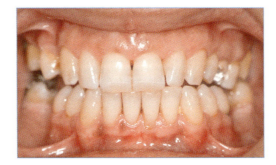 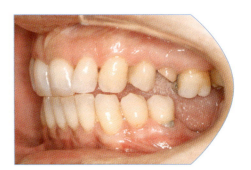

In the **maxillary arch**, the posterior quadrants made up the anchorage area, and the anterior teeth made up the movement area. The anterior teeth were buccalized with microscrews.

The areas were subsequently inverted.

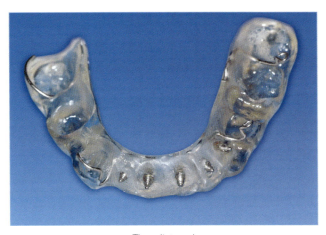

The splint used.

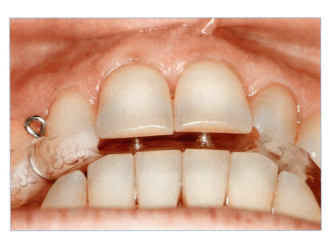

(Observe the microscrews)

Fixed appliances were fitted to both arches, partly to create the correct space for the implants. In the **mandibular arch**, the anterior district (specifically the flange) was used as the anchorage area to move the posterior teeth as required. In addition, the posterior wedge was progressively ground down to encourage the second molars to upright themselves axially with the other teeth.

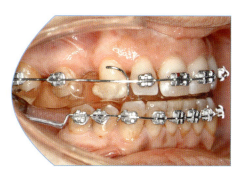
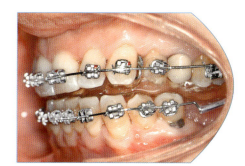

Preterminal records.

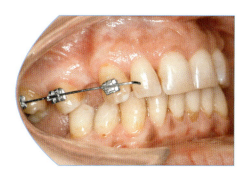
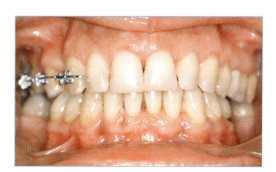
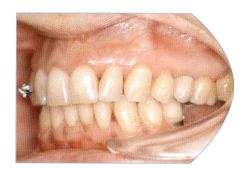

The patient continued to wear the splint throughout the entire orthodontic phase. Ongoing adjustments were made to aid tooth movement sequences in the sectorial treatment plan. **The position of the TMJs and mandible were kept consistent.**

As a result, the prosthodontist was able to work with a patient demonstrating stable repetitive mandibular excursions, correct articular structure placement, and good spaces for the implant work. It goes without saying that these conditions must be maintained both during and after prosthetic treatment.

Posttreatment TMJ tomograms show an improvement in condylar position. Less deformation of bony surfaces indicates some degree of remodeling. The patient had a slight increase in maximum mouth opening excursion.

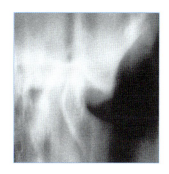
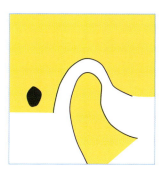
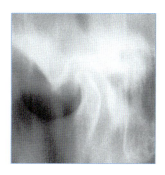
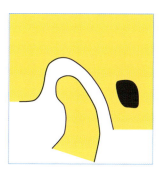

ORTHODONTICS: Provide occlusal finishing and preparation for implant-based restorations

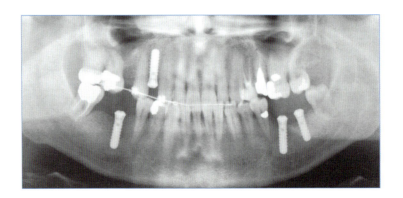

FINAL RECORDS WITH PROSTHODONTICS

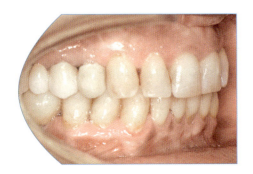 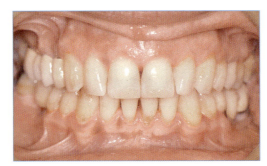 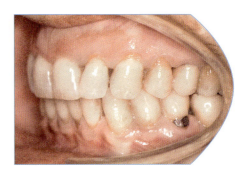

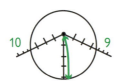

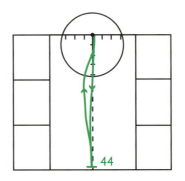

Conclusion: Posttreatment records confirm that the patient has reached a very satisfactory outcome and been cured of the many diagnosed complaints.

5-YEAR FOLLOW-UP

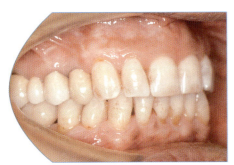 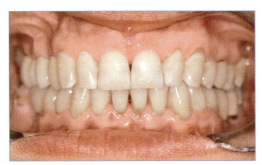 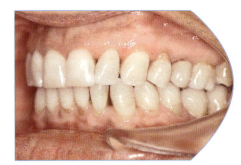

The outcome remains stable in both dental and articular terms.

COMPARISON BETWEEN PRE- AND POSTTREATMENT INVOLVING MUSCULOARTICULAR, ORTHODONTIC, AND PROSTHODONTIC TREATMENT

BEFORE | AFTER

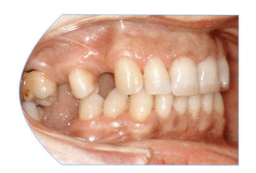 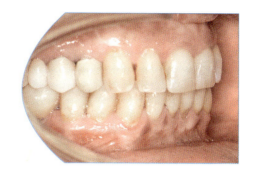

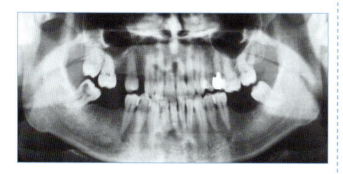 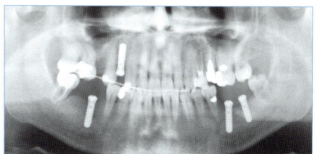

Right side, mouth closed

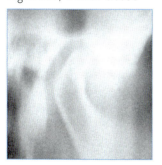 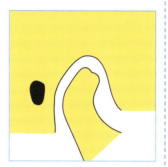 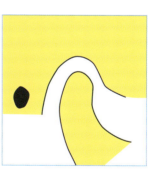

Left side, mouth closed

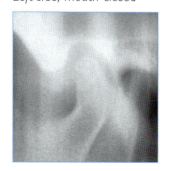 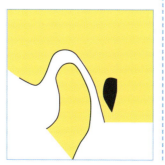 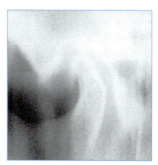 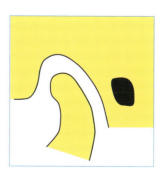

KEY POINT: VIRTUAL DIAGNOSTIC-THERAPEUTIC SET-UP IS USED TO PLAN POSITIONING OF IMPLANT AND PROSTHODONTICS

Patient: B. R. age 50

1. PRETREATMENT RECORDS

    Dual pathology: Condyle posteriorized and disc anteriorized with the mouth closed.
    In open-mouth position, the condyle is anteriorized, and the disc posteriorized due to ligamentous laxity.

2. MUSCULOARTICULAR TREATMENT (PHASE I)

    ORTHODONTIC OCCLUSAL FINISHING (PHASE II)

    PROCEDURES WERE NOT COMPLETED following the patient's involvement in a serious accident.

3. HYPOTHETICAL THERAPEUTIC SETUP PREPARING FOR IMPLANTS
    - In the upper jaw: With maxillary left and right sinus lift procedures.
    - In the lower jaw: To create proper spaces for replacements.

Although the case was, regrettably, not completed, details of this complex treatment plan are worth highlighting.

PRETREATMENT RECORDS

The patient has a skeletal Class I and dental Class II on the right side. Areas with a number of teeth missing caused bilateral posterior collapse and deviated midlines.

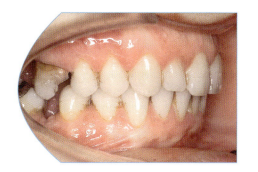
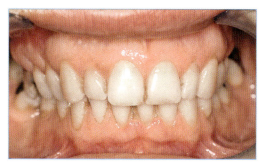
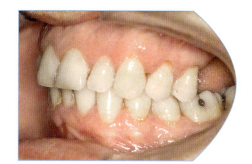

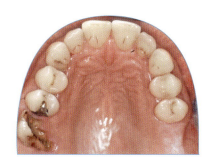
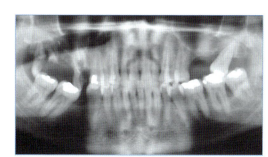
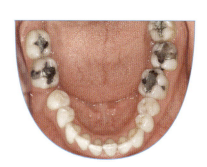

EVIDENCE OF TMJ DAMAGE WITH DUAL DISC POSITION ON THE LEFT SIDE

1) Anterior to the condyle with the mouth closed
2) Posterior with the mouth open

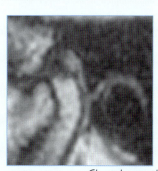
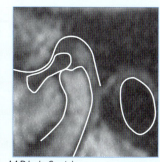
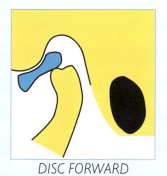

Closed-mouth MRI, left side   *DISC FORWARD*

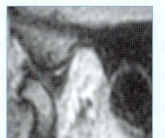
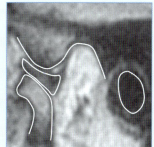
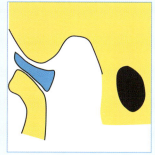

Open-mouth MRI, left side   *DISC BEHIND*

(Compare this case with the posterior dislocation case presented on page 190.)

275

Musculoarticular treatment was started with an ARS (PHASE I) and followed by fixed-appliance occlusal finishing (PHASE II). The mandible was treated first since it was assumed to be more complex and require longer treatment time.

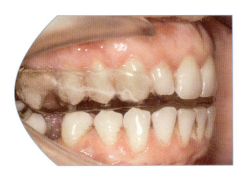 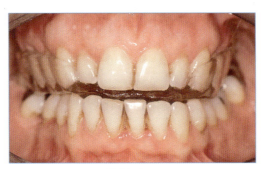 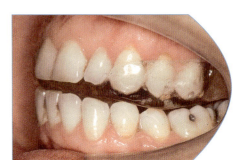

ARS in place.

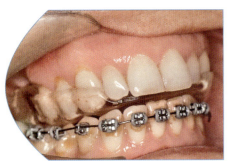 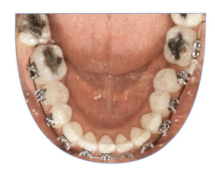 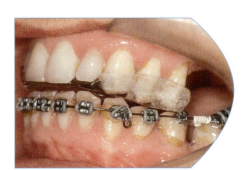

After a few weeks, a mandibular fixed appliance was fitted to provide simultaneous treatment.

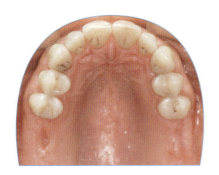

The mandibular fixed appliance was later followed by its maxillary counterpart to provide transversal maxillary expansion. The timing was planned to conclude the occlusal problems in both arches simultaneously. The appliances also created good spacing for implant placement in terms of correct relationships, both intra-arch and with their antagonists. The restored musculoarticular stability was consistently maintained throughout these procedures.

THERAPEUTIC SETUP ESTABLISHING CORRECT IMPLANT PLACEMENT

MANDIBULAR ARCH

Once the patient's own teeth were aligned (see photograph on facing page), a setup was made. The necessary space was created to model the right first molar replacement crown on its implant, once inserted.

MAXILLARY ARCH

The maxilla was in very bad condition. A great number of molars on the left and right sides had been lost,

leading to vertical and transversal collapse of the posterior alveolar areas.

Setup preparation had a dual purpose: (1) preparation for a surgical sinus lift and (2) expansion of the maxilla, which was considerably narrower than the mandibular arch. Without this preparatory work it would be extremely difficult if not impossible to insert implants that would intercuspate correctly with their mandibular antagonists. Correct anatomical interarch relationships had to be established by all means possible.

RIGHT SIDE   LEFT SIDE

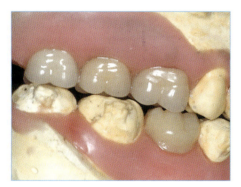

Implant uprighting checked on setup model.

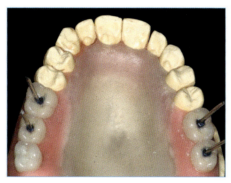

Occlusal view of arches showing replacement crowns and implant uprighting.

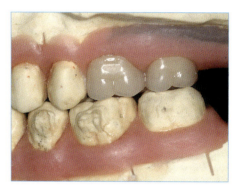

Checking implant uprighting on setup model.

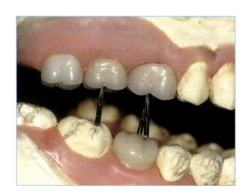

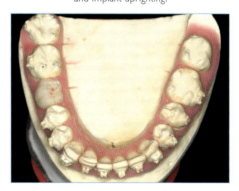

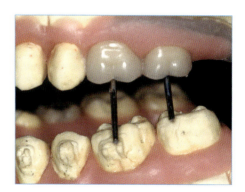

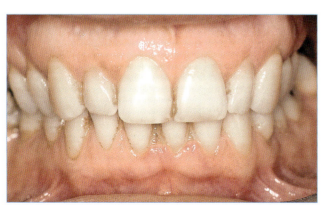

Deviated pretreatment midlines.

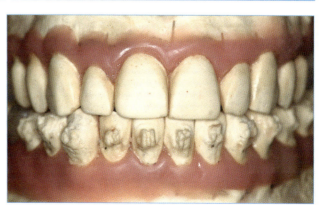

Midlines centered posttreatment

At this point, treatment was interrupted by external circumstances.

CONSIDERATIONS: PROSTHODONTICS, THE LAST STEP IN ORAL REHABILITATION

PROPOSED SEQUENCE OF THERAPEUTIC PROCEDURES

1. Motivation of the patient
2. Hygiene
3. Identification of dual bite or greater damage where applicable
4. Extractions
5. Conservative treatment
6. Endodontics
7. Periodontics
8. Orthodontics
9. TMD therapy
10. Surgery
11. Prosthodontics

Several decades ago, orthodontics stepped over the dividing line with prosthodontics by contributing to the preparation of replacements with new principles and techniques for treatment. The leading innovators, including Lucia, Thomas, Celenza, Amsterdam, and Cohen, to name but a few, promoted the importance of establishing a correct anatomical and functional gnathology involving all teeth in both jaws, even if replacing only a few teeth.

Any far-thinking orthodontist today is careful to prepare the way for prosthodontic work by ensuring not only good future alignment between both present and missing teeth with proper spacing but also a harmonic equilibrium between the teeth, muscles, and TMJs with the aim of achieving an anatomical-functional balance. It is then up to the prosthodontist to create replacements involving the fewest possible teeth while maintaining the musculoarticular and dental therapeutic position established by the orthodontist and therefore adapting the new replacements to this position.

CLINICAL IMPLICATIONS

On a practical note, an extremely simplified way to encompass dysfunctional features is to state that a patient may present with:

- **Dental, muscular, and articular equilibrium** without dislocation on final closing stages (therefore without dual bite), in which case treatment can proceed without specific therapy for the tooth-muscle-TMJ relationships.
- **Minor dental precontacts** that will be eliminated by replacements or by selective grinding, which may be accomplished in a single session.
- **Dental and muscular disorders starting to involve the TMJ.** Where this is the case, diagnostic-therapeutic intervention integrated with an SS may produce functional efficiency and therefore an acceptable compromise.

A considerably different approach is required when the pathology has gone beyond the teeth to involve the related muscles and TMJs at various levels:

- **Dislocation with reduction**
- **Dislocation without reduction**
- **Destruction (worst scenario)**

In these cases, any of the previously described procedures may be necessary to ensure functional efficiency and guarantee long-term anatomical and functional stability. It should be understood that every patient has normally been given treatment involving both musculoarticular recovery (PHASE I) and orthodontic occlusal finishing procedures (PHASE II). Only after these conditions have been met can the replacements be prepared and fitted. The tendency for clinicians to recommend implants creates additional problems that must be solved in cooperation with colleagues assisting in their respective specialties, such as periodontology, implantology, and others.

To conclude, full oral rehabilitation may require the collaborative efforts of a number of professionals, both in the choice of treatment plan and in the execution of various procedures. Ideally, they will work as a team according to a mutually agreed time frame and sequence.

CONSIDERATIONS ON OCCLUSAL REHARMONIZATION

The term occlusal reharmonization seems more appropriate than does selective grinding because it involves not only the precise removal of enamel as a subtractive procedure but almost always also involves additive procedures with remodeling of molar, premolar, and canine cusps as well as the incisal edges of the anteriors with composite or similar material.

Where gold, ceramic, or composite is used, preparatory work must be done in the laboratory following the same underlying principles applicable to what will then be done chairside.

Occlusal reharmonization, however it is achieved, may be considered as complete oral rehabilitation in that it involves all components of the stomatognathic apparatus. It is an extremely delicate procedure because it almost always results in removing enamel and is thus irreversible. For this reason, certain rules must be followed precisely.

The first is that nothing must be done to the patient's teeth without careful advance planning and a clear final aim in mind. Reduction of occlusal surfaces—in other words, flattening them—itself causes damage and may contribute to deterioration of existing pathology. An obligatory step is therefore careful articulator study on stone casts in a correct therapeutic function to ascertain which teeth are to be involved in the remodeling process. Case studies show a large variety ranging from treatment of a pair of teeth to the entire dentition. What matters is that the final result produces simultaneous contact between all teeth when the jaws are closed while ensuring correct disclosure dynamics.

OPERATIONAL TECHNIQUE

Once the procedures have been done with extreme precision on the articulator-mounted casts, they are then faithfully reproduced on the patient's real teeth by the same clinician who did the articulator work, with the lab technician acting as assistant only.

When reharmonization has been completed, the patient immediately feels the improvement. Negative interferences are eliminated as is the instability of flat surfaces that caused or risked causing bruxism.

COMPLETE PHASE I AND PHASE II CLINICAL CASE STUDIES

To simplify comprehension of the multiple sequences involved in complete oral rehabilitation of each individual patient, the cases described so far have been presented as separate units addressing single procedures in isolation. The next four cases are presented as complete sequences, a series of steps leading from one to the next. Three other cases are also presented later in the chapter:

• F. R. on page 336
• I. R. on page 358
• D. O. on page 380

The treatment plan for each of these patients follows the same progression with similar procedures in their complete therapeutic sequence. The individual characteristics of each patient are highlighted not only during diagnosis but also by the logical succession of the therapeutic procedures used to treat each patient's condition.

PHASE I followed by PHASE II

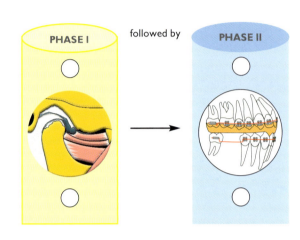

PHASE I and PHASE II simultaneously

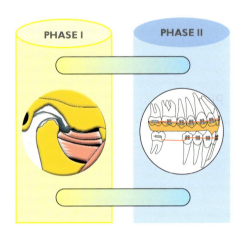

Orthodontic prephase II followed by PHASE I and PHASE II simultaneously

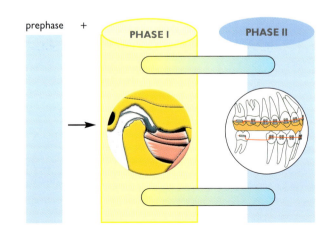

281

PHASE I followed by PHASE II WITH FIXED APPLIANCES

- R. M.   age 23   page 282

- D. C.   age 35   page 288

PHASE I and PHASE II simultaneously

- L. P.   age 30   page 294

ORTHODONTIC PREPHASE followed by PHASE I AND PHASE II SIMULTANEOUSLY

- S. G.   age 27   page 320

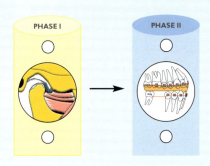

TREATMENT OF OPEN BITE IN AN ADULT PATIENT

PHASE I: MUSCULOARTICULAR THERAPY WITH AN SS AND SUBSEQUENT TREATMENT

PHASE II: OCCLUSAL FINISHING WITH ORTHODONTIC TREATMENT
INTRA-ARCH TREATMENT

Patient: R. M., age 23

DIAGNOSIS

This patient had a skeletal Class I with anterior and lateral open bite. Ligamentous laxity and bruxism were noted. Mandibular excursions were within normal limits.

TREATMENT

After the usual clinical records were taken, the patient was referred to a surgeon for consultation since it was felt that orthodontic treatment alone would not be sufficient. The surgeon recommended osteotomy combined with orthodontic treatment followed by a second operation to correct the open bite. The patient refused to undergo surgery, so orthodontic treatment alone was undertaken, albeit with reservations.

The first step was the use of an SS to establish correct muscular and articular mandibular position to provide normal functional conditions (PHASE I). Phase II then followed to provide orthodontic occlusal finishing with particular concentration on closing the anterior and lateral open bite.

The outcome was found to be stable at a follow-up visit 4 years posttreatment.

PRETREATMENT RECORDS

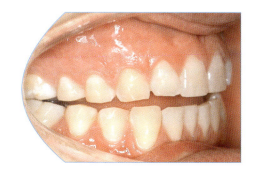
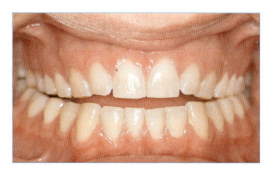
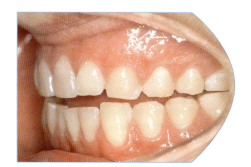

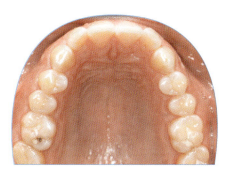
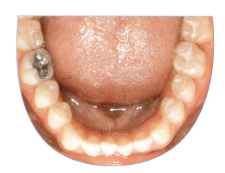

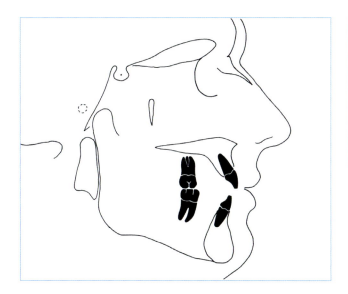

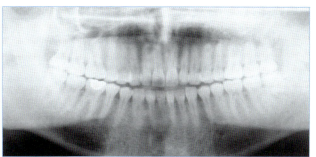

Pretreatment cephalometric outlines and OPT.

PHASE I: MUSCULOARTICULAR THERAPY WITH AN SS (laboratory work)

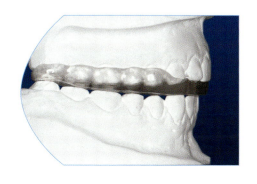
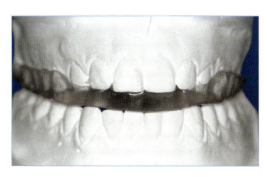
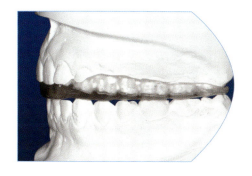

PHASE II: ORTHODONTIC OCCLUSAL FINISHING
with a fixed appliance

PHASE II proceeded with banding of the maxillary lateral areas. The canines and incisors were temporarily excluded both in the long-term interest of the patient's looks and because the priority was to gain bilateral expansion of the lateroposterior sectors with a plan based on reciprocal anchorage and movement areas.

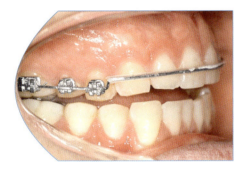 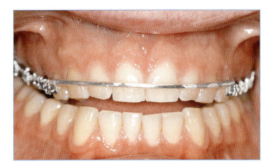 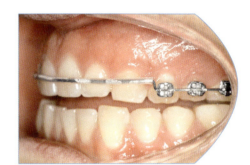

Transversal expansion.

An expanding rectangular wire was shaped to give ultra-active buccal root posterior torque with the aim of achieving bodily movement due to the combination of transversal crown expansion and buccal root movement.

Next, esthetic ceramic brackets were bonded to the six anterior teeth to advance and extrude them.

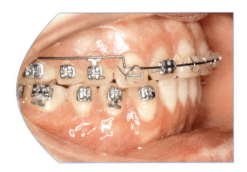 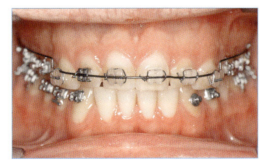

Closing the bite.

The patient's maxillary arch was subsequently fitted with a utility arch using a rectangular wire right back to the second molars.
Considerable posteroanterior pull was applied on the anterior teeth with bends facing distally toward the occlusal plane to close the open bite. Root-buccal torque was applied to the anterior teeth to ensure complete root control.

Next, wires were shaped for both arches, with mesial stops on the second molars and loops to extrude the canines beyond the first premolars.

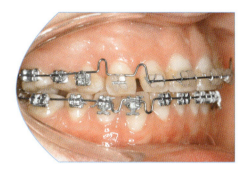
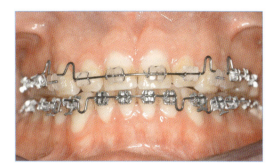
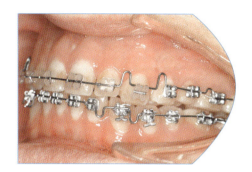

Additional loops were placed to extrude the incisors beyond the canines. This procedure is a prime example of intra-arch treatment with strict anchorage control and no need for compliance from the patient. At each appointment, the patient's muscle and TMJ stability were monitored and the next progressive movements of individual teeth planned for the separate arches, all with the aim of reaching correct reciprocal relationships.

END OF ORTHODONTIC TREATMENT

Mechanical treatment was integrated with myofunctional therapy, primarily to address the patient's swallowing movements. The results obtained confirmed that orthodontic treatment was successful in achieving a sufficient esthetic and functional outcome.

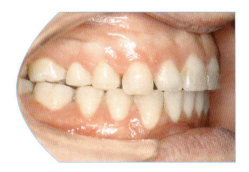
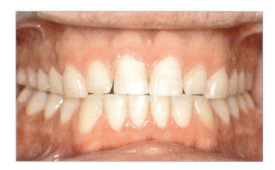
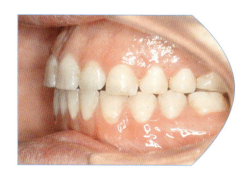

REMEMBER THAT THIS CASE WAS TREATED WITHOUT SURGERY
4-YEAR POSTTREATMENT FOLLOW-UP

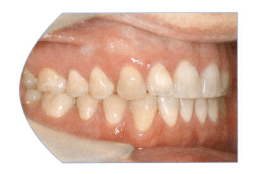
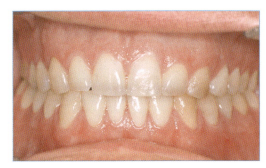
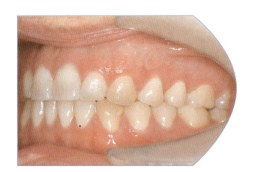

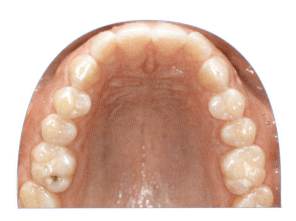
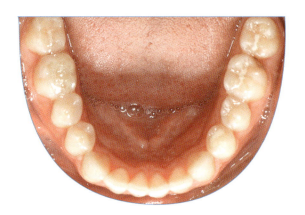

EXCURSIONS

RIGHT-SIDE VIEW | | LEFT-SIDE VIEW

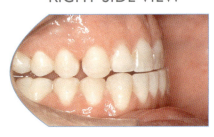
Protrusion
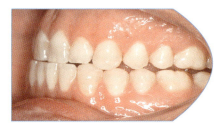

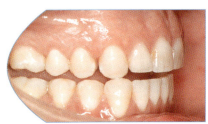
Right laterotrusion
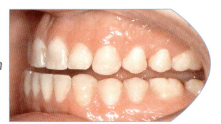

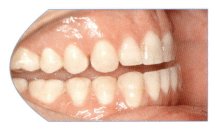
Left laterotrusion
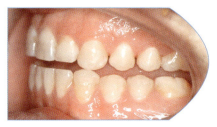

COMPARISONS

PRETREATMENT

4-YEAR FOLLOW-UP

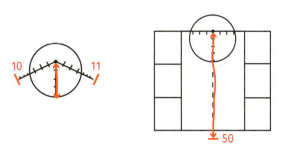

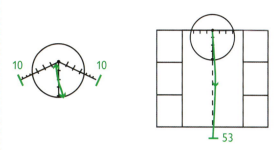

Although there was no significant difference in dynamic function, follow-up confirmed stability of the articular, muscular, and dental outcome.

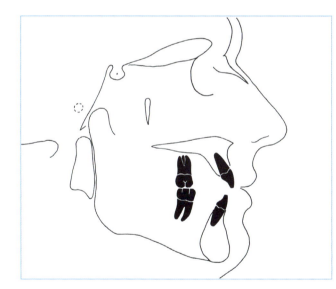

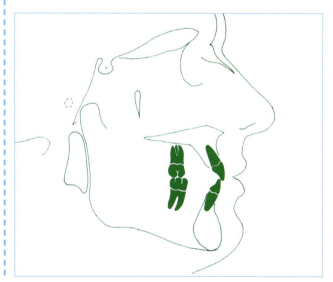

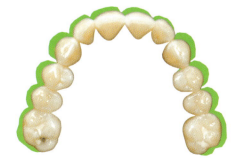

SUPERIMPOSED MAXILLARY ARCHES:
Observe the significant amount of expansion resulting from orthodontic treatment and myofunctional therapy.

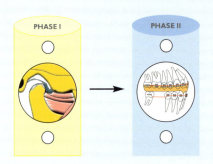

PHASE I: MUSCULOARTICULAR THERAPY WITH A STABILIZATION SPLINT AND SUBSEQUENT PAIN THERAPY

PHASE II: ORTHODONTIC OCCLUSAL FINISHING
(with the SS still worn)

Patient: D.C., age 35
Case treated by Dr Fabio Ciuffolo and Prof Felice Festa

DIAGNOSIS

The patient presented complaining of pain in the left part of her face. There was a significant discrepancy between muscle-led and dental occlusion, which was reproducible on the frontal plane with functional deviation toward the left. Other problems included:

- Left posterior crossbite
- Excessive posterior maxillary negative torque
- TMJ noise and click on the left side on late opening
- Limited mouth opening
- Painful muscles
- Bruxism
- Mandibular crowding
- Flat profile

TREATMENT PLAN

PHASE I

Physical treatments (ie, spray and stretch methods and biofeedback) were used to relieve the muscle pain. The functional mandibular deviation, caused by the crossbite, was corrected by fitting an SS.

PHASE II

With the patient still wearing her SS, the malocclusion was corrected with a fixed appliance. The primary goals were to expand the maxilla and solve the mandibular crowding, which necessitated interproximal stripping. Treatment yielded good results including an esthetic smile and profile improvement.

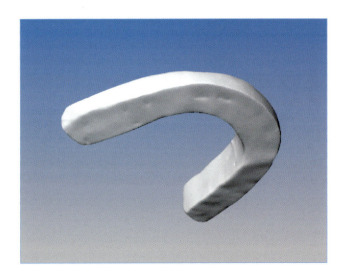

PHASE I: PRETREATMENT RECORDS

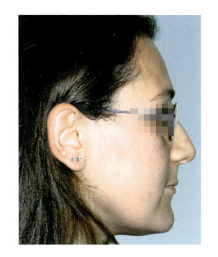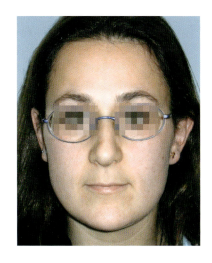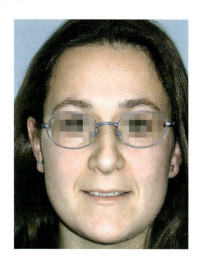

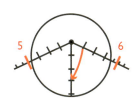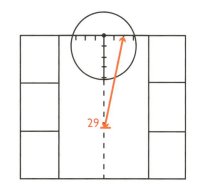

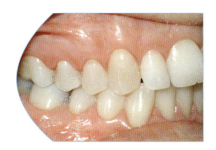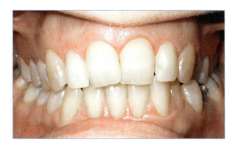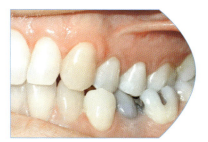

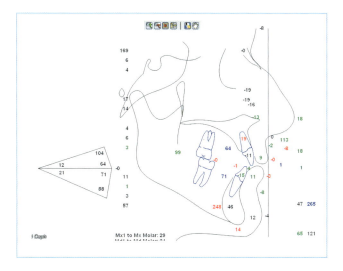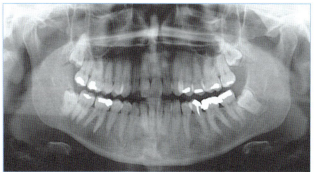

PRETREATMENT MRI

Mouth closed
Maximum intercusation

RIGHT SIDE   LEFT SIDE

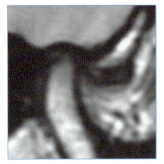 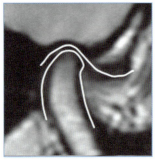 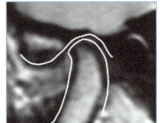 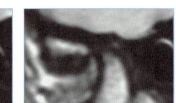

Mouth closed with splint

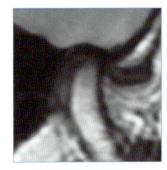 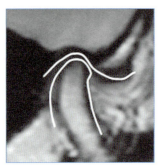 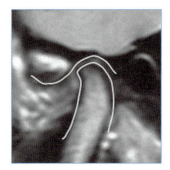 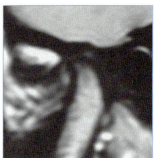

Mouth open

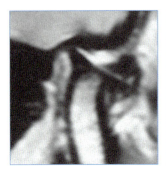 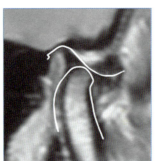 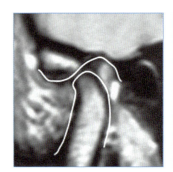 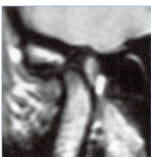

PHASE II

With the patient continuing to wear her SS, orthodontic occlusal finishing proceeds in both arches after a preliminary dental Visual Treatment Objective (VTO) study.

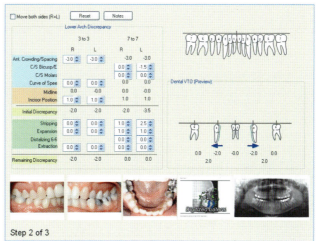

Analysis of space.

Step 2 of 3

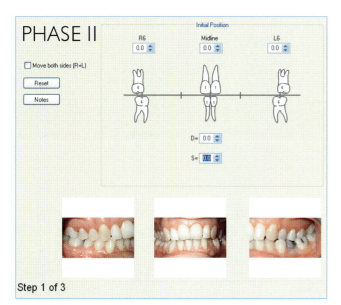

Step 1 of 3

Pretreatment.

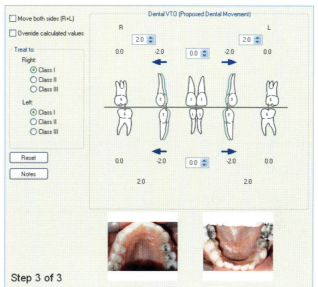

Planned movements.

Step 3 of 3

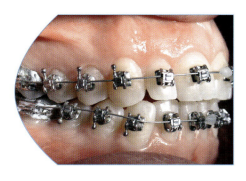
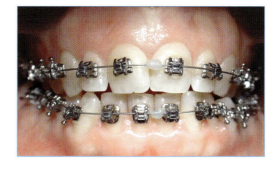
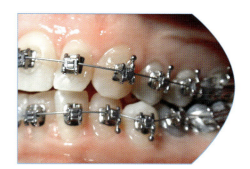

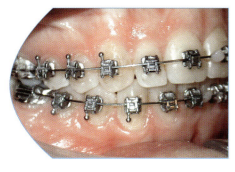
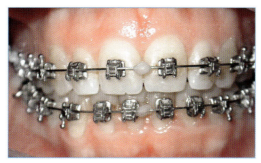
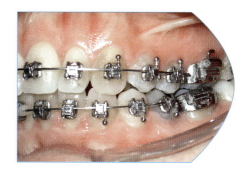

POSTTREATMENT RECORDS
Solution of the various problems reported during diagnosis

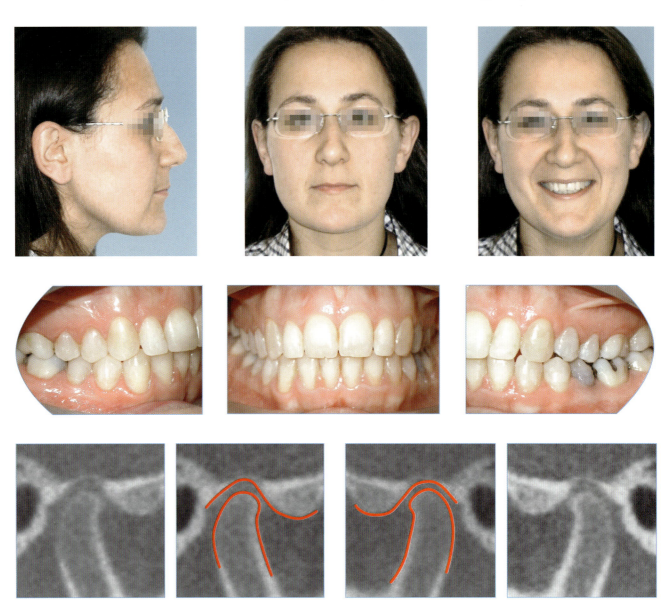

Closed-mouth cranial volumetric (cone beam) CT slices of the right and left TMJs.

Note: The patient declined a posttreatment MRI.

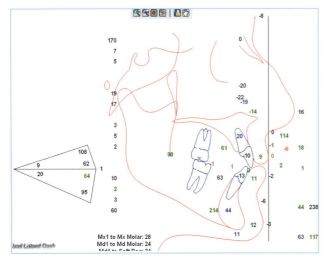

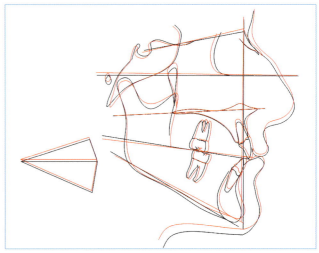

COMPARISONS

Pretreatment	Postreatment

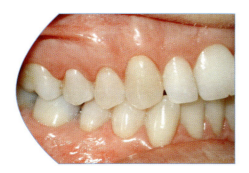

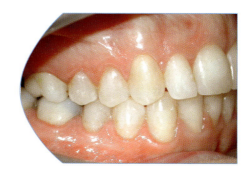

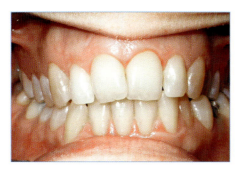

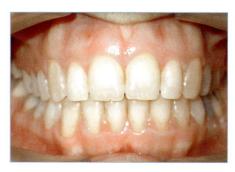

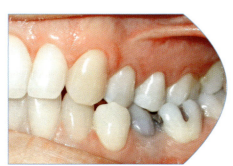

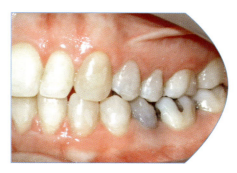

MRI	Volumetric (cone beam) CT

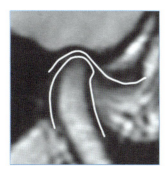

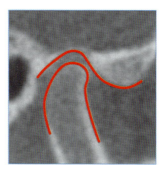

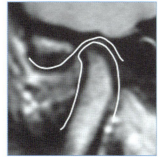

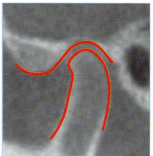

293

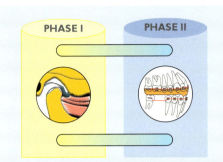

HIGHLY SIGNIFICANT DIDACTIC EXAMPLE
PHASE I AND PHASE II PERFORMED SIMULTANEOUSLY

KEY POINT: WEALTH OF RECORDS

Patient: L. P., age 30

DIAGNOSIS

The patient had a modest skeletal Class II and dental Class II on the right side only. Dual bite with mandible deviation in the final stage of jaw closure was present, and the maxillary right hemi-arch was transversally contracted. Transversal asymmetry was evident, with the interincisor line deviated inferiorly to the right. The patient had a deep bite accompanied by retroclined maxillary incisors and an accentuated curve of Spee, especially in the mandibular arch.

The patient complained of TMJ problems including nighttime grinding and muscle fatigue in the morning, intermittent facial pain, and pain in postural and thoracic muscles. Palpation revealed bilateral stiffness in the pterygoid and in the left-side trapezius and sternocleidomastoid. Observation of mandibular excursions showed deviation toward the left side on both opening and protrusion. Radiographic evidence indicated articular damage, predominantly on the right side.

ORGANIZATIONAL EXPLANATION The different therapeutic procedures are presented individually for the sake of clarity when in fact they were almost entirely done simultaneously.

PRETREATMENT RECORDS Features of pathology prevalent in the right condyle and noted during mandibular excursions were confirmed by CT.

ESSENTIAL CONDITION: Permanent ARS wear with progressive adaptations

I. MUSCULOARTICULAR THERAPY USING SKELETAL ANCHORAGE

Musculoarticular action acted mainly on the right side and also helped to stimulate the mandible. Skeletal anchorage was placed on the left side. CT and MRI findings were traced and compared in parallel. On completion of treatment, the patient had correct relationships among the articular components, especially regarding the right condyle, as clearly confirmed by posttreatment MRI.

II. ADVANCE OF THE MANDIBULAR RIGHT HEMI-ARCH USING DENTAL ANCHORAGE

The **Gi. Co. intra-arch system** (introduced for the first time with a description of its underlying concepts) was applied to achieve dental anchorage (together with skeletal anchorage) to advance the right hemi-arch and regain symmetry.

III. EXPANSION OF THE MAXILLARY RIGHT HEMI-ARCH

Anchorage in the left maxillary arch was stabilized with the left side teeth indented in the splint, which left the right side teeth free to be expanded with fixed appliances. Pre- and posttreatment results were compared.

IV. RECOVERY OF INCISAL GUIDANCE

From the start, microscrews were inserted in the superoanterior splint area, followed by a fixed appliance in the mandible and, later, in the maxilla to open the deep bite and obtain efficient incisal guidance.

V. OVERALL TREATMENT TIME: *LESS THAN 15 MONTHS* due to the patient's extraordinary compliance

POSTTREATMENT RECORDS
Posttreatment analysis showed that correct anatomy and efficient dynamic control in both incisal guidance and left and right side canine protection had been achieved.

FOLLOW-UP
Follow-up occurred 2 years posttreatment.

PRETREATMENT RECORDS

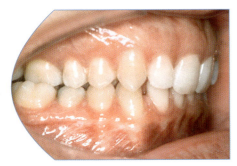

Right side: Dental Class II with crossbite.

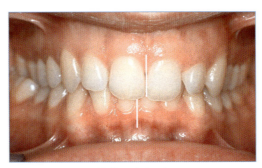

Midlines deviated.

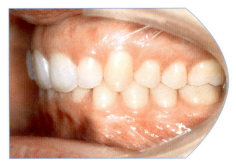

Left side: Correct dental relations.

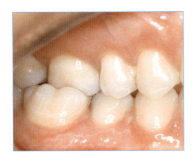

Crossbite.

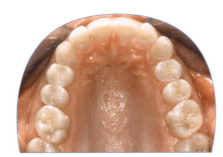

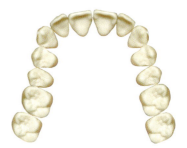

Right side contracted.

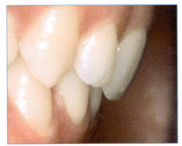

Interincisal angle accentuated, with deep bite.

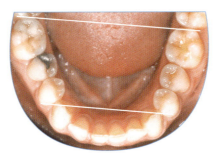

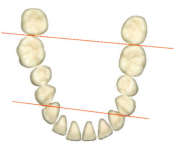

Right hemi-arch retracted.

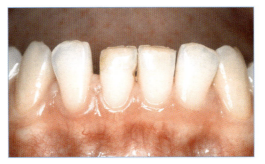

Spaces (subsequently used to center the midlines).

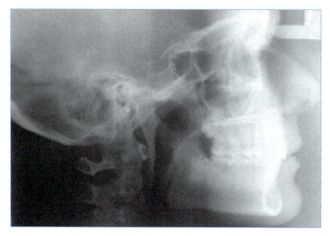

Modest skeletal Class II with relatively short upper lip.

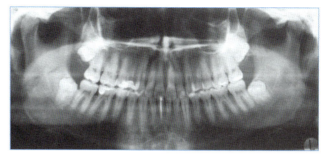

OPT: Eruption of third molars needs monitoring.

MANDIBULAR EXCURSIONS

Deviation with the midlines being musculoarticularly centered on both horizontal and transversal planes after initially departing from a deviated right side position.

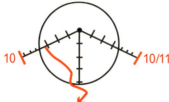

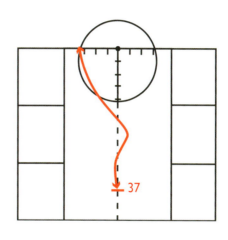

CT SCAN
Condylar position

Closed-mouth

Right side

Left side

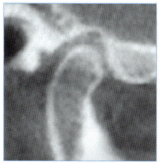

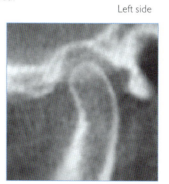

The condyle was anteriorized on the right side with modest flattening of the anterior surface.

Coronal section

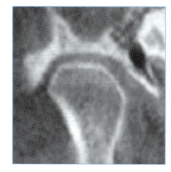

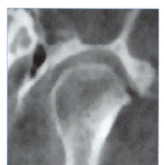

Reduced spacing on the external side.

MUSCULOARTICULAR THERAPY
USING SKELETAL ANCHORAGE

I.

Skeletal advance action on the right mandibular district was integrated with intra-arch orthodontic treatment (see pages 310 and 311).

While bringing about improvement, ARS treatment was unable to fully correct the right side dental Class II. For this reason, orthodontic treatment was started a few weeks later with the purpose of advancing the mandibular right hemi-arch to bring it into dental Class I. **Care was taken to maintain the therapeutic position of the articular structures and interarch relations established during initial bite registration and held in** place by the splint from the start of treatment through all subsequent steps until the very end of the program.

The patient tolerated her ARS well. She appreciated the considerable pain and muscle relief it provided as well as the greater mandibular protraction, which improved the deep bite and permitted lateral movements.

Microscrews were embedded into the splint area corresponding to the mandibular incisors, which required buccalization. This effect was subsequently completed with a fixed appliance.

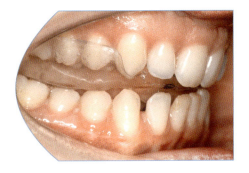
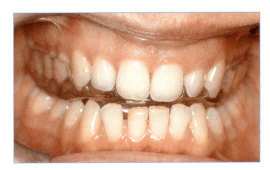
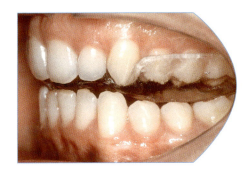

The splint was fitted, which placed the jaws in their therapeutic muscle position. Note how the acrylic blocks the maxillary teeth and improves the Class II relationships by advancing the right side more than the left and consequently also centering the midlines.

ANCHORAGE STABILIZATION BY THE ARS IS THE RESULT OF

1. **Indentation** in the acrylic of all maxillary teeth excepting only the incisors, where the microscrews are left to act.

2. The anterior flange on condition that **contact is limited to three mandibular left teeth**—the central and lateral incisors and the canine—to provide 3D mandibular position control. The corresponding teeth on the right side are involved in the protraction of the mandibular right district (see procedure II).
This is an intentional exception to the normal protocol in which all six mandibular inferiors usually interlock with the anterior flange, unlike the three affected in this case.

3. The splint's smooth **raised wedge** holding away the remaining mandibular teeth, which are moved one by one with the aid of dental anchorage.

SKELETAL ANCHORAGE ON THE LEFT SIDE

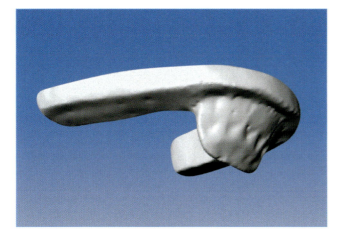

ARS used.

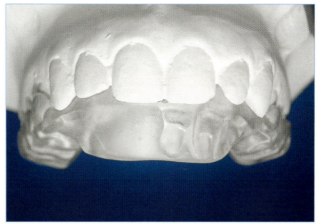

Front view of anterior flange.

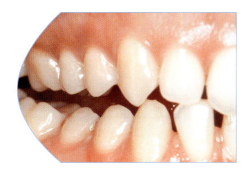

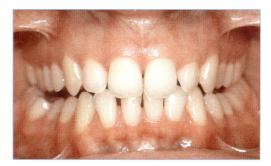

Therapeutic interarch position created by constant ARS wear.

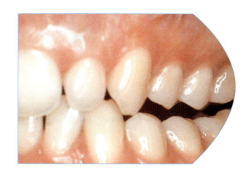

 Skeletal anchorage

KEY FEATURES OF ARS

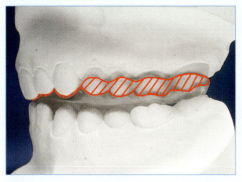

Maxillary teeth indented in the acrylic (viewed from the left side only).

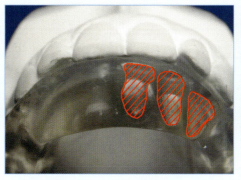

Contact points of -1, -2, and -3 on anterior flange, showing the key position for skeletal anchorage.

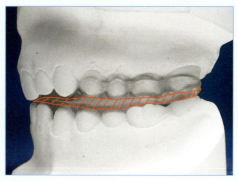

Side view of wedge acting on the mandibular arch.

This is the first of several pages illustrating how CT scans aid comparison of the patient's condylar position and shape. These images are integrated with MRIs offering interesting additional perspectives when compared with CT.

SAME-DAY PRETREATMENT COMPARISON: CLOSED-MOUTH CT WITH AND WITHOUT THE SPLINT FITTED

WITHOUT SPLINT	WITH SPLINT	SUPERIMPOSED

Right side

Left side

Coronal right side

Coronal left side

COMPARISON OF PRETREATMENT AND POSTTREATMENT CLOSED-MOUTH CT SCANS

PRETREATMENT	POSTTREATMENT	SUPERIMPOSED

Right side

Left side

Coronal right side

Coronal left side

POSTTREATMENT MRI

Right **Closed-mouth** *Left*

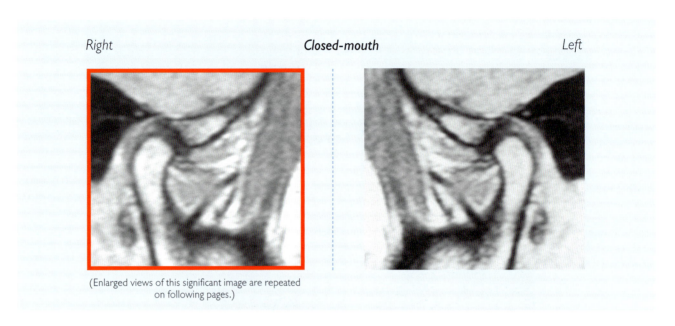

(Enlarged views of this significant image are repeated on following pages.)

Open-mouth

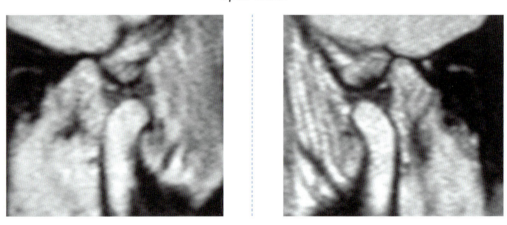

Coronal

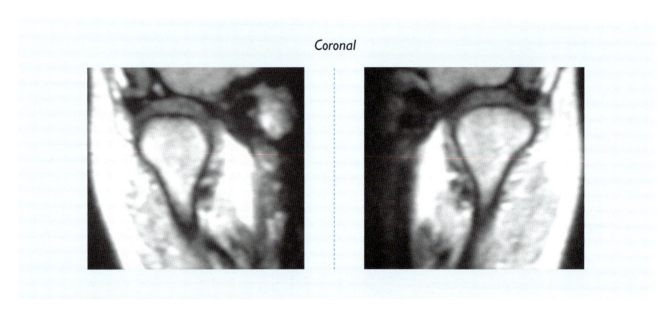

Although an **MRI was taken only posttreatment,** it is still valuable in highlighting a normal open-mouth and closed-mouth anatomy totally free of muscle inflammation or fluids.

POSTTREATMENT COMPARISON BETWEEN:
CT   and   MRI

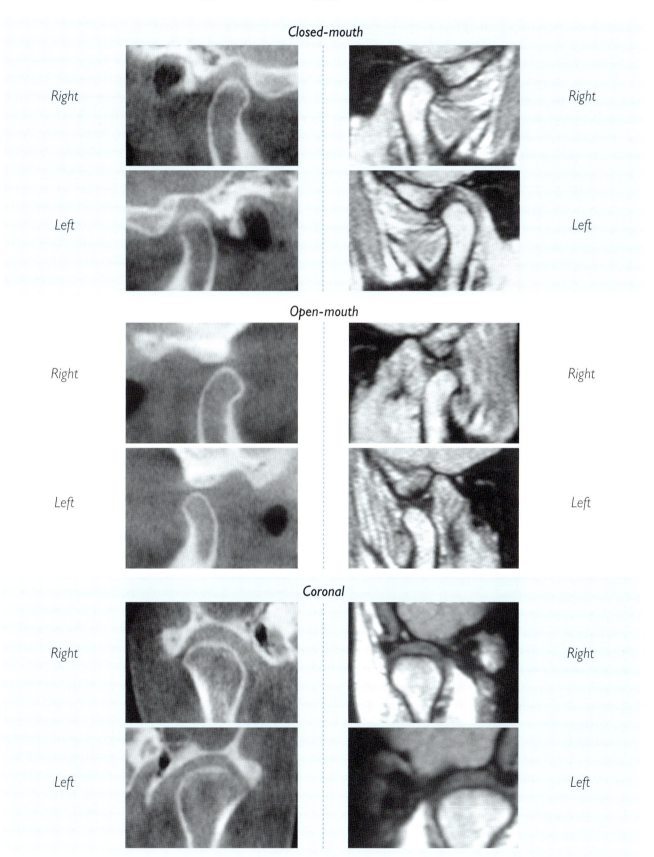

Closed-mouth

Right   Right

Left   Left

Open-mouth

Right   Right

Left   Left

Coronal

Right   Right

Left   Left

IMAGING SEQUENCES IN THE VARIOUS STAGES

CT

MRI

RIGHT SIDE

Pretreatment

With ARS fitted

Postreatment

Postreatment

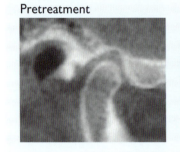
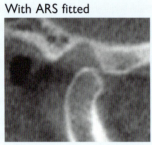
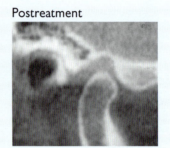
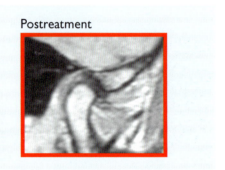

LEFT SIDE

Pretreatment

With ARS fitted

Postreatment

Postreatment

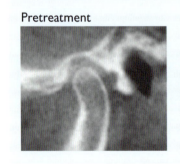
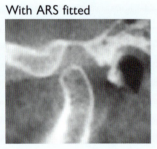
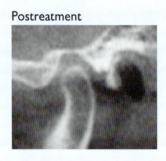

PREFERABILITY OF MRI VERSUS CT

Posttreatment CT sequences show condylar position as being lower and forward but apparently at a short distance from the fossa, which creates some doubt as to correct disc position. MRIs taken within the same time frame clearly show the correct anatomical position of the disc between condyle and fossa, which is further confirmation of a successful treatment outcome (see significant detail in enlargement on facing page).

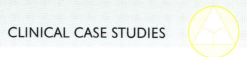

CORRECT ANATOMY OF ARTICULAR STRUCTURES
SHOWN BY RIGHT SIDE, POSTTREATMENT MRI
(greater enlargement)

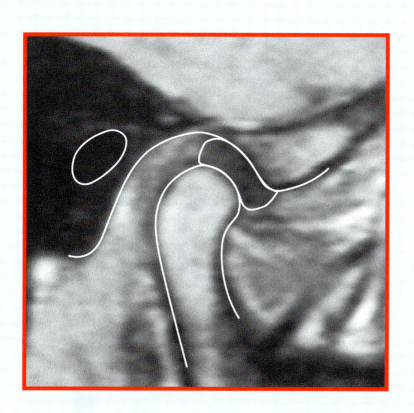

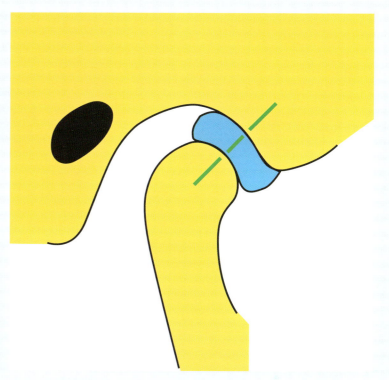

This result confirms the correct anatomical relationships in terms of functional efficiency between condyle, disc, and articulating surface despite the protrusive stimulus provided by the ARS and protraction of the teeth in the mandibular right hemi-arch, the latter being a positive action difficult to interpret.

II.

PROTRACTION OF MANDIBULAR RIGHT HEMI-ARCH: ACHIEVED PARTLY WITH DENTAL ANCHORAGE
(in addition to ARS skeletal anchorage)

Further recovery of symmetry in the mandibular arch was achieved with dental anchorage based on the **GI intra-arch system**, which integrates mandibular advance for simultaneous application of skeletal anchorage.

A *metal plate* was used to observe the inter-arch relationships in greater detail, with special reference to the curves of Spee.

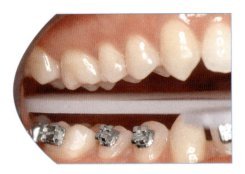
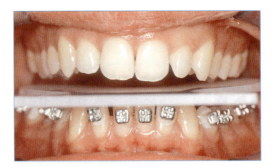
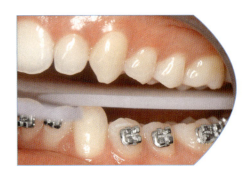

This showed that it was necessary to flatten the mandibular curve of Spee bilaterally by intruding the mandibular anterior teeth and extruding the premolars and first molars as far as possible. Because of the patient's exceptional compliance, repeatable movements were obtained. Within the first few weeks, microscrews were added to the splint over the central and lateral incisors, which required buccalization. This meant that orthodontics commenced almost at the same time as orthopedic-articular therapy.

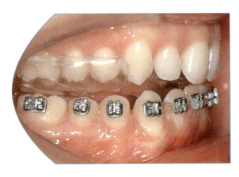
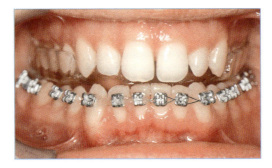
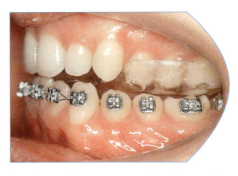

Further confirmation of synchrony between orthopedic and dental action (ie, PHASE I and PHASE II) came after approximately 2 months after the start of ARS treatment. A fixed appliance was fitted to the mandibular arch since it was judged that this area would require longer treatment than would the maxilla.

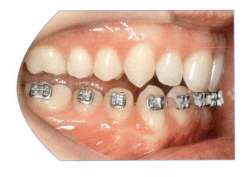
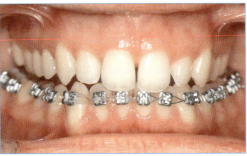
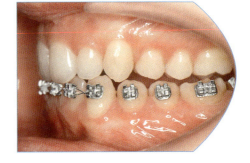

Without splint.

Systematic monitoring occurred throughout treatment. The patient was splint-free so that the repetitive stability of the musculoarticular position could be checked and ongoing simultaneous procedures could be planned to reduce overall length of treatment.

To correct the right side Class II relationships, the mandibular hemi-arch, considered to be retracted, was protracted. This option was chosen instead of retracting the maxillary equivalent since it was considered to already be correctly positioned.

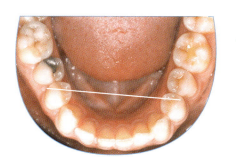 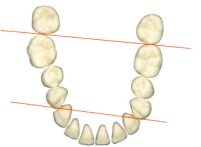 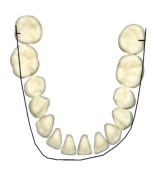

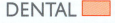 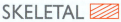

ANCHORAGE: DENTAL SKELETAL

LEFT SIDE:
SKELETAL ANCHORAGE

- On maxillary arch posterolateral districts, excluding anterior teeth where microscrews are fitted
- On the ARS raised wedge contacting the occlusal surface of mandibulars -4, -5, -6, and -7
- On -1, -2, and -3 lingual surfaces

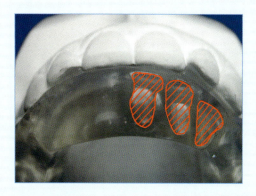

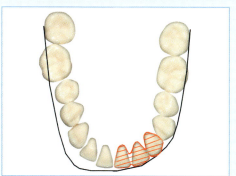

1-2-3 are involved in both skeletal and dental anchorage.

SIMULTANEOUS TREATMENT OF RIGHT AND LEFT SIDES:
DENTAL ANCHORAGE

One tooth is moved progressively at a time while all the other teeth provide anchorage (Gi.Co. intra-arch system).

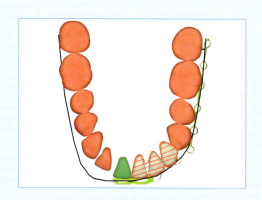

INTRA-ARCH TREATMENT: UNDERLYING PRINCIPLES

In the case of L.P., use of an ARS designed in part to create protractive orthopedic action predominantly on the right side of the mandible improved the patient's skeletal Class II and made it necessary to protract the lateroposterior right district by means of orthodontic dental anchorage.

For continuation of treatment, a mandibular archwire was shaped with mesial stops on both the left and right second molars. The wire was deliberately left approximately 5 mm longer than the span between the second molars to create extra space in the area of the mandibular right canine for mesial movement of the right premolars and molars.

A crucial factor was the proper tooth **ligature sequence**:

- On the left side, ligature departed from the first molar forward, tooth by tooth as far as the lateral incisor.
- On the right side, the teeth were ligated starting with the second molar, followed by the first molar, and then the second premolar.

This left an arch-shaped protruberance in the lateroanterior district of the archwire, along which the teeth requiring mesialization were shifted in a logical progression. Dental anchorage was stabilized by ligating together -7 with -6 and, in succession, -6 with -5, and so on, until blocking -1 with -2. An elastic ligature was then created to mesialize 1-, thus closing the space between the central incisors and centering the midlines (see drawing 4 on page 311). Once 1- and -1 were locked together, 2- was also mesialized. To stabilize the anchorage, it was necessary to secure -4 to the archwire (see drawing 5 on page 310).

The existing space created by the additional archwire length is noticeable in the area of the canine, and ligation of this tooth to the wire forced it to move mesially and buccally.

This was precisely what was required to give symmetric balance between the two canines, where the right canine had formerly been in a more distal position (see drawing 6 on page 310), to improve the discrepancy between the upper and lower arches. The right side Class II became a skeletal and dental Class I as a result of the combined skeletal action of the ARS and dental action with progressive forward movement of the teeth on the right side. The 4- was moved forward with the same procedure, as were the other teeth.

To deal with the 7-, the last tooth requiring mesialization, the archwire was changed to eliminate its mesial stop. The new wire had a stop distal to 6- and was bent behind -7 to anchor all the teeth in the arch together, thereby forcing 7- to mesialize under pressure from elastic ligatures with **all the remaining teeth pulling against the last one needing to move.** This completed remodeling of the entire mandibular arch (see illustrations on pages 310 and 311).

Each tooth needing to be moved was ligated with elastic to its anchorage neighbor, which in turn was anchored to all the other teeth on that side. In addition, movements were speeded up with an open coil spring of the appropriate length inserted into the archwire and acting on the tooth requiring moving. This created a further movement force and was used for all the teeth except the last one. This procedure could be called a **"push and pull"** method (see illustration 12 bottom of page 311).

GI. CO. INTRA-ARCH SYSTEM PRINCIPLES

This last procedure as developed in this patient's treatment plan can be classified as an example of the **GI intra-arch system** (greater detail on page 395).

1. The possibility of creating the space necessary to move teeth (greater wire length and suitable ligatures).

2. Use of traditional fixed and removable orthodontic appliances on the buccal surfaces only and acting within a single arch.

3. Anchorage is dental, involving all the teeth in the arch (or hemi-arch), with the exception of the tooth being moved in its turn.

4. The possibility of applying more than one therapeutic procedure simultaneously, thus drastically reducing the length of treatment.

5. **Anchorage with orthodontic mini-implants**
    The book contains many suggestions regarding new therapeutic approaches and their many potential clinical applications, while following the rule of demonstrating these with real patients.
    On the subject of anchorage in Gi.Co. System, we would like to break this rule by referring in theory alone to an interesting project yet to be defined: insertion of palatal orthodontic mini-implants in the gap between canine and premolar in Class II patients, and between first and second molar in Class III patients.
    A rectangular wire with appropriate ligatures is used to create a solid unit between the abutment and brackets bonded to the palatal faces of the two teeth providing anchorage, somewhat as if treating ankylosed teeth.

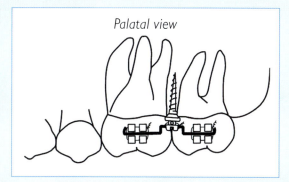

Palatal view

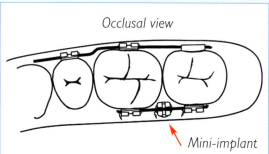

Occlusal view

Mini-implant

Advantages: by avoiding bulky appliances this makes the technique straightforward. The clinician can therefore apply the buccal brackets of choice and implement a personal series of solutions to move the teeth as required, and may if necessary insert mini-implants in other positions after having removed these first ones.

INTRA-ARCH TREATMENT: SEQUENCE OF PROCEDURES

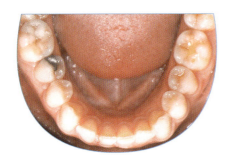

1. Pretreatment mandibular arch.

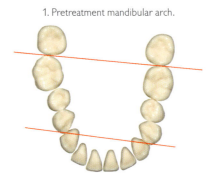

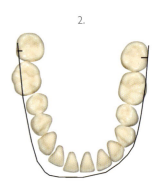

2.

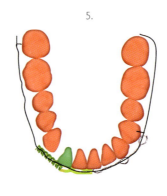

5.

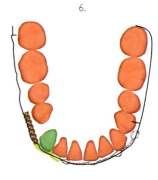

6.

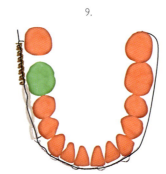

9.

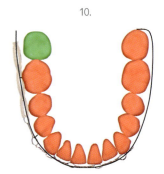

10.

MOVING ONE TOOTH AT A TIME: THE *"PUSH AND PULL"* SYSTEM

Each tooth needing to be moved is pulled toward its proper position as planned to correct the malocclusion, using elastic ligatures and the pressure of the compressed spring, while all the remaining teeth are ligated together in a single anchorage unit.

In greater detail, the tooth (in this case, the mandibular right first premolar) is forced forward by the combined action of the compressed spring placed between the second and first premolars and the active elastic pulling from the anchorage canine, which is fixed in the main arch and mesially ligated to the bracket on the first premolar.
THE PROCEDURE IS SYSTEMATICALLY APPLIED TO REDUCE TREATMENT TIME.

DENTAL ANCHORAGE

3.
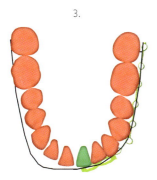

4.
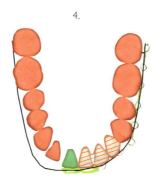

7.
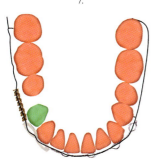
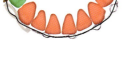

8.
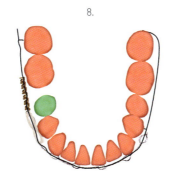

11. Posttreatment situation.
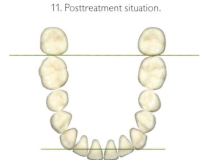

Posttreatment mandibular arch.
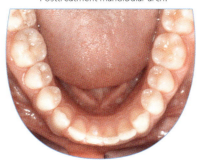
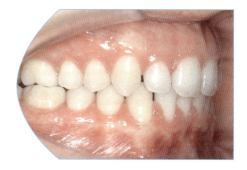

"PUSH AND PULL" PROCEDURE

12.
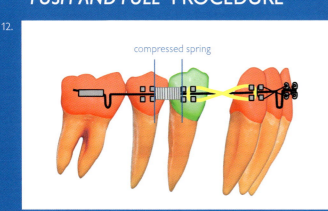

compressed spring

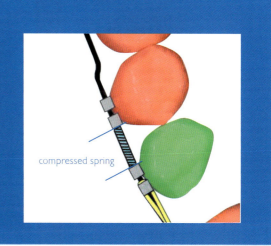

compressed spring

III.

EXPANSION OF MAXILLARY RIGHT HEMI-ARCH

Approximately 6 months after the start of ARS therapy, the patient demonstrated consistently repetitive opening and closure movements, so expansion of the maxillary right hemi-arch was started.

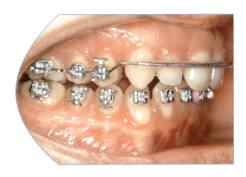 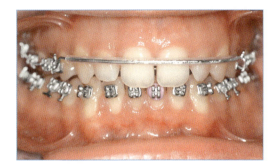 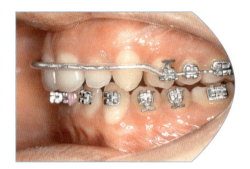

Brackets were bonded from the first premolars back to the second molars on both sides. A rectangular archwire was shaped with root-buccal torque programmed to expand, with reciprocal anchorage and movement areas. The teeth on the left side were indented into and held in place by the splint acrylic. On the right side, acrylic was ground away to leave the teeth free to slide outward.

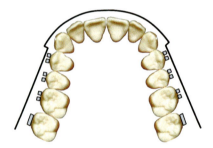

Expanding archwire viewed occlusally.

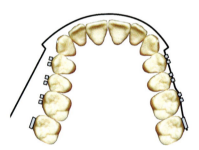

Archwire ligated on the left with teeth anchored in the splint.

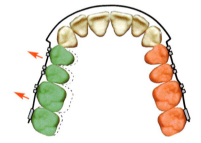

Teeth on right side free to expand.

Right side: Teeth are free to move (acrylic eliminated from smooth external side and on occlusal plane).

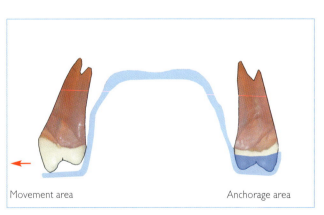

Movement area   Anchorage area

Left side: Crowns are indented in splint acrylic.

It was decided not to bond brackets to the maxillary canines and incisors to postpone as long as possible this young woman's esthetic problems. For the same reason, the anterior straight archwire segment was raised as high as possible toward the gingival line (see photographs at top of page).

EXPANSION OF MAXILLARY RIGHT HEMI-ARCH
COMPARISONS

PRETREATMENT

POSTTREATMENT

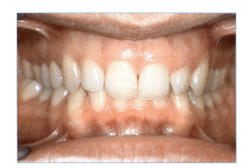
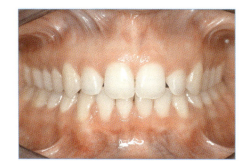
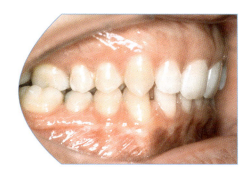
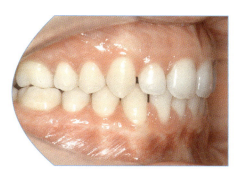

COMPARISON OF MAXILLARY ARCH

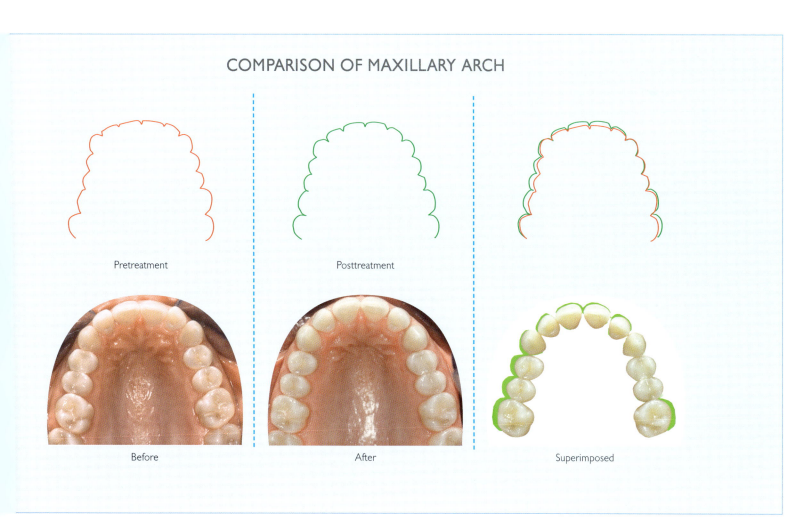

Pretreatment

Posttreatment

Before

After

Superimposed

IV. RECOVERY OF INCISAL GUIDANCE

Correction of the patient's incisal guidance commenced in the early weeks with palatal miscroscrews applied to the ARS to buccalize the maxillary anteriors while the mandibular counterparts were anteriorized by pressure from the flange. A complete fixed appliance was subsequently applied in the maxillary arch to expand the right side as a continuation of the action previously described and to improve incisal guidance by buccalizing and intruding the anterior teeth. This procedure was also done in the mandibular arch (again with a fixed appliance) where it was necessary to buccalize, intrude, and align the mandibular anterior teeth and move them

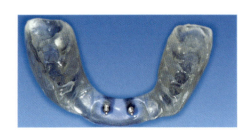

to the left to align the midlines (intra-arch treatment). Changes in the upper and lower anterior districts brought about good incisal guidance, both static and dynamic (see page 317).

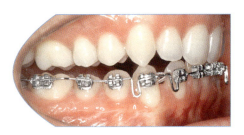
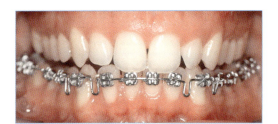
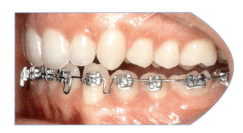

Wires used to restore correct incisal guidance.

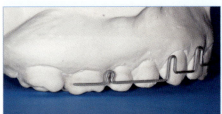
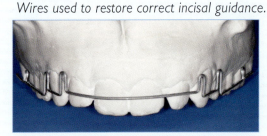
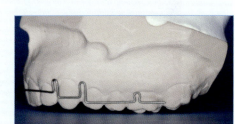
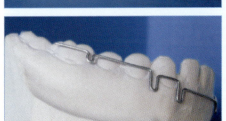
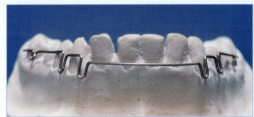
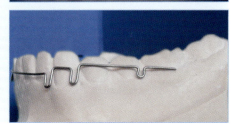

During the final stages of treatment, the appliances were progressively removed, with the mandibular anterior area being removed last.

Because this type of case is prone to relapse, a fixed lingual retainer is often applied, though not in this patient.

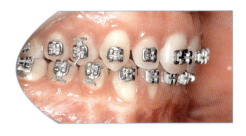
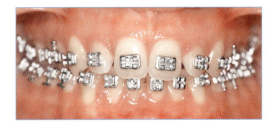
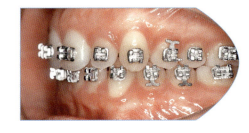

COMPARISONS

| PRETREATMENT | POSTTREATMENT |

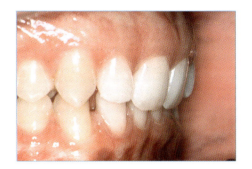
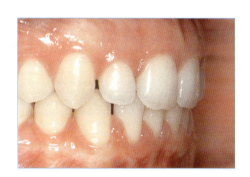

CROSS-SECTION OF STONE CASTS

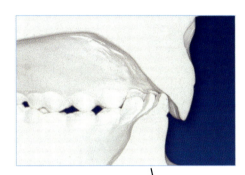
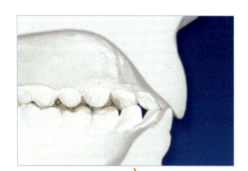

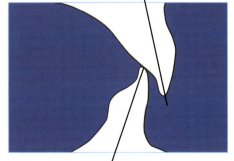
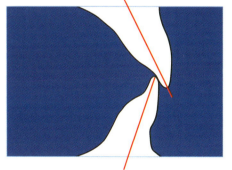

OUTLINES

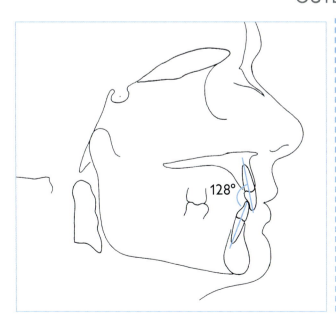

128°

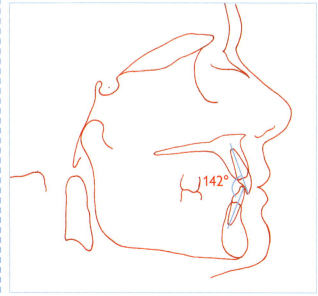

142°

V. OVERALL LENGTH OF TREATMENT: LESS THAN 15 MONTHS
due to the patient's extraordinary compliance

POSTTREATMENT RECORDS

Correct anatomy key to functional efficiency

Recovery of the different dental districts is done, as far as possible, with the aim of reducing treatment time while achieving an acceptable result. The upper right crossbite was corrected together with the right side Class II and anterior deep bite. Occlusion was stable. No fixed retainer was applied, and the patient wears a customized ARS only at night.

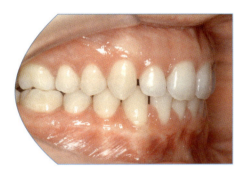
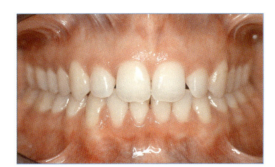
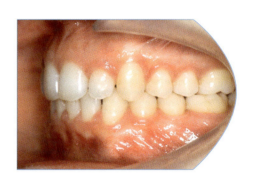
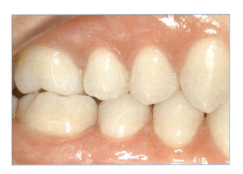
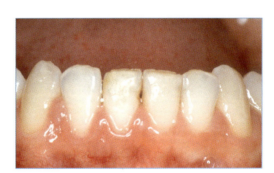
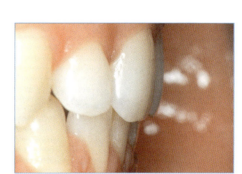

ON COMPLETION OF TREATMENT
The faults found during diagnosis have been resolved.
Subjective parameters
- The patient no longer has dual bite.
- The interincisor midlines coincide.
- The patient no longer has pain affecting her TMJs, head, and chest, and she is pleased that she has stopped grinding her teeth at night.

Objective parameters
- The posttreatment documentation, including CTs and MRIs, shows considerable improvement, especially in the right TMJ, which shows every sign of an ideal anatomy.

The patient's splint was removed at every appointment to check the spatial stability of her muscoloarticular apparatus in the position ascertained with initial bite registration. It was held steady with the ARS while the teeth were progressively moved into a correct dental anatomy, therefore moving the teeth to fit the requirements of the muscles and TMJs.

START: 18 September 2004
END: 29 November 2005

DISCLUSION

Protrusive:

Viewed from right   *Viewed from left*

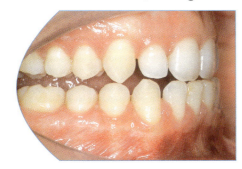
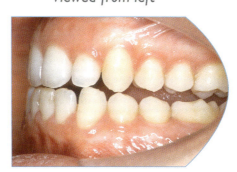

Right cuspid rise:

Viewed from right (working side)   *Viewed from left (nonworking side)*

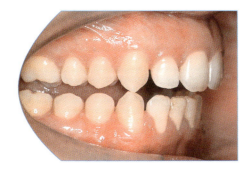
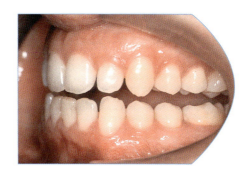

Left cuspid rise:

Viewed from right (nonworking side)   *Viewed from left (working side)*

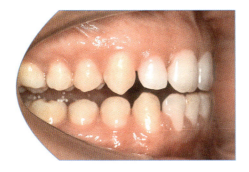
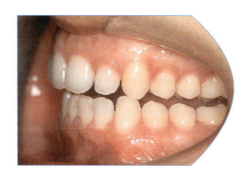

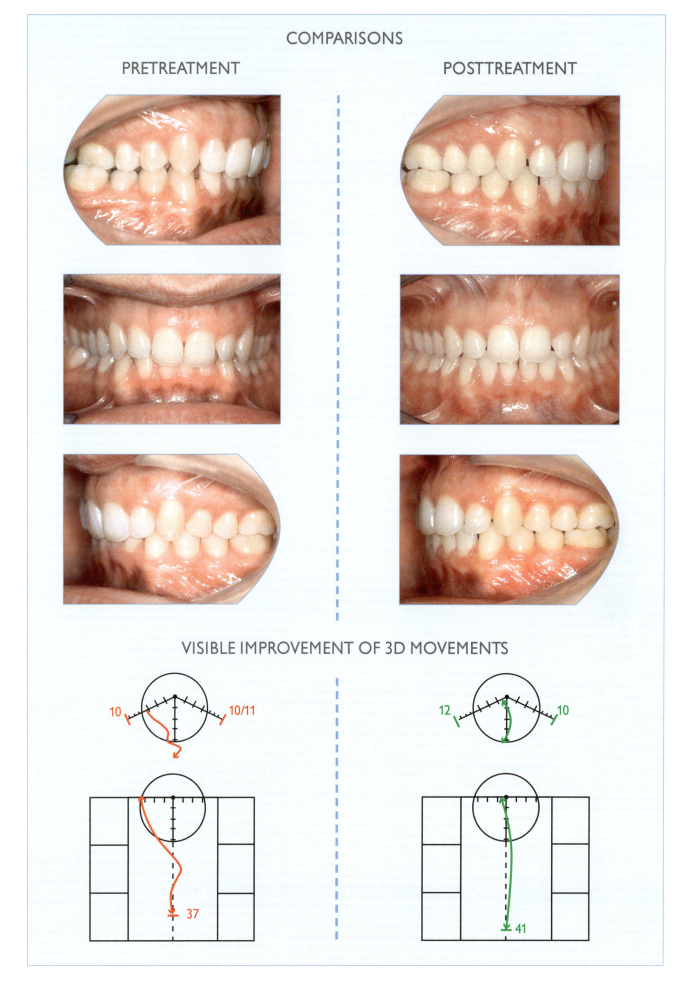

COMPARISONS

PRETREATMENT   POSTTREATMENT

VISIBLE IMPROVEMENT OF 3D MOVEMENTS

FOLLOW-UP 2 YEARS posttreatment: 2007

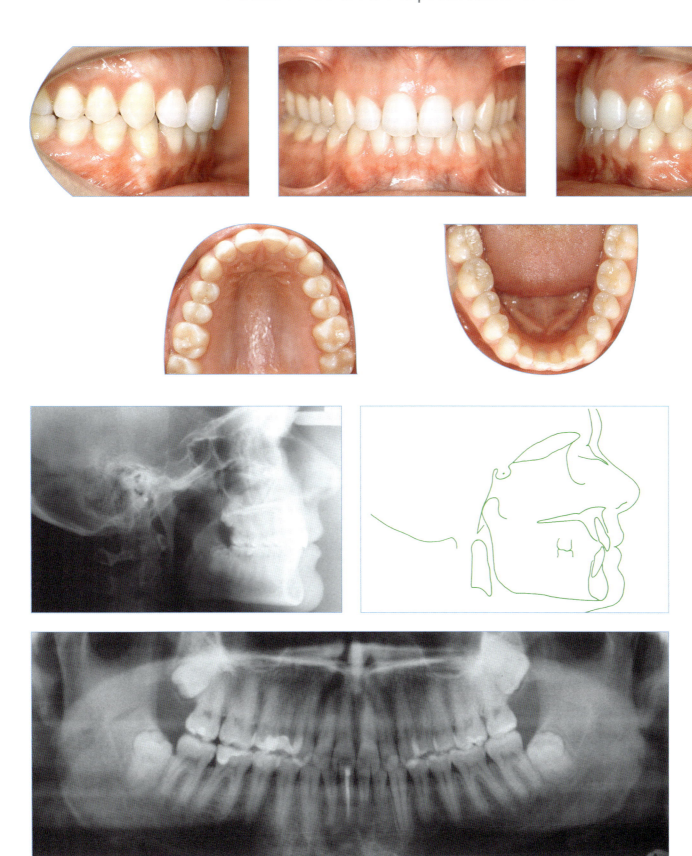

Extraction of mandibular third molars was recommended (and subsequently done) because of difficulties in maintaining hygiene. The maxillary antagonists will be extracted after eruption.

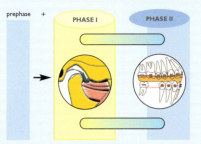

KEY FEATURE:
ORTHODONTIC PREPHASE
FOLLOWED BY
PHASE I AND PHASE II SIMULTANEOUSLY

This adult patient presented with severe deep bite, noticeably prominent maxillary incisors, and anterior crowding in both the maxillary and mandibular arches. Prior to musculoarticular therapy (PHASE I), it was decided to proceed with decisive orthodontic treatment with fixed appliances to significantly correct the interarch relationship. Failure to do so would have meant an excessively bulky ARS with considerable discomfort for the patient.

This preliminary correction provided a number of benefits:
- Less effort for the patient to wear the ARS
- Simplification of phase I and phase II treatment as a result of the dental movements already done in the orthodontic prephase
- Reduction of total treatment time

Patient: S. G., age 27

DIAGNOSIS

This patient presented with an unattractive appearance due to a Class II malocclusion and considerable overjet and overbite. TMJ damage was evident. The left TMJ had anterolateral dislocation of the disc with recapture when the jaws were open. Ligamentous laxity was also present, with the condyles translating beyond the eminence in the open-mouth position.

THERAPY

Orthognathic surgery was planned but refused by the patient. It was therefore decided to commence orthodontic treatment for esthetic compensation. A fixed maxillary appliance was applied first, followed shortly afterward by a mandibular appliance to open the bite and improve crowding. After approximately 4 months, ARS musculoarticular therapy was started at the same time as orthodontic occlusal finishing, giving an overall treatment length of 19 months.

PRETREATMENT RECORDS

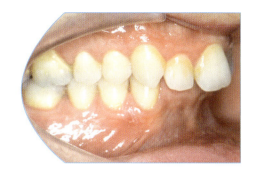
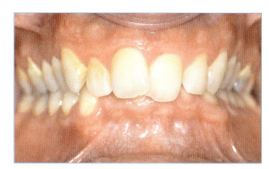
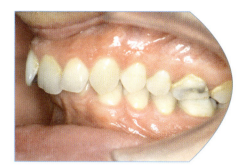

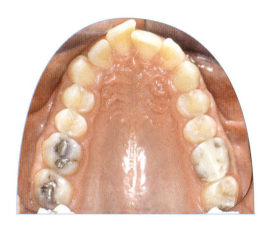
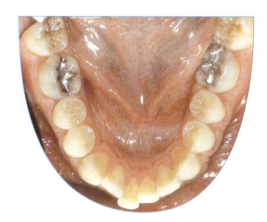

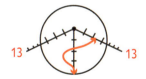

13   13

The left condyle
dislocates later than the
right and follows an
altered path.

Slight
crepitus,
stronger
on opening
on the
right side.

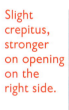
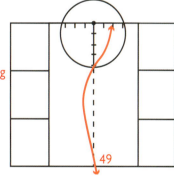

Slight
crepitus on
the left side
on opening
and closure.

49

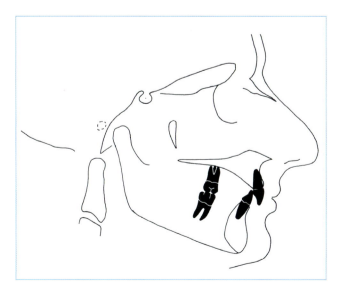
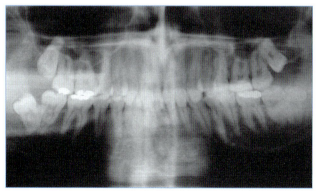

Pretreatment head film outline and OPT.

PRETREATMENT CT SCANS

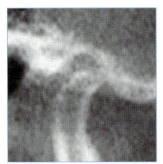 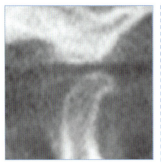 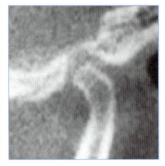 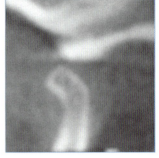

Right side, mouth closed and open
(condyle anterior to eminence).

Left side, mouth closed and open
(condyle anterior to eminence).

PRETREATMENT MRI

Right side: Within normal limits

Left side: Anterolateral dislocation of disc with recapture on opening

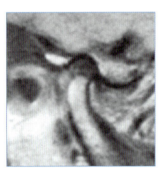 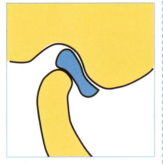 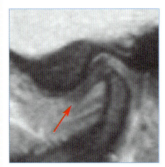 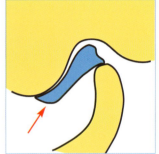

Closed-mouth right condyle with disc in normal position.

Closed-mouth left condyle with disc dislocated anteriorly.

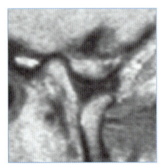 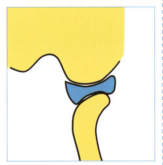 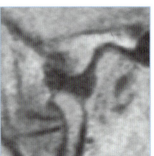 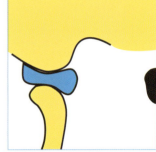

Open-mouth right condyle with disc in normal position.

Open-mouth left condyle with disc in normal position (recaptured).

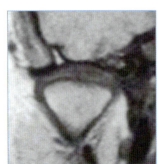 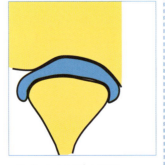 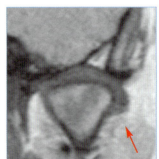 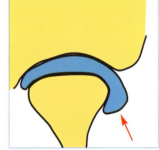

Right condyle, coronal section, with disc in normal position.

Left condyle, coronal section, with disc slipping laterally.

322

PREPHASE: ORTHODONTIC TREATMENT

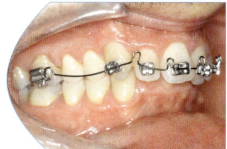
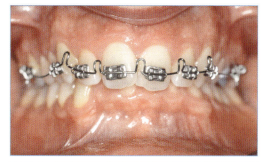
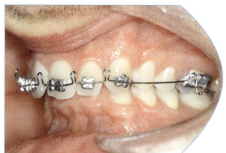
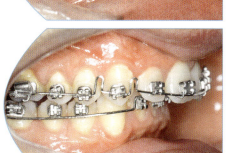
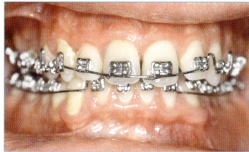
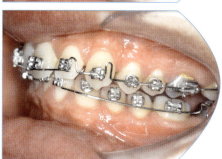

PHASE I AND PHASE II PERFORMED SIMULTANEOUSLY

The ARS was fitted approximately 4 months after the start of the orthodontic prephase. The splint actually worn (see left photograph) was far less bulky than it would have been (see right photograph) without the initial preparatory phase.

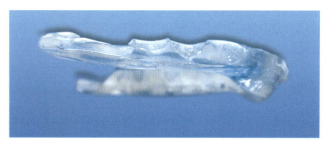
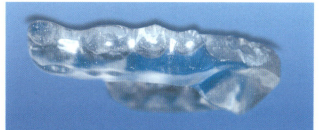

Fig. 1 Splint actually fitted.

Fig. 2 Hypothetical larger splint needed in the absence of the orthodontic prophase.

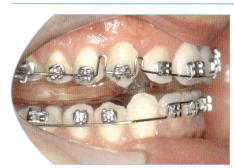
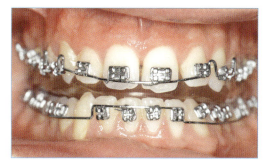
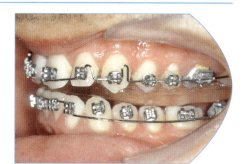
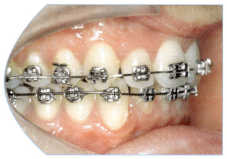
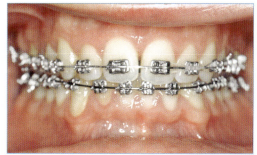
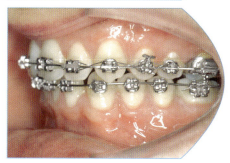

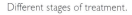

Different stages of treatment.

POSTTREATMENT RECORDS

The patient was extremely satisfied with the final esthetic and functional outcome, which was obtained in less than 20 months. Unfortunately, he declined a posttreatment MRI. Nevertheless, the available posttreatment documentation is considered useful and is therefore presented.

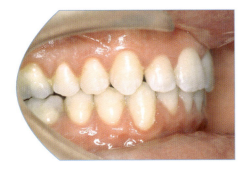
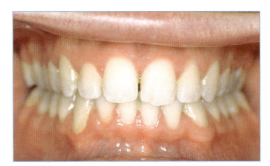
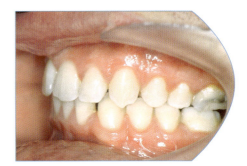

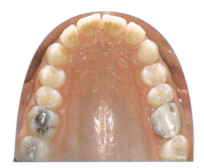
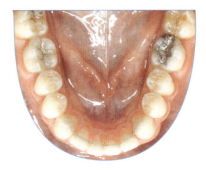

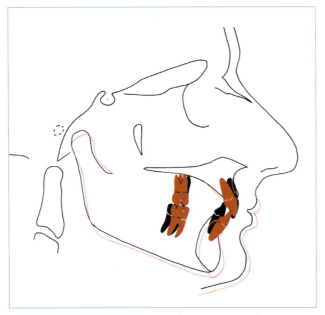

Superimposed pretreatment and posttreatment outlines.

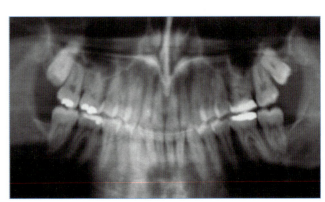

Posttreatment OPT.

COMPARISONS

PRETREATMENT	POSTTREATMENT

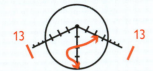

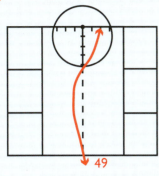

The left condyle dislocates later than the right condyle.

A slight crepitus, present at both dx and sx on closure and opening, is stronger on opening on the right side.

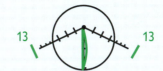

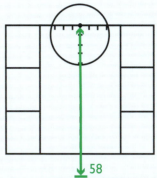

A slight crepitus is present in the final closing stage on the right side and the final opening stage on the left side.

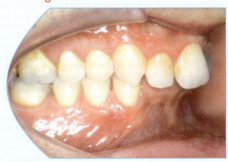

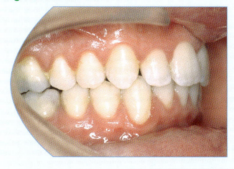

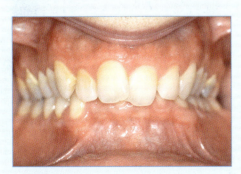

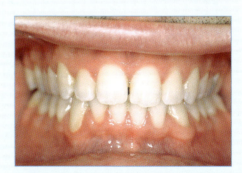

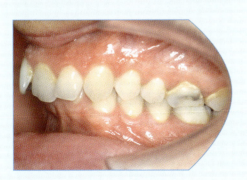

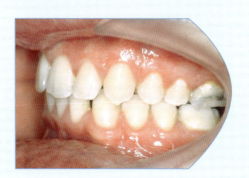

SPORTS-RELATED TMD

Damage caused by dysfunctional problems can lead to anatomical and functional alterations not only to the stomatognathic apparatus in isolation but also to different areas of the body including the locomotor apparatus. This realization opens up a new area of study with much still to be learned and defined.

Although research-based evidence is lacking, empirical experience has shown that athletes can improve their individual performance by receiving musculoarticular treatment, when needed, integrated with other therapy. For instance, athletes from differing specialties can be helped by a generic splint acting on occlusal discrepancies. In much the same way that an SS relieves muscle stress and potentially improves TMJ tone, a splint can contribute to an individual's overall wellbeing and sports performance.

The case studies presented here deal with competitors in the fields of tennis, soccer, and swimming. In all of these, changes were noted through imaging and other tests. In addition, the athletes demonstrated enhanced performance as a result of musculoarticular therapy. These examples suggest that more accurate guidelines are warranted. Data collection with more selective clinical examination and imaging diagnostics such as MRI, stabilometry, electromyography, and pain charting, may contribute to forming more accurate diagnoses and more targeted therapies.

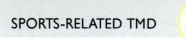

V. CLINICAL CASE STUDIES ON ATHLETES

TEEN TENNIS PLAYER: INITIAL EXAMINATION REVEALING BADLY INFLAMED EXTERNAL PTERYGOID
(pretreatment records only)

Patient: M. V., age 14
Tennis player

KEY FEATURES

The patient had loss of strength in his left arm, altered mandibular excursions, and inflammation of the external pterygoid—the first muscle to suffer negative resonance and the last to relax.

PRETREATMENT RECORDS ONLY

In addition to loss of strength in his left arm, this left-hander also complained of reduced service speed and pain in his left deltoid after a few minutes of play.

THERAPY

The patient was fitted with an ARS, which he wore continuously except at mealtimes and during matches.

RESULTS

Partly due to the player's eagerness in wearing his splint regularly, the pain disappeared. The patient's overall play improved, and he achieved prestigious wins for his age.

LIMITATION

Follow-up continued for only the first 4 months.

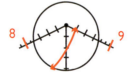

Evidently altered mandibular dynamics.

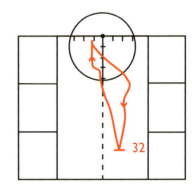

MAGNETIC RESONANCE IMAGING

T2-weighted, fat-suppressed, closed-mouth sequences were taken so that fluids could be visualized. The sections crossing the lateral pterygoid muscles show hyperintense stripes typical of muscle edema.

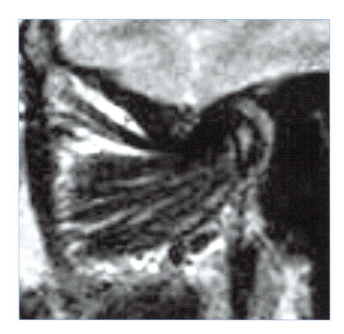

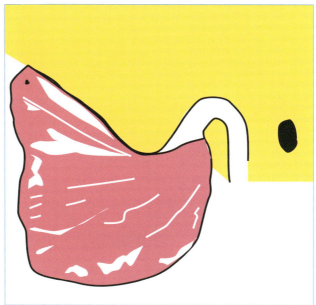

ORAFACIAL PAIN CHART FILLED OUT BY THE PATIENT
Chart kindly provided by Prof Felice Festa (G. D'Annunzio University, Chieti, Italy)

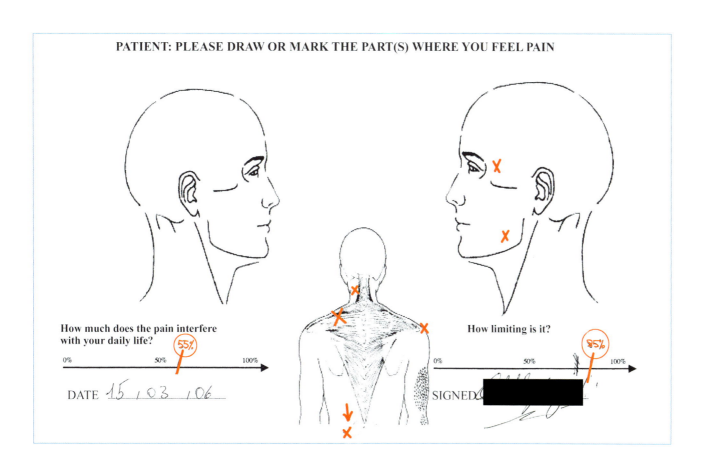

PROFESSIONAL SOCCER PLAYER

PHASE I ONLY: COMBINED THERAPY AND ARS

Patient: L. R., age 30
Patient treated by Dr. Fabio Ciuffolo
(G. D'Annunzio University, Chieti, Italy, Prof Felice Festa)

DIAGNOSIS
The patient presented with a dental Class II on the right side, a deep bite, and deviated midlines.

REASON FOR PRESENTING
The patient complained of pain in the inferior trapezius that interfered with his play.

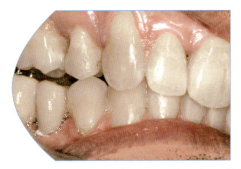 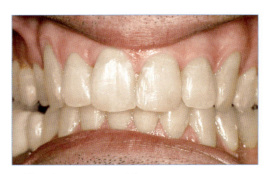 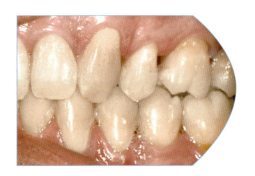

Attempted various forms of local treatment without success.

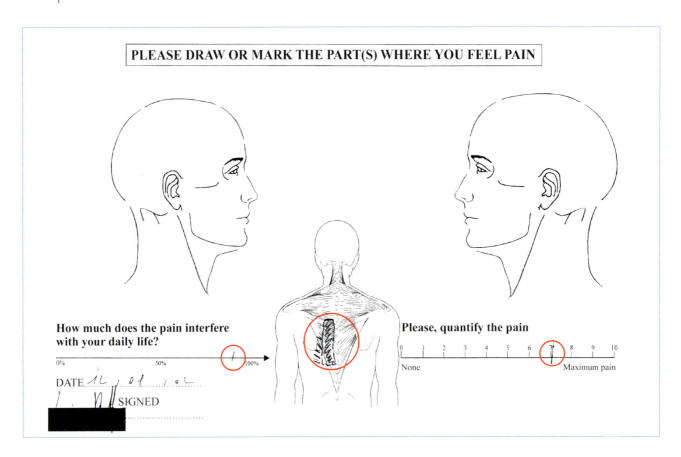

HEAD AND NECK MUSCLE ELECTROMYOGRAPHY PATTERNS WITHOUT ARS

Widespread electromyography (EMG) signal hyperactivity and asymmetry were seen in the masticatory area and anterior neck muscles, while the posterior neck district and upper back area gave results that were within normal values.

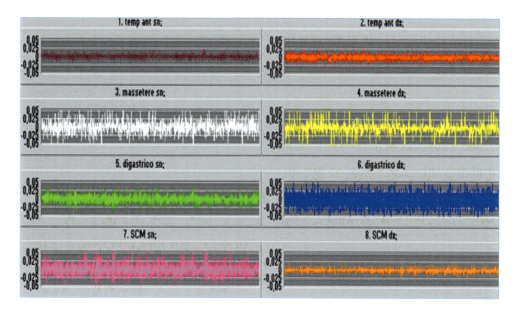

COMBINED THERAPIES

- Support manipulation therapy
- Biofeedback EMG
- ARS producing positive results from the start that motivated the patient to wear it consistently, excepting only mealtimes and when playing sports

STABILOMETRIC PATTERN

There was an absence of postural blindness. Signs of a significant stabilizing effect on body posture, especially in the mandible-advancement position, were evident (see TMD and postural disorders, pages 110 and 111).

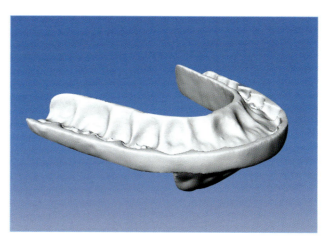

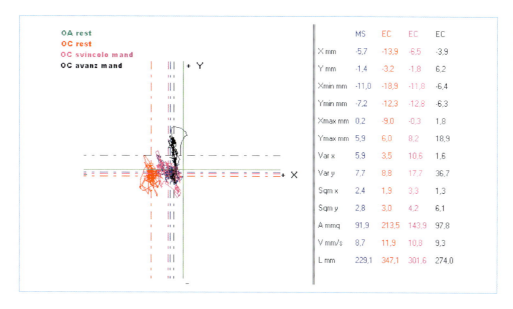

Key:
OA = eyes open
OC = eyes closed
Rest = mandible in habitual rest position

	MS	EC	EC	EC
X mm	-5,7	-13,9	-6,5	-3,9
Y mm	-1,4	-3,2	-1,8	6,2
Xmin mm	-11,0	-18,9	-11,8	-6,4
Ymin mm	-7,2	-12,3	-12,8	-6,3
Xmax mm	0,2	-9,0	-0,3	1,8
Ymax mm	5,9	6,0	8,2	18,9
Var x	5,9	3,5	10,6	1,6
Var y	7,7	8,8	17,7	36,7
Sqm x	2,4	1,9	3,3	1,3
Sqm y	2,8	3,0	4,2	6,1
A mmq	91,9	213,5	143,9	97,8
V mm/s	8,7	11,9	10,8	9,3
L mm	229,1	347,1	301,6	274,0

OA rest
OC rest
OC svincolo mand
OC avanz mand

COMPARISON: CONDITIONS BEFORE TREATMENT

Pretreatment orofacial pain chart

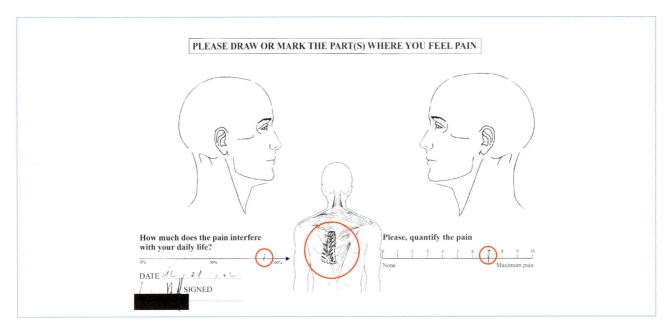

HEAD AND NECK EMG PATTERN

Pretreatment: Widespread EMG signal hyperactivity and asymmetry were seen in the masticatory area and anterior neck muscles while the posterior neck district and upper back area gave results that were within normal values.

Pretreatment EMG right side

Pretreatment EMG left side

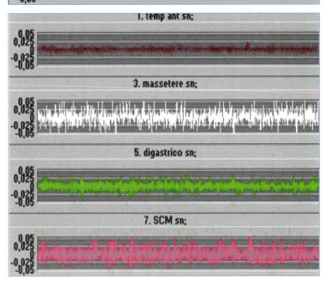

AND POSTTREATMENT

Disappearance of pain and noticeable overall improved performance on the playing field
(Posttreatment orofacial pain chart)

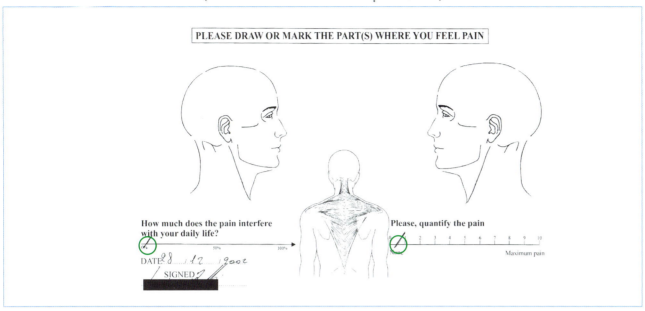

HEAD AND NECK EMG PATTERN

Posttreatment: Posttreatment tests yielded normal (significantly reduced) EMG signals compared with pretreatment hyperactivity.

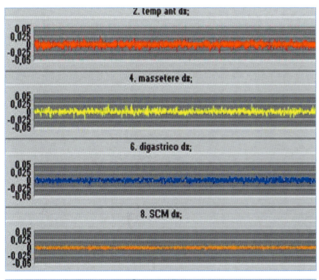

Posttreatment EMG right side

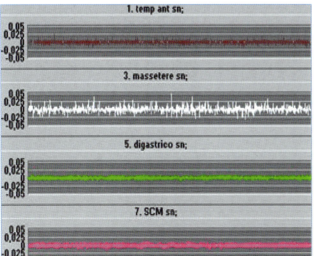

Posttreatment EMG left side

PROFESSIONAL SOCCER PLAYER

 PHASE I ONLY: MUSCULOARTICULAR THERAPY WITH A SIX-POINT SPLINT AND SUBSEQUENT STABILIZATION SPLINT

Patient: A. G., age 22

KEY FEATURE

After a series of interruptions due to muscle problems, splint wear allowed this patient to resume his profession without further incident.

DIAGNOSIS

This patient experienced such severe tension and torn muscles with sharp leg pains while playing soccer that he stopped playing altogether. He presented with mandibular dislocation and dual bite.

THERAPY

The patient was initially given a six-point split to wear during the daytime for just 3 weeks, after which it was transformed into an SS (see page 129) to be worn at night and when playing soccer. Two months later, the SS was again modified with the addition of cuspid rise and incisal guidance features to turn it into a Michigan Plate. The patient was able to resume his normal activities with no further complaints, and after 18 months of treatment, he no longer felt the need to wear the splint. In addition to pretreatment and posttreatment records showing how the problems were eliminated, the patient's own account of the facts is included here as well.

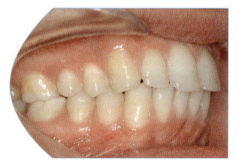 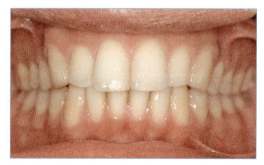 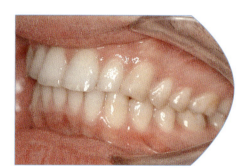

Initial situation: Dental closure in maximum intercuspation but with muscle stress.

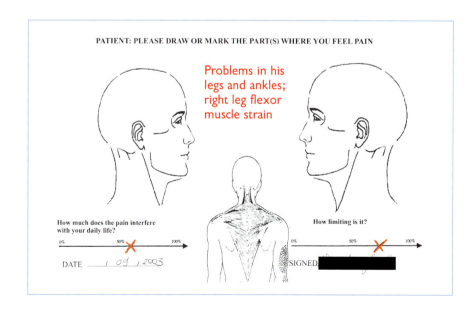

Alessandro's version

I've played soccer since the age of 6 and turned professional when I was 18. In February 2002, I had my first soccer accident with a badly sprained right ankle that had me laid up for a month with the ankle in a cast. What seemed like minor mishap turned into a series of problems.

When my ankle was better I thought I was ready for the 2002–2003 soccer season, only to have my right leg flexor tear no less than three times in 5 months between September and February. Never before having suffered muscle problems, I started treatment and a series of medical appointments to try to find out why the same leg kept having problems. I went from massage therapists to physiotherapists to chiropractors until I finally discovered that it all started in my mouth.

The problems that seemed to explode after that sprained ankle had never shown up before. Anyway, I was given a customized splint to wear at night and while training and playing because I didn't have any symptoms during my everyday life. Unbelievable as it may seem, from the day I first wore that splint in April 2003, I never had another muscle problem, and my nightmare was over. I wore my splint for a year and a half when I played, then only at night as I didn't feel I needed it so much, and finally I stopped wearing it altogether.

It is now May 2006, and I feel great.

Alessandro

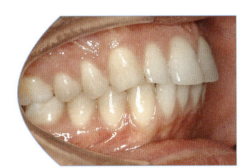 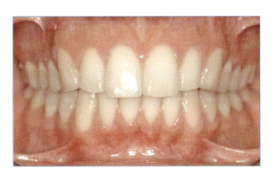 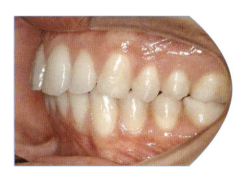

Follow-up: Minor changes in interarch relationships, especially in lateral districts.

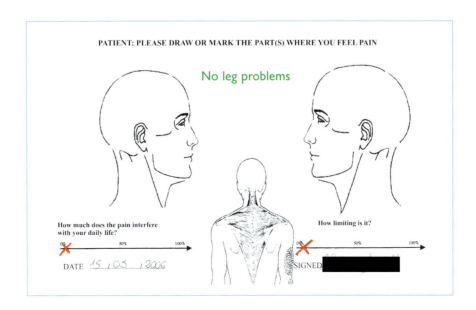

PROFESSIONAL WATER POLO PLAYER

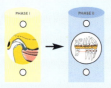

PHASE I: MUSCULOARTICULAR ARS THERAPY
followed by
PHASE II: OCCLUSAL FINISHING WITH ORTHODONTICS

KEY FEATURE: Splint wear gave the patient immediate relief with subsequent noticeable increase in her performance at the top level of her sport.
Final outcome: COMPROMISE (her mandibular left first premolar is still rotated).

Patient: F. R.	age 37	COMPROMISE

DIAGNOSIS

The patient presented with a dental Class II on the right side, deviated midlines, and bilateral transverse contraction of the maxillary arch. She had anterior crowding in the maxilla and the mandible and edge-to-edge bite between several teeth. Her mandibular excursions were limited and deviated to the right. Palpation revealed that the right condyle dislocated less and after the right.

THERAPY

An ARS was prescribed (PHASE I) until the patient had regained stability in her mandibular excursions and dental closure final contacts. The patient continued to wear the splint during orthodontic treatment (PHASE II).

PRETREATMENT RECORDS (CENTRIC OCCLUSION WITH MUSCLE TENSION)

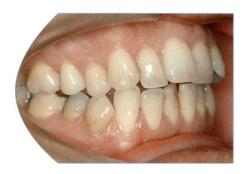
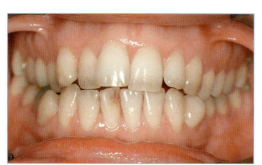
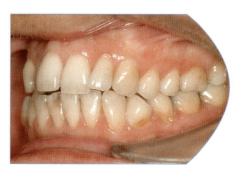

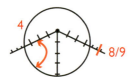

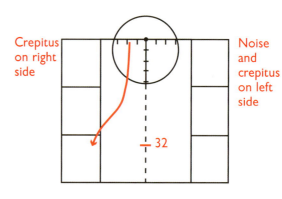

PRETREATMENT CT

Right and left closed-mouth TMJ sagittal CTs and related drawings.

RIGHT   LEFT

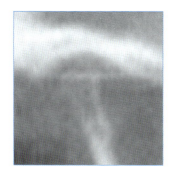
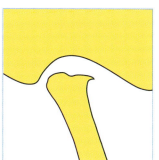
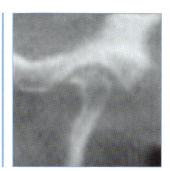
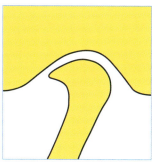

Right and left TMJ transversal TMJ CTs and related drawings.

RIGHT   LEFT

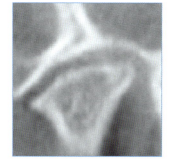
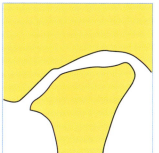
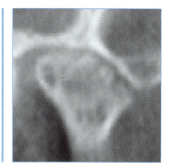
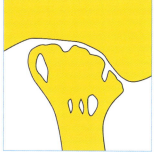

PHASE I   MUSCULOARTICULAR THERAPY

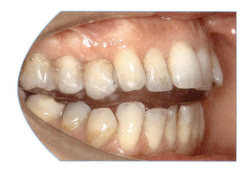
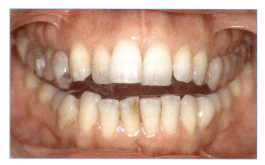
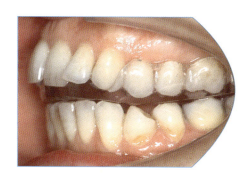

Photographs with splint fitted, showing poor dental order.

ARS worn for a total of 10 months.

PHASE II ORTHODONTIC OCCLUSAL FINISHING

A first fixed appliance was fitted in the maxillary arch, followed by another in the mandibular arch.

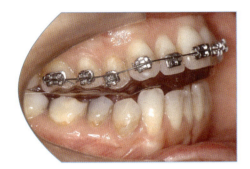 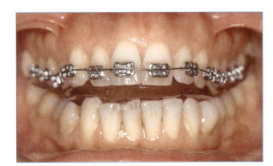 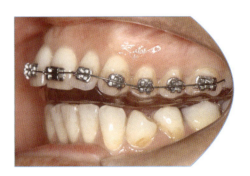

POSTTREATMENT

There is a remaining dental imperfection on the left side. This represents a compromise since it does not cause functional or esthetic alterations.

Objective improvements:
- Dynamic excursions: Opening and closure occur within normal limits
- Posttreatment CT scans: Evident improvements in both position and shape (see facing page)

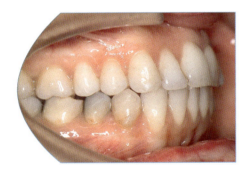 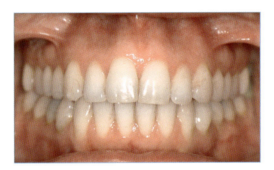 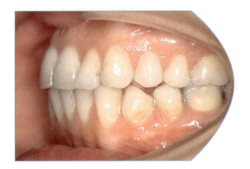

COMPARISON OF PRETREATMENT AND POSTTREATMENT DYNAMIC EXCURSIONS

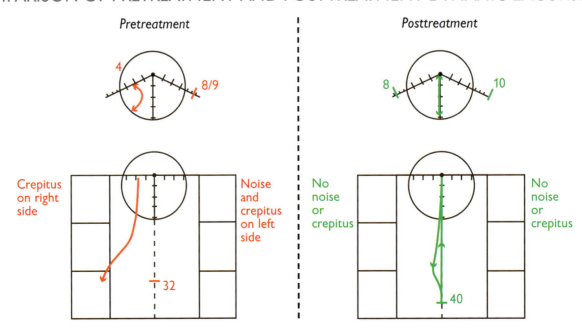

Pretreatment

Posttreatment

Crepitus on right side

Noise and crepitus on left side

No noise or crepitus

No noise or crepitus

COMPARISON OF CT SCANS

PRETREATMENT	POSTTREATMENT

Right sagittal

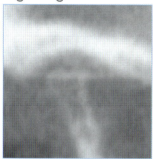 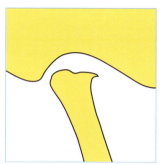 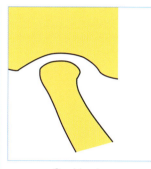 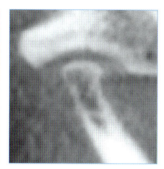

Condylar shape more regular, rounded, and centered.

Left sagittal

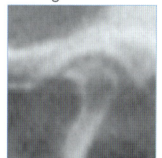 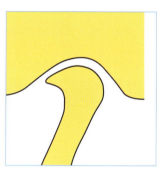 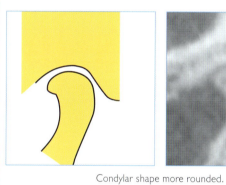 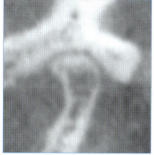

Condylar shape more rounded.

Right coronal

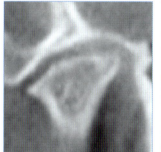 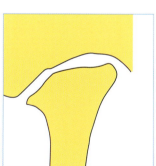 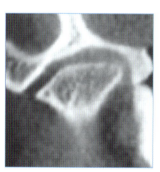

A small external bone spur remains, but the internal bone structure appears noticeably more regular.

Left coronal

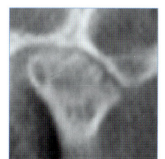 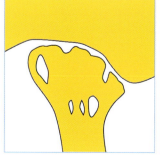 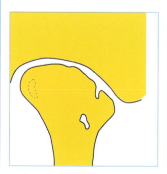 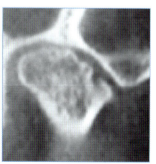

Improvement in both fossa contour and condylar osseous structure.

COMPARISON OF OROFACIAL PAIN CHARTS

PRETREATMENT

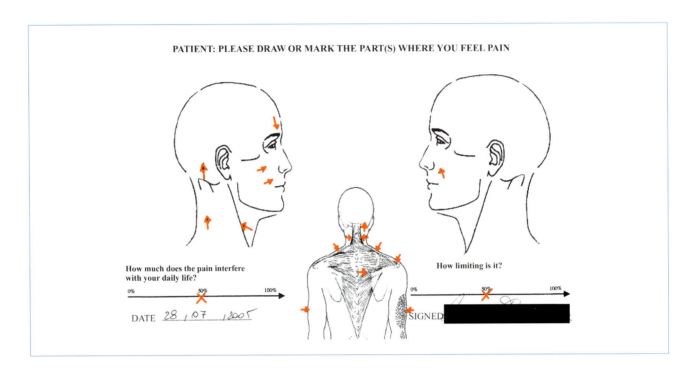

POSTTREATMENT

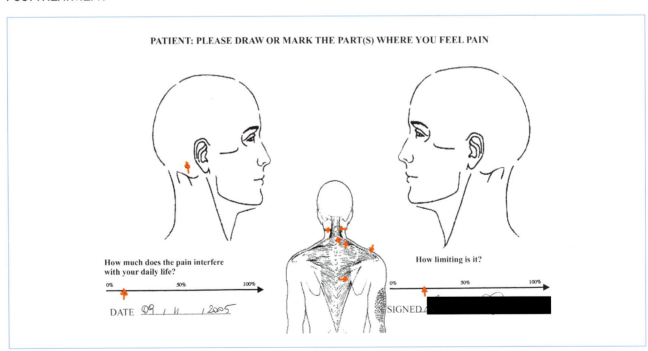

As with the account given on page 335, this patient has also commented on how her pathology was resolved and its effect on her professional life.

A SHORT HISTORY OF MY ACHES AND PAINS

I started competitive swimming at a very young age and took up water polo at 18 (4 years in division B, 10 years in division A1, 6 years in division A2). Today, in 2006, I am 38 years old. These are the health problems that arose during my career.

1994: For the first time in my life I felt really dizzy. I went to the hospital of a provincial town in Tuscany where they told me I had vertigo but were unable to ascertain the cause. However, they did exclude labyrinth problems or anything severe affecting the brain. I did water polo training 3 hours per day, 5 days per week, and took part in the division A1 championship.

1995 to 1996: More bad attacks of vertigo. A hospital in a coastal town admitted me for tests that lasted a week, at the end of which I was told there was nothing wrong with my labyrinth, central nervous system, or cervical spine. But no diagnosis. I was then on the National Water Polo Team, training 6 hours per day, 6 days per week, and taking part in the division A1 championship.

1996 to 2003: My vertigo attacks were more and more frequent. I was seen by two leading orthopedic specialists, neither of whom understood the cause. It was suggested that there could be a connection with my sport due to neck trauma and strain to my right shoulder, which in the meantime had become so painful that I could no longer swim freestyle properly or throw the ball hard. I started to get bad headaches and pain in my muscles of mastication, trapezius, and right sternocleidomastoid muscles. I had to reduce training to 2 hours per day, 5 days a week, and go down a category into division A2 (in 2000) because I could not make full use of my right shoulder or move my neck properly.

2004: The vertigo and headaches were making my life a misery. They were really frequent (4 to 5 times a

week) and excruciatingly painful. I was seen by another famous orthopedic specialist who prescribed magnetic resonance, ultrasound scans, and dynamic cervical spine radiography, none of which revealed anything important (no osseous morpho-functional alterations, slight initial metameric rigidity on hyperflexion). He recommended a physiotherapist, but my problems did not go away. I went back to Tuscany where I was examined by another orthopedic specialist and a physician whose only findings are enlarged lymph nodes in my neck, both left and right sides (laterocervical and posterocervical lymphadenomegaly, of hyperplastic reactive aspect; no musculotendinous alterations), indicating inflammation. I trained even less than before, but the problems persisted through the summer, even when we take a break from training.

2005: The National Water Polo Team had a new physiotherapist, who examined me and found that I had badly tensed masticatory muscles, right sternocleidomastoid, and trapezius muscles, with areas of major contracture. She recommended a specialist in temporomandibular disorders who is also an orthodontist. After thorough examination and tests, he told me I have seriously damaged temporomandibular joints with considerable bone loss and gave me a splint to correct the joint structures and improve muscle tone prior to fitting fixed appliances to correct my dental interrelationships. I started by wearing the splint religiously. After 1 week, my headaches went away, and after another week, I no longer suffered from vertigo. I was able to train more frequently, although my right shoulder and neck still hurt.

May 2006: My vertigo and headaches have disappeared. There is still a bit of tension in my right sternocleidomastoid, which is a little tender, and in my trapezius. Instead of swallowing Nimesulide (Helsinn Healthcare) and painkillers, I now wear a splint. At the age of 38, I can get into the pool and swim 50 meters freestyle in times I hadn't made since I was 18. My arms and shoulders are much stronger, even if my right shoulder still hurts when I play. Needless to say, I wear my splint when I train and compete.

Francesca

CONSIDERATIONS ON COMPROMISES

Even the most careful attempts to repair damage may not be 100% successful, and a compromise may have to be accepted, meaning that each party has to give way a little. In other words, a good outcome may mean considerable improvement, albeit with minor incongruencies that in practical terms do not detract from the overall success. It may be that the clinician is unable to completely satisfy the many requirements presented by the case in question or the patient is unwilling to pursue treatment beyond certain limits of time and commitment or there are individual anatomical and functional limits.

Compromises may be:

- *Acceptable though debatable:* Dental relationships may show a complete Class II (or even a complete Class III) with simultaneous terminal contacts on closing but without static or dynamic muscle tension even though incisal guidance may be completely lacking.

- *Unacceptable:* No orthodontic treatment may be concluded if the patient presents with dislocation in the final stages of closure (dual bite) or incorrectly correlated teeth and muscles that generate muscle tension and pain and may cause further deterioration of the pathology.

Clearly, a compromise is never an objective to aim for, yet for various reasons it may be necessary. Without these cautious considerations and all the limitations they imply, this book would be incomplete. When addressing clinicians who deal with patients every day, it would be unrealistic to deny the compromises that occur in every practice despite the practitioner's most painstaking efforts and care.

WHIPLASH-ASSOCIATED DISORDERS

A whiplash injury following a sudden distortion of the neck is considered a mechanism of traumatic hyperflexion and hyperextension of the cervicofacial region. The trauma may cause damage of varying degrees to the musculoarticular structures of the TMJs, with dislocation of the disc and ligamentous distraction. Other pathologies, including those affecting the spine, are not addressed in this work except as part of a differential diagnosis.

Damage to the relationships between condyle, disc, and articulating surface may affect one or more components in a number of different ways and conditions. A careful clinical examination may help establish the diagnosis and differential diagnosis with other pathologies. Since there may be very subtle differences, it is essential to seek accurate information with CT and, more importantly, with MRI.

If used properly, **manipulation** (see pages 72 to 82) can be of primary importance in reestablishing correct axial alignment among the various joint structures, thereby improving muscle tone and relieving pain. The patient will almost always require an ARS to ensure that the suddenly deranged parts are held in place for as long as necessary to guarantee healing.

Choosing among manipulation techniques is not easy, and the clinician must select the most suitable for each individual case. When in doubt, it is advisable to start with the simplest. Many whiplash cases exhibit severe functional damage and require complex treatment, especially for patients affected by ligamentous laxity. (See ARS adaptation B, pages 350 and 406.)

V. CLINICAL CASE STUDIES WITH COMPROMISE OUTCOMES

VIRTUAL EXAMPLE OF WHIPLASH THERAPY: UNDERLYING LIGAMENTOUS LAXITY

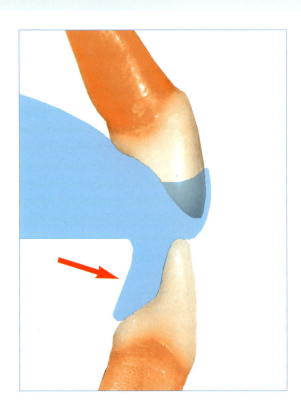

MUSCULOARTICULAR THERAPY

TRADITIONAL SPLINT WITH ANTERIOR FLANGE TO STIMULATE CONDYLAR AND MANDIBULAR ADVANCE

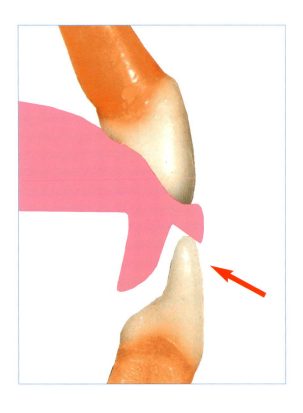

WHIPLASH THERAPY

CUSTOMIZED SPLINT TO RETRUDE THE CONDYLES AND MANDIBLE

The mandible slides against the oblique plane of the splint.

TRADITIONAL MUSCULOARTICULAR THERAPY
SPLINT WITH ANTERIOR FLANGE TO STIMULATE CONDYLAR AND MANDIBULAR
ADVANCE

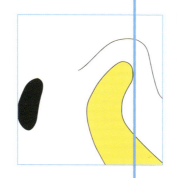

I. Pathologic pretreatment situation: Condyle posteriorized.

CONDYLAR ADVANCE

II. After hypothetical phase I (musculoarticular therapy): Functional efficiency is reached.

WHIPLASH THERAPY
CUSTOMIZED SPLINT TO RETRUDE CONDYLES AND MANDIBLE

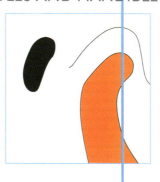

III. Theoretical whiplash causing a return to a pathologic state: Condyle anteriorized.

CONDYLAR RETRUSION

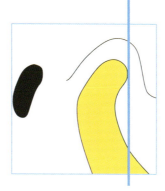

IV. After hypothetical new phase I with ARS modified with retaining anterior flange: Functional efficiency regained.

THREE CONSECUTIVE WHIPLASH INJURIES

KEY FEATURE: POSITIVE RESULTS WERE OBTAINED AFTER THE FIRST TWO INJURIES, BUT A MORE DUBIOUS OUTCOME FOLLOWED THE THIRD INJURY

Patient: C. T., age 29
Joint instability with ligamentous laxity

FIRST WHIPLASH: November 27, 2004

Type of impact: The patient was sitting upright in the driver's seat. She had momentarily stopped her car when it was rear-ended hard.

On examination
THE PATIENT HAD ACUTE PAIN.
IMMEDIATE MANIPULATION
Carrying out tests would have delayed the pain relief immediately provided by the manipulation techniques.

Benefit
Subjective: The patient felt much better.
Objective: The patient's examination results were within normal ranges with the exception of excessive opening excursions.

Because of her considerable ligamentous laxity, the patient was advised to limit her opening movements. The patient's situation returned to normal without other particular problems.

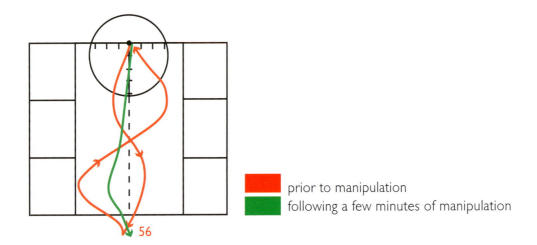

prior to manipulation
following a few minutes of manipulation

56

SECOND WHIPLASH INJURY, FEBRUARY 9, 2005 (APPROXIMATELY 3 MONTHS AFTER THE PREVIOUS ACCIDENT)

Type of impact: The patient was sitting in the passenger seat with her head turned to the right when the car was struck by another vehicle with a hard impact on the rear left side. At her second examination, the patient was seen to have altered excursions; however, these were less pronounced than on the previous occasion.

Traditional manipulation again gave subjective and objective improvement.

This time, although the whiplash did not appear to have caused as much damage as on the previous occasion, the patient was advised to be extremely cautious in opening her jaws and to do so as little as possible because of her severe ligamentous laxity. Given her determination and compliance, it was considered acceptable not to prescribe a therapeutic splint, especially since her profession as television host would have suffered.

THIRD WHIPLASH INJURY: MAY 27, 2006

Type of impact: **The patient was involved in another rear-end collision**. She presented at the office wearing a soft collar fitted at the hospital. The rear neck pain she had suffered from prior to the accident had moved to the right side of her neck near the shoulder, and she now had lower back pain.

The patient was fitted with an ARS, after which she felt immediately better, even after removing the collar, since her dental contacts improved. Her physician recommended various forms of medication that gave temporary relief. She went for relaxation and postural physiotherapy and had custom orthotic insoles made.

Of all the forms of treatment, the patient's ARS gave highly satisfactory results including **significant relief.** Unfortunately, her profession prevented her from wearing it as often as it should be. After several months,

she felt better and stopped wearing the splint. The pain in her neck and arm had disappeared, and throughout the entire summer and autumn she experienced only occasional muscle stiffness, which medication solved. Regular swimming improved her overall fitness and gave greater muscle relaxation and tone, partially compensating for the consequences of her sedentary lifestyle during an 8-hour working day. The patient sensibly used an adjustable height chair with good back support.

After some months in an acceptable condition, the patient's situation **deteriorated subjectively** and objectively. She suffered frequent attacks of intense throbbing pain in her neck, especially at the base, and in her face, where the pain was worst near the TMJs. No apparent reason was found for the symptoms although it was observed that she was more prone to the attacks in cold, damp weather and when menstruating. The patient attempted to cure her symptoms with muscle relaxants and pain relief medication but without success. The pain became more acute in the following months. She was careful not to open her jaws more than 20 to 22 mm as advised from the start.

After a series of postural therapy treatments, the patient decided to resume splint therapy, which resulted in a better response to arm movements and a definite overall improvement. The pain still returned at times but in a less intense and more bearable manner.

A groove was made in the patient's ARS to retain her mandibular anterior teeth and stabilize the mandibular position (see adaptation "B," page 350). As a result, the pain in the base and upper nape of her neck almost completely disappeared. She took medication just once more, unlike the previous months during which she had regularly been taking pain relief medication.

The success of this new splint was confirmed by an absence of the acute pain the patient had previously suffered from. Even potentially critical factors such as a change in mattress, unavailability of an orthopedic pillow, or long, tiring journey causing unnatural and uncomfortable positions did not trigger the pain.

PRETREATMENT CT PRIOR TO MANIPULATION (SEPTEMBER 2005) (MAJOR LIGAMENTOUS LAXITY)

Right side: Open mouth

Complete CT series

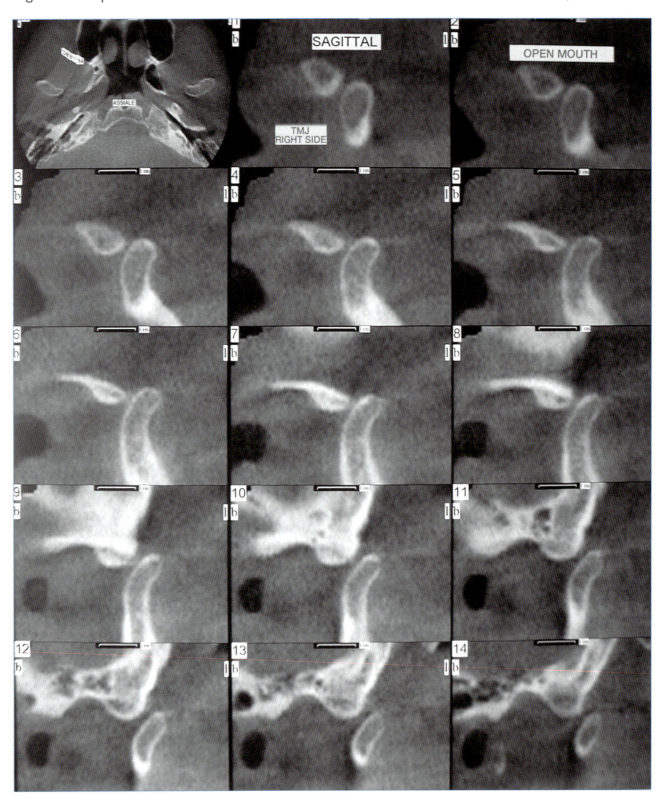

PRETREATMENT CT FOLLOWING MANIPULATION (SEPTEMBER 2005) MAJOR LIGAMENTOUS LAXITY

Left side, open mouth

Complete CT series

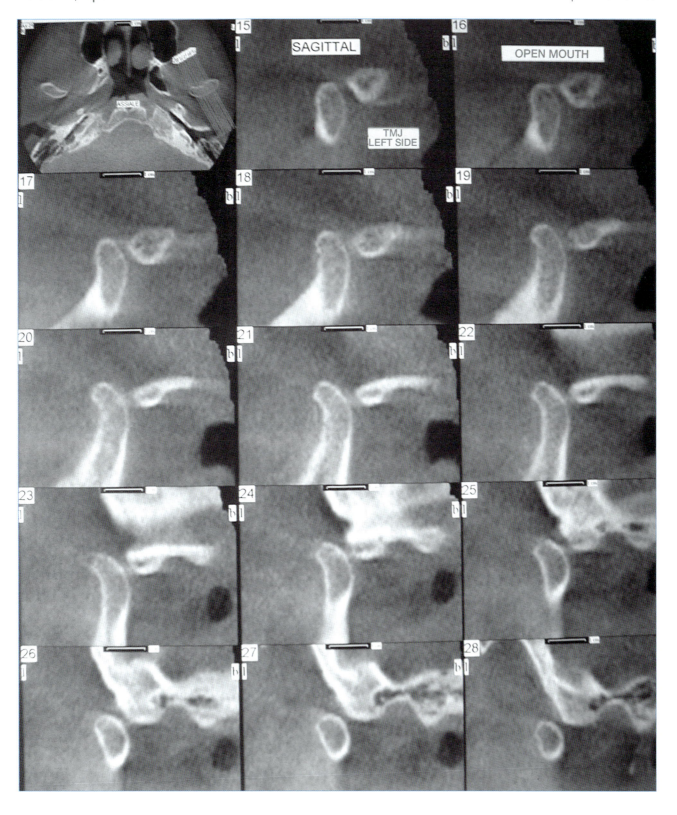

As stated previously on several occasions, ligamentous laxity may contribute to musculoarticular pathology. Where this condition is combined with whiplash, the pathology is likely to be serious, especially if the trauma occurs repeatedly as it did for this patient who suffered three whiplash injuries in little more than a year. Although the complex therapy based on an ARS integrated with medication and psychotherapy gave some benefit, her problem was not entirely solved.

A patient with ligamentous laxity must first of all be advised to limit mouth opening to not more than 20 to 22 mm. This advice is sufficient in a good percentage of mild cases at helping patients to avoid pain.

Nevertheless, the basis of treatment remains that of limiting mandibular excursions on all three spatial planes, the opening movement being the most frequent. This requirement is addressed by a custom ARS with a horizontal groove for the mandibular anterior teeth and

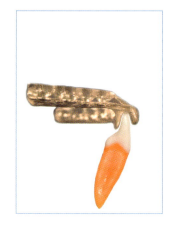
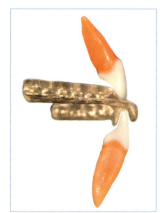

with the traditional lingual flange integrated with a buccal flange giving greater mandibular stability in even the smallest movements (**see ARS adaptation "B," mandibular stability splint, page 406**). Wearing this version of the splint gave the patient noticeable relief of her symptoms.

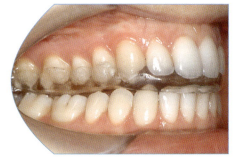
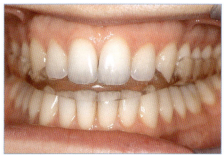
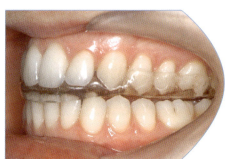
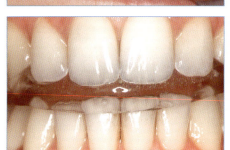

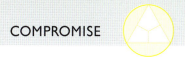

PHASE I ONLY: SPLINT WORN INDEFINITELY

KEY FEATURES:
- The invalidating nature of the pathology, which had persisted for years.
- The extreme simplicity with which immediate relief was given, and which lasted long-term.
- The fact that the treatment plan was not completed, with the case consequently coming under the category of "COMPROMISE" outcomes.

Patient: M. G.	age 54	COMPROMISE

PATIENT HISTORY

The patient came to the office with a friend because she felt unable to face the journey alone. She complained of violent head pain affecting the left side of her face. She had difficulty in opening her mouth, had almost abandoned social interaction, and was unable to teach singing as she had previously done. She spent most of her time in a dark room because light was painful for her.

The patient was disappointed that numerous consultations had failed to provide satisfactory treatment, and she had been advised not to open her mouth to avoid making matters worse.

She drew a pension on the grounds that her pathology was officially recognized as permanently debilitating.

Following her anamnesis, the patient was examined under the standard new patient procedure. The most significant findings were that her maximum mouth opening was limited to a mere 25 mm and there was obvious mandibular deviation to the left by several millimeters.

Full tests were required to complete the assessment of her condition although the new patient clinical examination was sufficient to reasonably suspect left TMJ lock. The patient was in such pain that she requested immediate help by any means possible. Mandibular manipulation (see page 78 onward) was proposed and accepted even though this meant there would be a lack of records documenting the true pretreatment situation. The manipulation was highly successful with the patient feeling a noticeable reduction in her widespread pain. Her maximum mouth opening increased to 38 mm while her deviation to the left was reduced to a mere 2 mm.

An ARS was fabricated in a matter of hours. Tinted acrylic was added to the left side to distract the compressed condyle significantly and hold it well away from the fossa in a stable manner. To reduce treatment time, orthodontic occlusal finishing orthodontic was started just a few weeks later starting with the mandibular arch, which was in worse condition than the maxilla.

After 6 months, the patient opted not to follow the entire treatment plan proposed, which should have included prosthodontic work. She was given a splint to wear indefinitely. Consequently, the case was reluctantly closed as a less-than-perfect compromise.

PRETREATMENT RECORDS

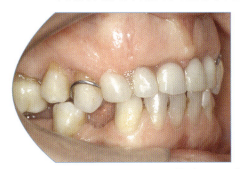

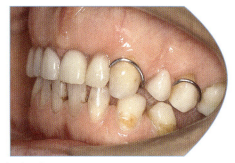

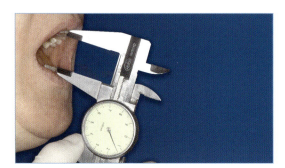

Teeth missing from both arches.

Maximum mouth opening, 25 mm.

PHASE I: ARS MUSCULOARTICULAR THERAPY

A wedge was added to the ARS on the left side to distract the more seriously damaged left condyle.

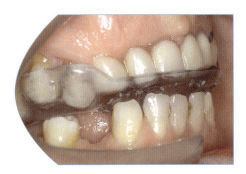

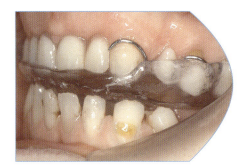

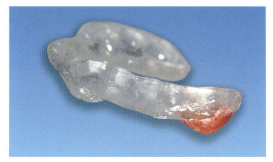

Tinted acrylic wedge.

START OF PHASE II: ORTHODONTIC OCCLUSAL FINISHING

A fixed appliance was bonded to the mandibular arch, which required more correction. After a few months, however, the patient decided she was unable to continue the treatment.

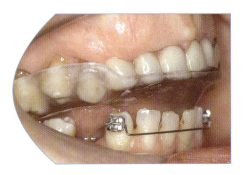

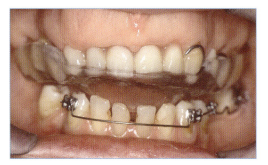

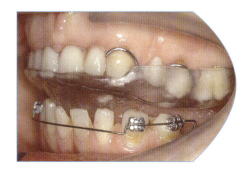

Initial orthodontic treatment of the mandibular arch.

The treatment applied brought about significant functional changes and enabled the patient to resume her normal life. Unfortunately, she chose not to finalize the result with complete orthodontic treatment and prosthodontics but chose instead to wear a splint indefinitely.

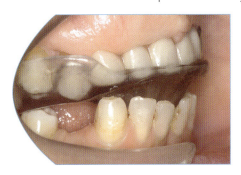

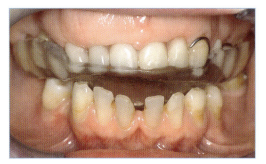

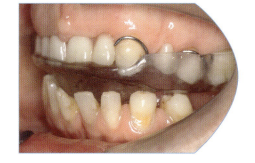

Treatment interrupted.

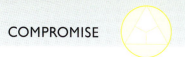

COMPARISON

BEFORE	AFTER
(not a real pretreatment situation since a first treatment with manipulation had already been carried out)	*(at the start of the orthodontic finishing stage, which was almost immediately interrupted) (approximately 9 months later)*

Left side open mouth tomograms

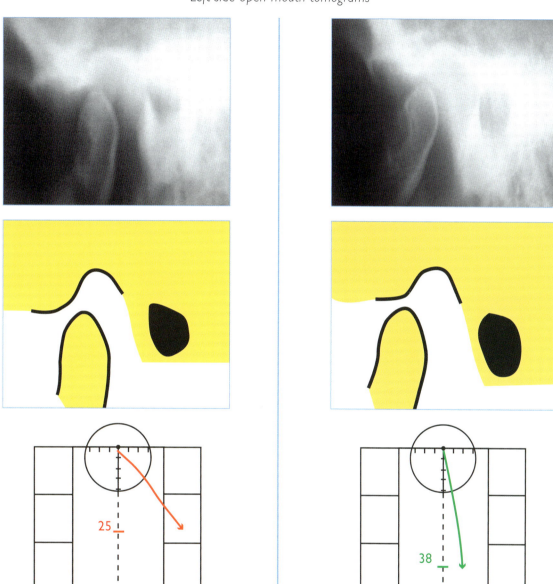

Since the patient declined full treatment, a splint is applied "for indefinite wear."

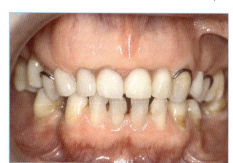

Before.

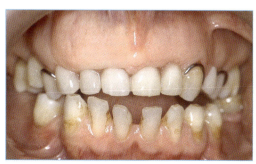

After ARS wear.

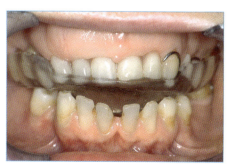

With the splint.

PHASE I: MUSCULOARTICULAR SS THERAPY
PHASE II: DENTURES FITTED WITHOUT ORTHODONTIC FINISHING

KEY FEATURES: TMJ therapy with SS and wedges were added to temporary partial dentures to hold and maintain the therapeutic position. The patient's refusal to go through with orthodontic occlusal finishing made it necessary to conclude the case with the partial dentures, as a compromise outcome.

Patient: L. S.	age 42	COMPROMISE

(Treated by Dr Pietro Petroni)

DIAGNOSIS

The patient presented following an automobile accident injury. He complained of TMJ pain, predominantly on the right side, with widespread headache and neck pain. The patient had dental and skeletal Class II with deep bite, reduced vertical height, and some missing teeth.

His mandibular excursions were deviated in all three spatial planes, and he had noise and clicks on the right side when opening. His closed-mouth, right-side MRI showed the condyle to be posteriorized with consequent discal dislocation.

PROCEDURE

Treatment with an all-point split (SS) to reduce muscle tension and increase vertical height yielded positive results. After approximately 3 months, not only had the patient's symptoms almost disappeared but also his mandible had slid forward, the joint noise was no longer heard on auscultation, and his opening and closing movements had returned to normal. However, it was obvious that his mandibular position could not remain stable.

An orthodontic treatment plan was created with the aim of leveling and aligning the dental arches, opening the bite, creating satisfactory incisal guidance, and preparing correct spaces for subsequent prosthodontic work. The patient initially agreed to the treatment plan but later changed his mind and refused orthodontic treatment on personal grounds.

It was decided to accept a dental compromise but to proceed with articular treatment.

The condylar and mandibular positions were checked with MRI. To do this, the patient was given two removable temporary partial dentures without metal clasps but with posterior wedges to maintain the position given by the initial splint. The MRI response was positive. The right condyle had moved forward and downward, and the condyle-disc fossa relationships also appeared to be within normal limits. The patient was sent on to the prosthodontist for his definitive removable partial dentures, which were designed to maintain therapeutic position.

PRETREATMENT RECORDS

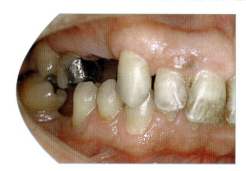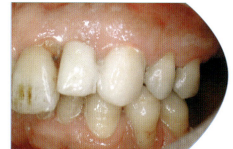

MRI, right side   *MRI, left side*

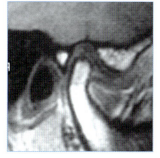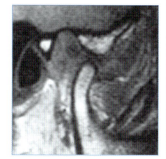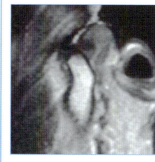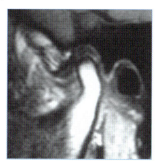

Mouth closed.   Mouth open.   Mouth open.   Mouth closed.

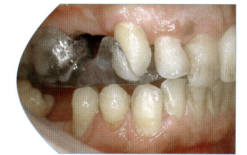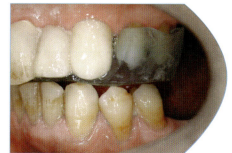

Application of the SS.

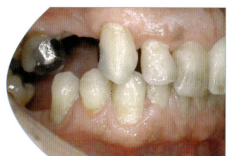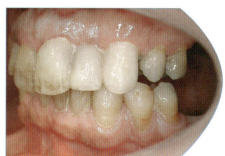

Note how the patient spontaneously slides his mandible forward.

Two metal-free removable partial dentures were fabricated for the purpose of:

- Maintaining the therapeutic position reached with the splint
- Improving the patient's comfort
- Being able to keep them for the follow-up MRI

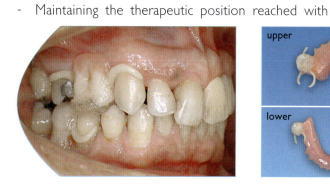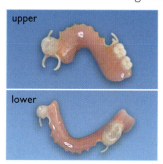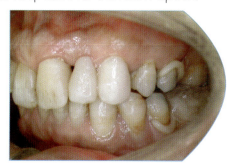

upper

lower

MRI with removable partial dentures: Position prior to definitive finishing with dentures, as compromise outcome.

MRI, right side

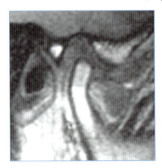
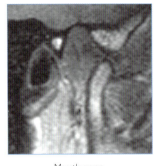

Mouth closed.   Mouth open.

MRI, left side

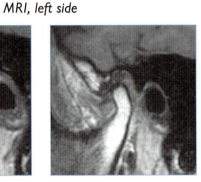

Mouth open.   Mouth closed.

Compared with his initial situation, the patient demonstrated evident clinical and symptomatologic improvement, which was confirmed by the MRI results.

The patient was referred to the prosthodontist for his definitive dentures, which are to maintain therapeutic position.

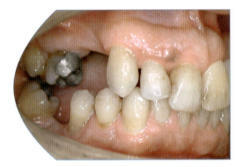
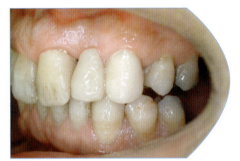

The prosthodontist was given the therapeutic position for the preparation of permanent dentures.

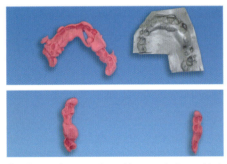
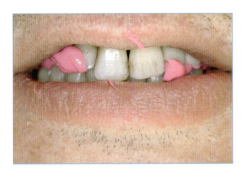

One impression was taken with a wax similar to Alminax (Kemdent) and another with silicone. More silicone was used to register the position of the arches separately so that they could be used alone.

POSTTREATMENT RECORDS

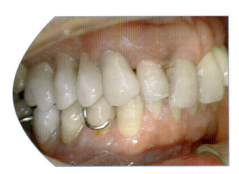
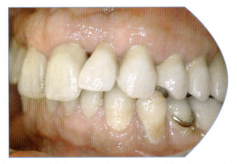

Dr Serena Ferrara, an external specialist, completed the case with a removable lower partial denture and fixed upper denture.

COMPARISONS

PRETREATMENT	POSTTREATMENT

Right side

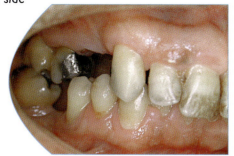 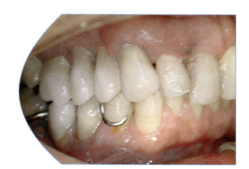

Left side

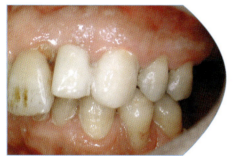 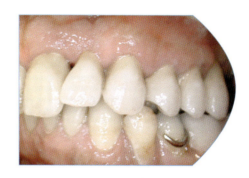

Right side, closed mouth

PRETREATMENT	POSTTREATMENT

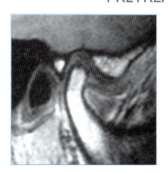 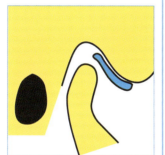 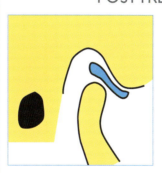 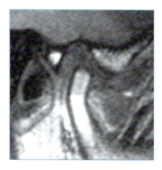

Left side, closed mouth

PRETREATMENT	POSTTREATMENT

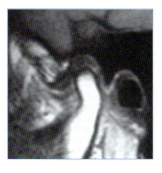 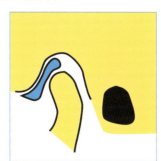 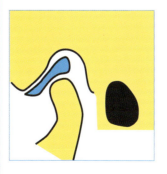 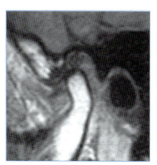

Observe the change in position within the two TMJs. Particularly in the right TMJ, the condyle is definitely further downward and forward, giving improved condylar-disc-articulating surface alignment.

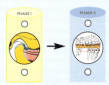

COMPROMISE (ALSO IN YOUNG PATIENTS)
PHASE I AND PHASE II

KEY FEATURES:
EXCELLENT MUSCULOARTICULAR RECOVERY
(WITH CONDYLAR REMODELING)
DENTAL COMPROMISE: SURGERY NOT ACCEPTED
(teeth require further work including orthodontics once the patient has finished growing)

THERAPEUTIC PROCEDURE

This young girl arrived at the office in tears complaining of acute widespread pain in her head, neck, and whole body. Loud clicks came from the left condyle, and considerable ligamentous laxity was noted.

1) At the first appointment, the patient was immediately given manipulation, which provided instant relief, significant pain reduction, and improved function.
2) ARS therapy (PHASE I).
3) While continuing splint wear continuing, the patient was treated simultaneously with fixed appliances (PHASE II: occlusal finishing).
4) Results: Condylar remodelling occurred, and mandibular dynamics returned to near normal. The pain completely disappeared. The family did not accept the maxillary surgery recommended to correct the patient's skeletal and dental discrepancies and consequently to help her esthetics.
5) The problem remains of how to prepare for subsequent prosthodontics in the edentulous area.

Patient: I. R.	age 13	CORRECTED, DENTAL COMPROMISE

DIAGNOSIS

The patient presented with a severe Class II with deep bite and an inexplicable loss of the left mandibular second premolar and first molar. She had a short upper lip that aggravated her overjet. The most immediate problem however was TMJ lock and pain.

Immediate manipulation eliminated the TMJ lock and increased her maximum mouth opening from 22 to 43 mm. All mandibular excursions were improved, and much of the pain was eliminated. An ARS prepared and fitted later on the same day contributed to improved therapeutic movements. Some months later, fixed appliances were fitted for occlusal finishing, although the case remained a debatable compromise.

PRETREATMENT RECORDS

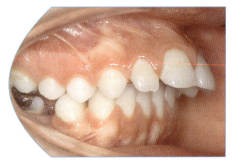
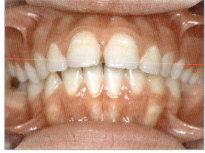
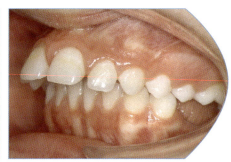
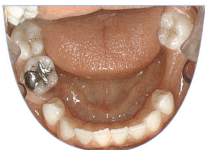

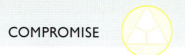

PRETREATMENT RECORDS

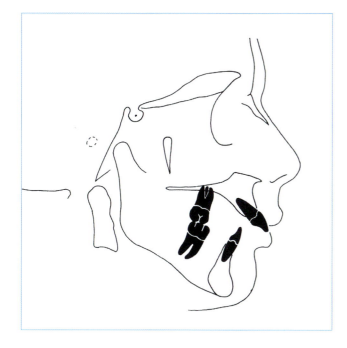

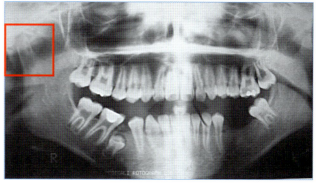

Pretreatment cephalogram outline and OPT.

Detail of pretreatment OPT, right side: Large "crater" below condylar apex.

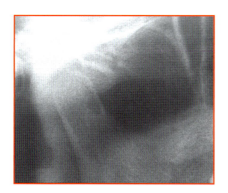

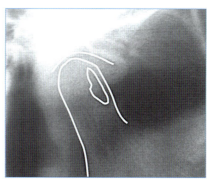

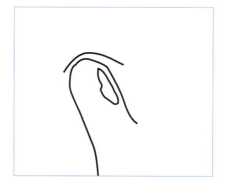

PRETREATMENT DYNAMIC EXCURSIONS

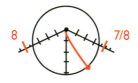

8   7/8

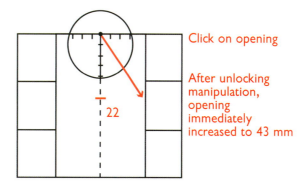

Click on opening

After unlocking manipulation, opening immediately increased to 43 mm

22

PHASE I: MUSCULOARTICULAR THERAPY
An ARS was fitted.

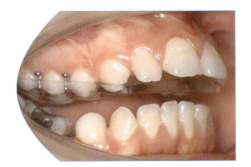 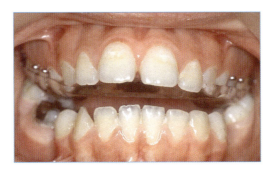 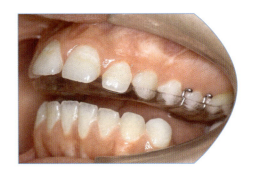

PHASE II: ORTHODONTIC OCCLUSAL FINISHING

After 8 months, all the mandibular teeth were banded since this arch required greater correction. The left side was badly collapsed, and a more logical arch shape was needed in all three spatial planes. On the right side, the impacted 4.5 was recovered while overall mandibular advance contributed not only to improving the patient's looks but also toward partial correction of her skeletal Class II.

After 12 months of treatment the patient was able to open her mouth 50 mm, indicating a ligamentous laxity that had probably contributed to her pathology.

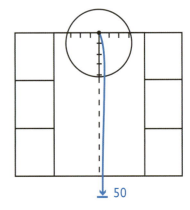

After 16 months, the patient was given a new ARS with a central expansion screw. Observe the incorrect way in which the patient closes her mouth in these photographs.

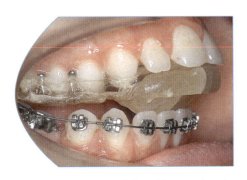 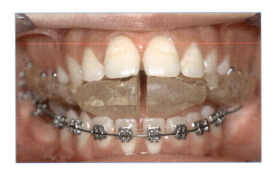 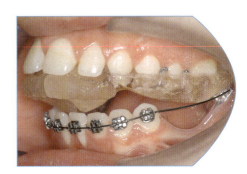

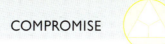

Bands and brackets were fitted in the lateral maxillary districts with a utility archwire to provide bilateral expansion through reciprocating areas of anchorage and movement. Extrusion of 3.7 continued.

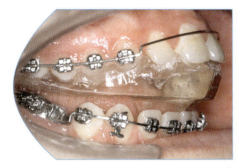
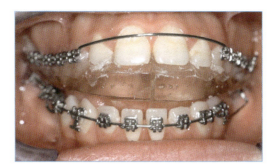
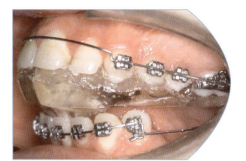

Particularly bulky splint and orthodontic appliances were worn simultaneously.

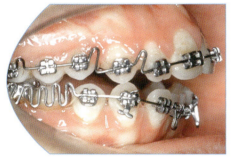
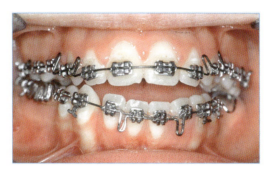
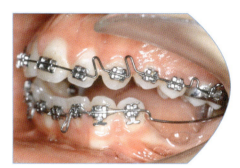

Brackets were bonded to the maxillary anterior teeth to add to the treatment by closing the patient's bite.

The patient continued to wear the splint, and it was progressively adapted for the various tooth movements. After 30 months, the maxillary appliance was completed by bracketing the anterior teeth to retract them.

To control tooth movements, the progressive elimination of acrylic was combined with archwire activation. As a result, interarch relationships gradually improved and came closer and closer to the consistent muscle-led closure which was the ultimate goal of treatment.

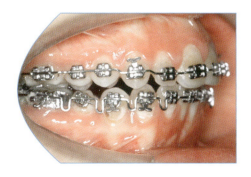
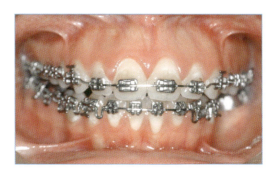
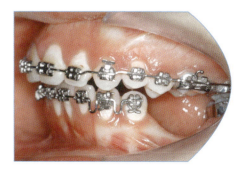

After 36 months, the posterior teeth were properly aligned and extruded, which noticeably improved both the curve of Spee and the skeletal relationships between maxilla and mandible.

TEMPORARY POSTTREATMENT RECORDS

This treatment represents a compromise in dental terms. There was no compromise regarding the TMJs; both anatomical and functional recovery were achieved.

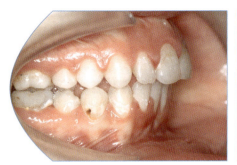
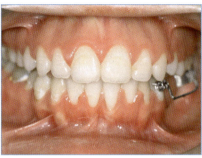
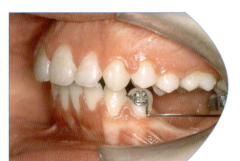
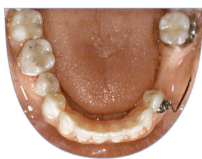

POSTTREATMENT DYNAMIC EXCURSIONS

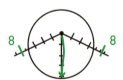
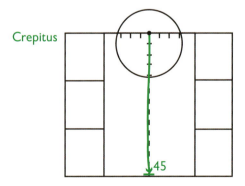

A further ARS was fabricated to maintain the results achieved up to this point—that is, elimination of the terrible pretreatment pain and correct articular alignment. Since the patient's skeletal and dental relationships remain Class II, it is to be hoped that the logical solution of surgery may be accepted later. Failing that, the alternative will be to proceed with further orthodontic treatment, seeing the results already achieved. This should commence at least 1 year prior to prosthodontic work on the edentulous area so that the complex series of procedures put into practice over the years can be completed at the same time and in the best possible manner.

POSTTREATMENT RECORDS

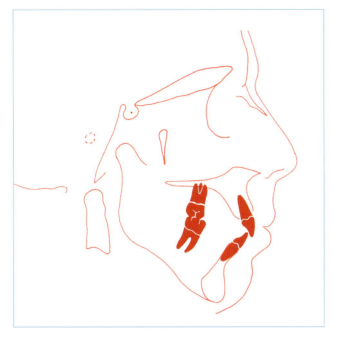

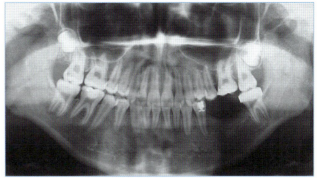

Posttreatment cephalogram outline and OPT.

Posttreatment closed-mouth, right-side CT scan: NO MUSCULOARTICULAR COMPROMISE.
The pretreatment crater has been completely filled in.

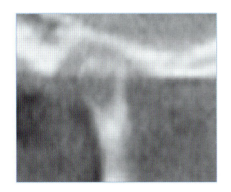

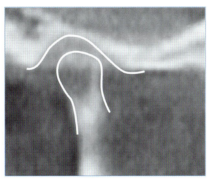

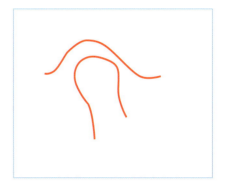

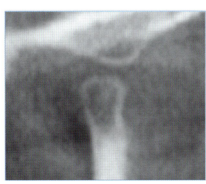

Open-mouth, right-side CT scan. Note the acceptable condylar excursion.

The case will be completed once the patient has finished growing.

COMPARISONS

PRETREATMENT	POSTTREATMENT

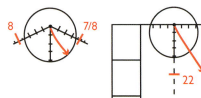
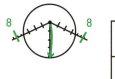
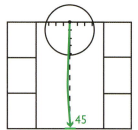

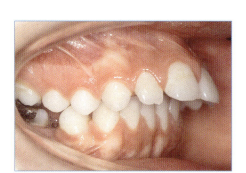
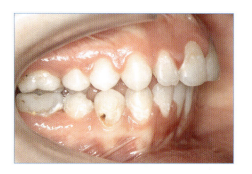

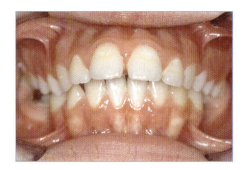
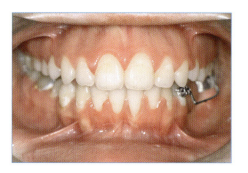

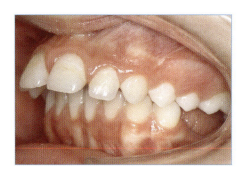
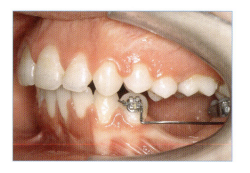

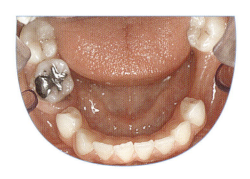
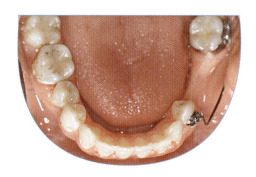

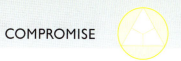

COMPARISON OF RIGHT CONDYLE PRE- AND POSTTREATMENT

Although the comparison is made between two different types of radiography (pretreatment OPT and posttreatment CT), disappearance of the crater is undeniable.

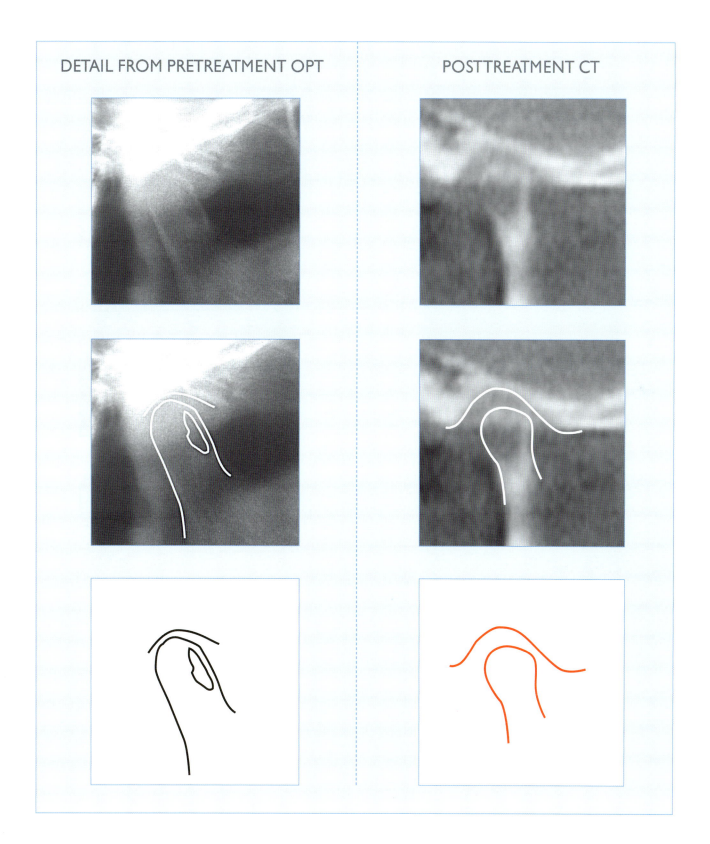

DETAIL FROM PRETREATMENT OPT

POSTTREATMENT CT

REFERENCES

1. Tsukiyama T, Kazuyoshi B, Glenn TC. An evidence-based assessment of occlusal adjustment as a treatment for temporomandibular disorders. J Prosthet Dent 2001;86:57–66.
2. Farrar WB. Differentiation of temporomandibular joint dysfunction to simplify treatment. J Prosthet Dent 1972;28:629–636.
3. Gianelly A. Evidence-based therapy: An orthodontic dilemma. Am J Orthod Dentofacial Orthop 2006;129:596–598.
4. Luhr HG, Schauer W, Jager A, Kubein-Meesenburg D. Changes in the shape of the mandible by orthodontic surgical technics with stable fixation of the segments [in German]. Fortschr Kieferorthop 1986;47:39–47.
5. Luhr HG, Kubein-Meesenburg D. Rigid skeletal fixation in maxillary osteotomies. Intraoperative control of condylar position. Clin Plast Surg 1989;16:157–163.

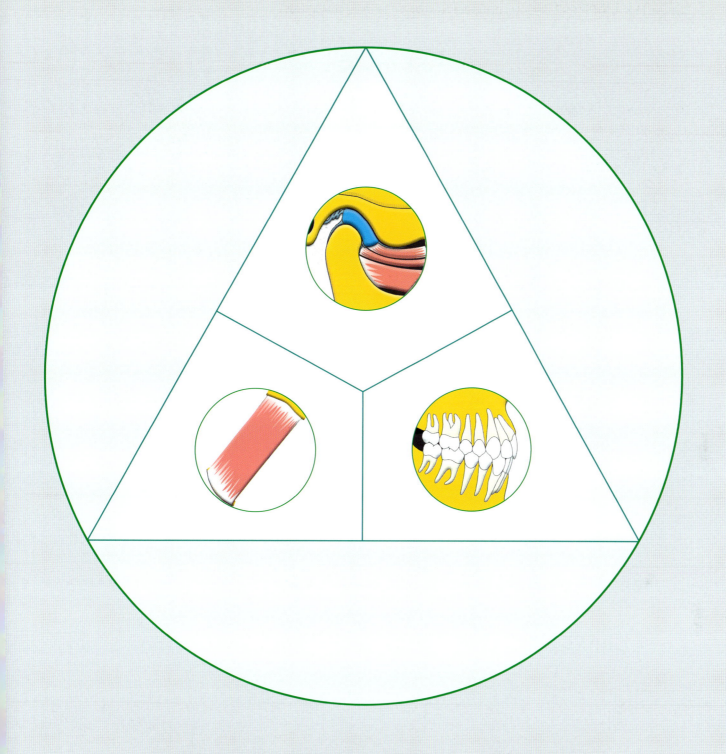

CHILDREN AND TEMPOROMANDIBULAR DISORDERS

Damage to teeth, muscles, and temporomandibular joints (TMJs) is not limited to adults but may be found in children and teenagers as well. Anatomical and functional alterations similar or identical to those seen in adults are frequently observed even in very young patients and equally affect different parts of the apparatus. Muscular problems resulting in unprovoked tension, pain, or discomfort on palpation are prevalent. They may be caused by medical pathology or dental situations such as missing incisal guidance, open bite, monolateral or bilateral crossbites, and deep bite. Altered anatomical shapes and interrelationships of articular structures—the result of excessive pressure on organs that are not yet fully developed—occur less frequently. As in all areas of medicine, early assessment of the damage is critical in establishing effective prevention.

When examining a child, it is advisable to use the same record charts and diagnostic procedures used with adults:

- Take a complete case history. In particular, investigate trauma to the head, mandible, and anterior jaw, and note any tooth fracture and scars, even from accidents that occurred years earlier. It is not uncommon, for instance, for an 8-year-old patient to show signs of an accident that that took place when she or he was 2.
- Check for mandibular excursions that may indicate limitations and/or alterations.
- Palpate the muscles of mastication. Pay particular attention to the external pterygoid area and the muscles of posture. Legs of a differing length are frequently observed in patients with crossbite on one side.
- Look for habits indicating the presence of any factors detrimental to a correct anatomy.

Case studies

Manipulation eliminating pathologic symptoms, including clicks, in three-dimensional mandibular excursions:
Patient: G. L., age 10   page 370

Dislocation of the disc with recapture achieved via an anterior repositioning splint (ARS):
Patient: S. F., age 9   page 372

Single TMJ lock:
Patient: F. D., age 10   page 374

Conditioning of growth in a very young patient:
Patient: A. T., age 3 years 6 months   page 376

Treating a damaged condylar head in two phases with articular remodeling, improved excursions, and resolution of Class II malocclusion:
Patient: D. O., age 11   page 380

Remodeling the condylar head:
Patient: I. R., previously described on page 358

MANIPULATION ELIMINATING PATHOLOGIC SYMPTOMS, INCLUDING CLICKS, IN THREE-DIMENSIONAL MANDIBULAR EXCURSIONS

Patient: G. L., age 10 years

The patient was brought for systematic checkups over several years following diagnosis of Class I malocclusion and crowding in both arches. At the age of 10, fixed-appliance orthodontic treatment was started during exfoliation of the patient's last primary teeth to correct the crowding without premolar extraction. The third molars, not yet visible on the orthopantomography film, would be extracted subsequently if the need arose.

Orthodontic treatment was completed in approximately 2 years, and the patient continued to return for checkups every 6 months.

More than 2 years after completion of treatment, the patient presented with a click on opening the left TMJ and with widespread head pain. Her maximum mouth opening was limited to about 30 mm and deviated to the left, with the click occurring in the final stages. On the horizontal plane, her lateral excursions were 6 mm to the right and 10 mm (almost within normal range) to the left. See pages 66 and 67.

The patient's jaws were manipulated a few times laterally, both to the left and right, and opened and closed on protrusion, which was sufficient to normalize the situation.

Postmanipulation, the patient exhibited straight opening and closing of the mouth. Her maximum mouth opening measured 38 mm, and both her left and right lateral excursions were 9 mm. The click and the pain disappeared. No negative symptoms were observed over the following 5 years.

CONSIDERATIONS

This example indicates that children may present the same conditions as adults. Therefore, the three-dimensional checking of mandibular excursions should never be omitted when examining any patient, no matter how young. Observations of initial dysfunctional signs in younger patients are becoming increasingly frequent, especially in those with ligamentous laxity or who have suffered head trauma (especially from the front), even if it occurred several years earlier.

It may be hypothesized that in this case, early anterior disc dislocation with recapture on opening was entirely resolved with simple diagnostic-therapeutic manipulation that lasted a matter of minutes and caused little or no discomfort for the patient. Straightforward manipulation may provide a simple solution in uncomplicated conditions and may help to improve the symptoms in more severe situations.

ON THE SAME DAY

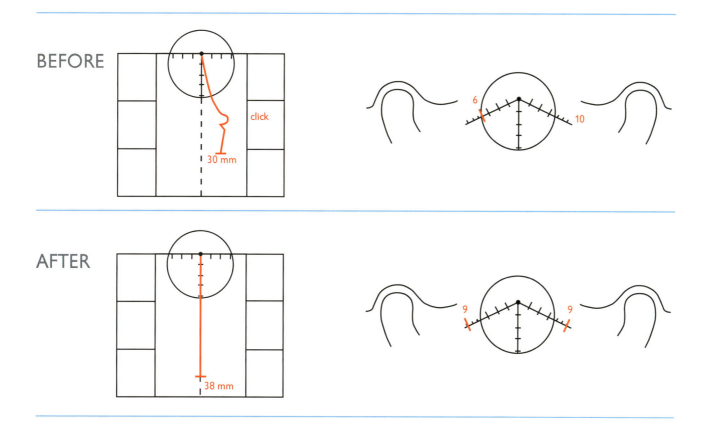

BEFORE

click

30 mm

6

10

AFTER

38 mm

9

9

DISLOCATION OF THE DISC WITH RECAPTURE OBTAINED VIA AN ARS

Patient: S. F., age 9 years

Although the patient's history was not entirely clear, trauma at the age of 2 was reported with fracture of the maxillary primary teeth. At the age of 9, the patient had a difficult Class II malocclusion with bilateral crossbite and TMJ noise. Because of the noise, magnetic resonance images (MRIs) of both TMJs were taken under three different conditions: with the mouth closed, with the mouth open, and with the ARS fitted. The MRIs confirmed what the clinicians suspected: disc dislocation with reduction, both with the jaws open and with the splint fitted.

Although TMJ disorders are often thought of as a phenomenon affecting only adults, this case is further evidence that these disorders commonly occur in children as well. It also highlights the importance of using diagnostic imaging, under certain conditions, on children to aid in the selection of future interceptive therapy.

PRIOR TO SPLINT WEAR

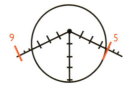

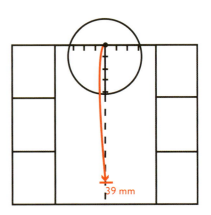

FOLLOWING SPLINT WEAR

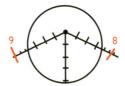

MRI

Right side

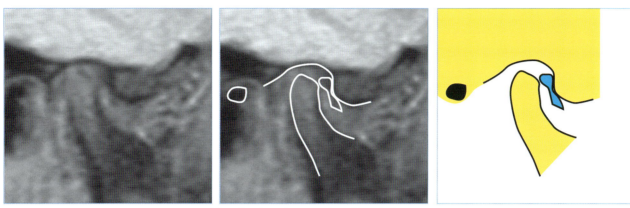

Mouth closed: anterior disc dislocation.

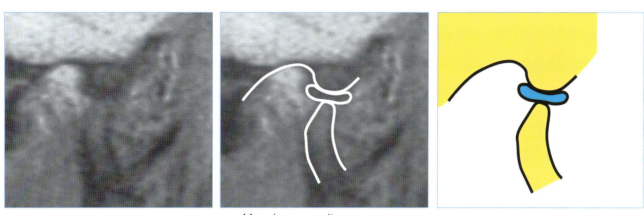

Mouth open: disc recapture.

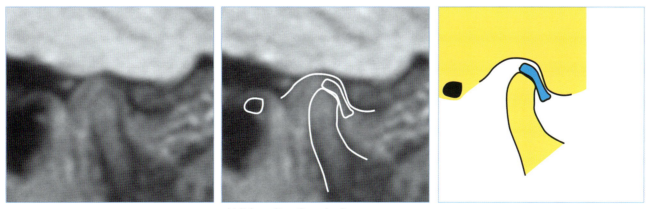

With splint fitted: disc recapture.

SINGLE TMJ LOCK

Patient: F. D., age 10 years

The patient presented with mild pain affecting his left TMJ and limited mouth opening. His mandibular excursions were typical of those associated with monolateral joint lock: mouth opening limited to 26 mm with 5-mm deviation toward the left. Horizontal movements were 9 mm to the left, which is almost normal since the locked joint acts as fulcrum, but only 3 mm to the right because of locking of the rotating (left) joint. See pages 66 and 67.

MOUTH CLOSED
Condyle posteriorized and disc anteriorized (left TMJ).

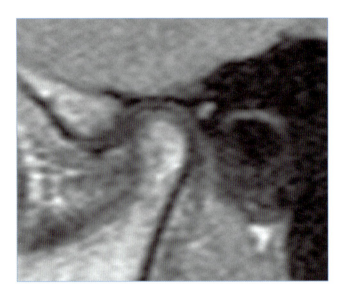

MOUTH OPEN
When the jaws are opened, the condyle fails to recapture the disc, thus remaining in a posterior position behind the disc.
Condition of severe pathology.

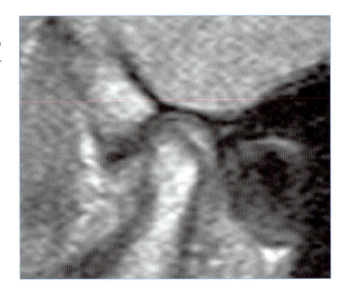

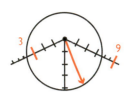

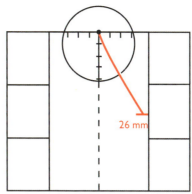

26 mm

Note that the excursions follow the same path with the mouth both open and closed.

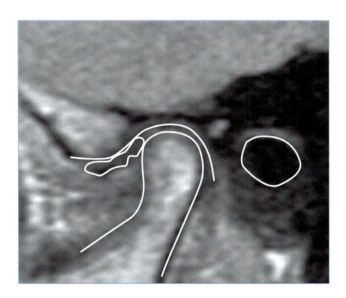

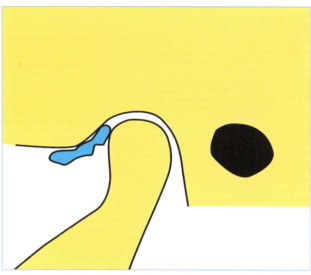

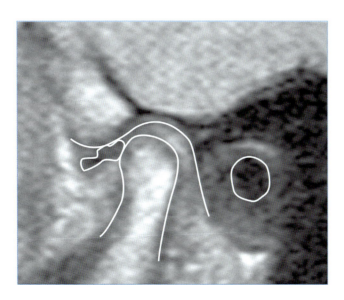

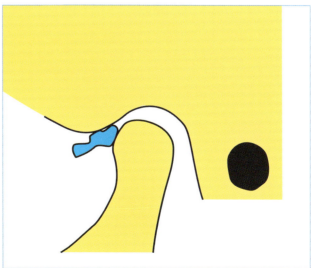

CONDITIONING OF GROWTH IN A VERY YOUNG PATIENT

KEY FEATURE
Is it possible to correct potentially negative condylar and mandibular growth in a severe Class III malocclusion?

Patient: A. T., age 3 years 6 months
The patient presented with a severe skeletal Class III with complete anterior crossbite. No dislocation was observed during the final stage of mouth closure, so the patient has only muscle-led bite without dual bite. The highly negative skeletal situation causes dental discrepancy.

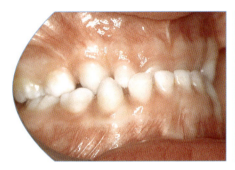 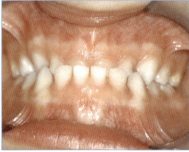 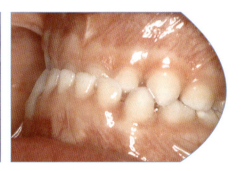

FATHER'S QUESTIONS	CLINICIAN'S REPLIES
Is it possible to alter the growth potential of a highly prominent mandible of a little girl aged three and a half??	With absolute certainty, no. But, yes, I have very reasonable grounds for believing it possible.
At what age would you start orthodontic treatment?	As soon as possible.
As young as three and a half?	Yes, on two conditions. First, both parents must be in agreement. Second, the child must be able to keep still with her mouth open for a few minutes while the appliances are fitted.
With fixed or removable appliances?	Fixed, of course. Once they are fitted, practically no compliance is required from such a young patient.
Can appliances be bonded to primary teeth?	Certainly. This is a normal procedure.
How long might the treatment last?	Many factors contributing to treatment length and outcome. Unless major difficulties arise, we can reasonably presume that treatment will last from 6 months to 1 year.
Can x-rays be avoided?	Orthopantomography is not indicated since it is typically not used until after the age of 6 or 7 years, except under particular circumstances. A pretreatment head film would be very helpful, with further shots taken to confirm modifications and highlight progressive skeletal and dental changes.* *At the parents' request, no x-rays were taken.

USE OF GI.CO. INTRA-ARCH SYSTEM (see page 308 onward)

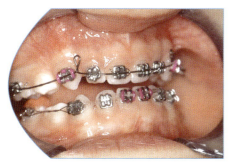
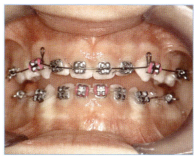
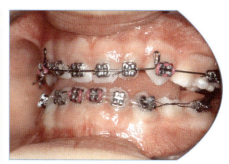

MAXILLARY ARCH

Brackets were placed directly on the patient's primary teeth, including the second molars. The first molars were excluded since they are affected even without the application of brackets.

Anchorage areas

On both the right and left sides, the first and second molars and canines were anchored with .018 Australian wire, with a stop mesial to both first molars and with powerful expanding loops mesial to both canines.

Movement areas

We created a very open loop mesial to the canines so that the archwire ligated to the four anterior teeth would stimulate their advancement.

MANDIBULAR ARCH

Brackets were bonded to the right and left second molars and canines but not to the first molars, where they are unnecessary.

Anchorage areas

All brackets were actively ligated together with normal ligature wire to create anchorage areas.

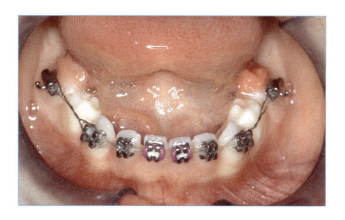

Movement areas

Elastic wire was placed from canine to canine to retract the anterior teeth and to close diastemas between teeth (these being physiologic but momentarily eliminated). Acrylic was added to the occlusal surfaces of the mandibular second molars to raise the patient's excessive deep bite. This procedure is rarely applied. In this case, however, it was used to help the maxillary anterior teeth "jump" into a correct bite. The maxillary loop was activated after 3 weeks and again after 7 weeks to complete this process.

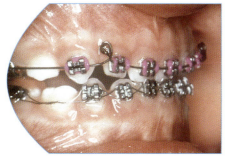
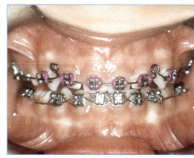
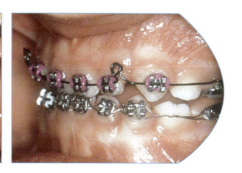

END OF TREATMENT

All appliances were removed **after 74 days.**

According to the patient, the nastiest part was the removal of the acrylic from her mandibular primary molars.

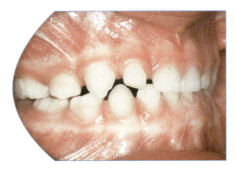
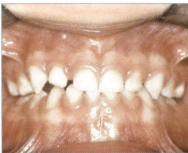
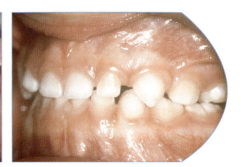

FOLLOW-UP: 2 YEARS AND 3 MONTHS AFTER TREATMENT

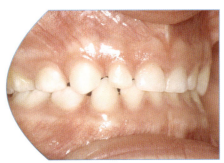
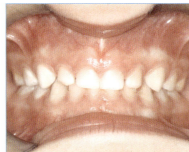
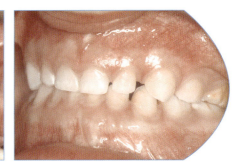

FOLLOW-UP: 4 YEARS AFTER TREATMENT

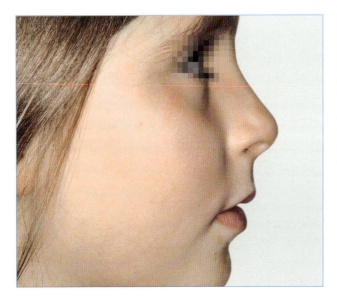
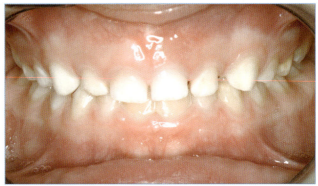

COMPARISONS

Pretreatment

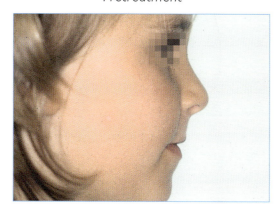

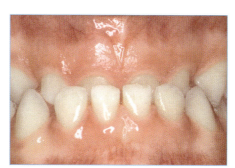

Posttreatment (after 74 days)

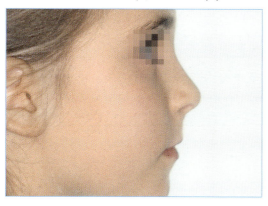

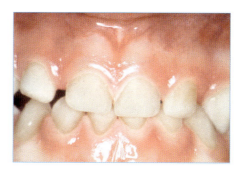

Four years later

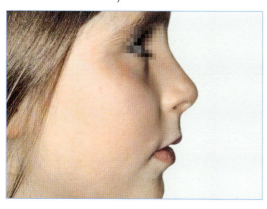

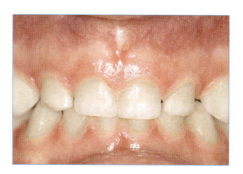

Result: Treatment validity and effectiveness were confirmed. It may be supposed that drastic changes were made in jaw growth giving control—thus far—of occlusal relationships. There was no need for compliance from the patient, and no negative condylar-distalizing forces, such as Class III elastics and/or a Delaire face mask, were used.

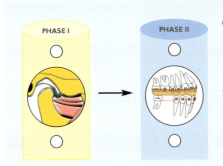

TREATING A DAMAGED CONDYLAR HEAD IN TWO PHASES with ARTICULAR REMODELING, IMPROVED EXCURSIONS, AND RESOLUTION OF CLASS II MALOCCLUSION

KEY FEATURE Significant damage to the condylar head at a very young age

Patient: D. O., age 11

DIAGNOSIS

The patient presented with a Class II malocclusion, deep bite, crowding, and anatomical damage to the condylar head.

THERAPY

Treatment consisted of two phases. In PHASE I, an ARS was used for musculoarticular therapy and bone growth stimulating therapy, resulting in positive changes in skeletal relationships.[1] In PHASE II, use of the ARS was continued, to maintain musculoarticular therapeutic action and skeletal stimulation, and fixed braces were added to integrate with orthodontic occlusal finishing.

PRETREATMENT RECORDS

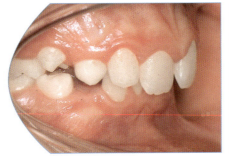
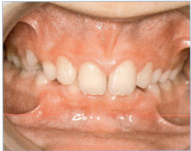
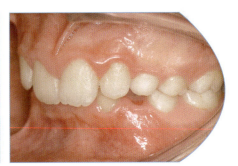

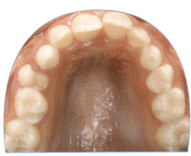
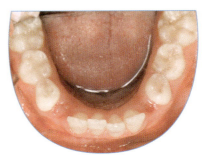

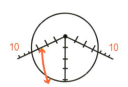

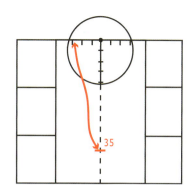

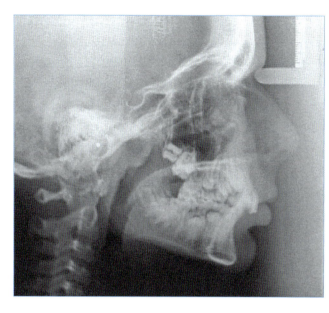

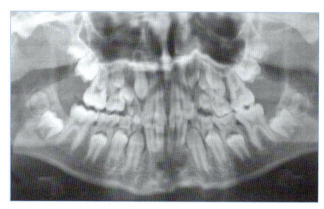

Pretreatment head film and orthopantomography.

PRETREATMENT COMPUTED TOMOGRAPH (CT)

MOUTH CLOSED   *RIGHT SIDE*   *LEFT SIDE*

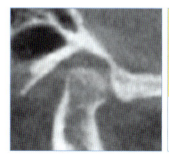
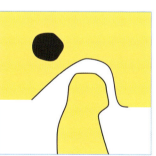
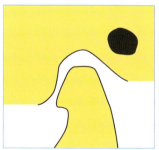
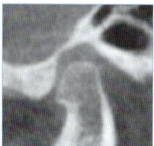

MOUTH OPEN

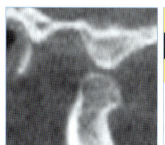
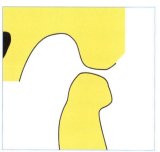
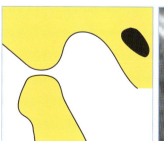
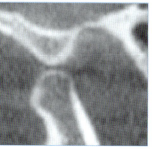

PHASE I: ARS FITTED IN THE MOUTH

(September 2001)

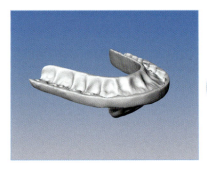 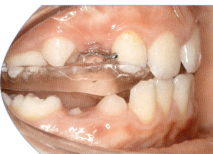 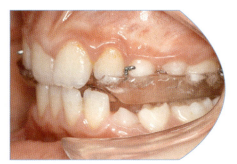

ARS fitted in the mouth

(February 2002)
Brackets bonded to the upper and lower lateral incisors permit night-time vertical elastics to attached to ensure better splint stability for permanent action.
Note: This procedure is often applied with children and sometimes with adults, if accepted. With adults, acrylic is often used in place of brackets. The acrylic is scored with a horizontal groove; the groove is positioned higher on the maxillary teeth and lower on the mandibular teeth.

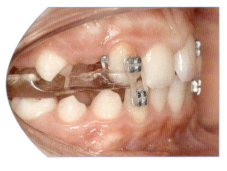 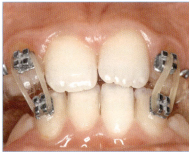 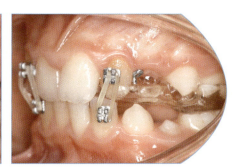

The splint is ground down where necessary to allow extrusion of the mandibular premolars, flatten the curve of Spee, and produce any other desired results.

During this stage, orthodontic treatment without fixed appliances may be done by adapting the ARS according to dental changes.

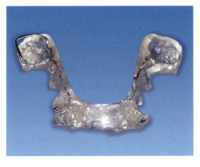 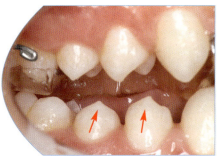 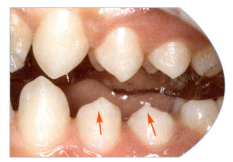

PHASE II: ORTHODONTIC OCCLUSAL FINISHING

Fixed appliances are bonded throughout both arches for phase II orthodontic occlusal finishing. The patient continues to wear the adapted ARS (always) to maintain the stability of the correct musculoarticular and mandibular position.

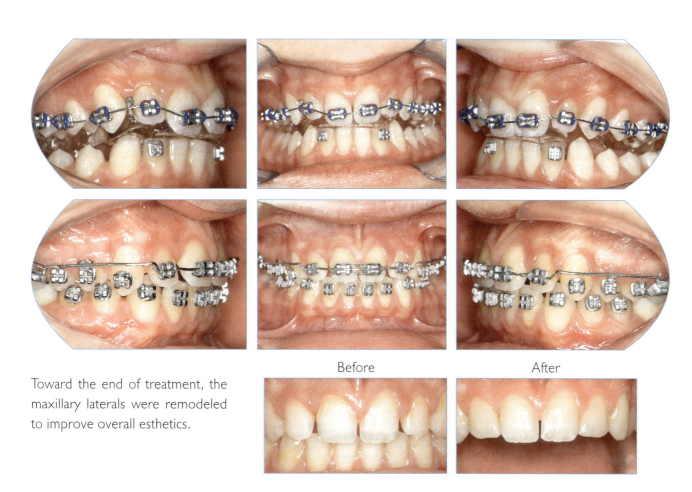

Toward the end of treatment, the maxillary laterals were remodeled to improve overall esthetics.

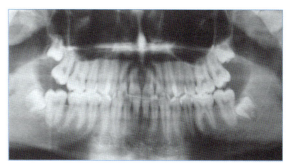

Before   After

End of treatment (2005). Extraction of mandibular third molars was recommended but postponed a number of times.

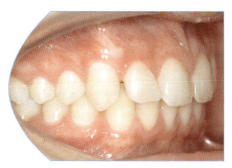
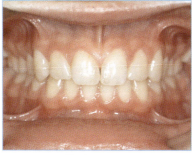
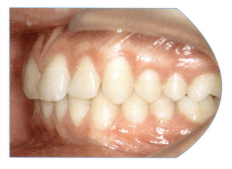

Final outcome.

COMPARISON

BEFORE	AFTER ARS

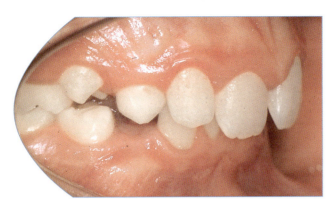 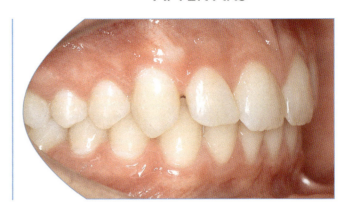

CT closed-mouth, left TMJ: improvement in condylar head.

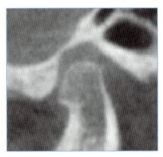 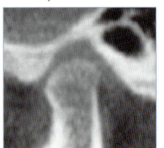

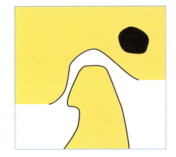 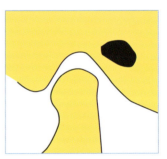

CT open-mouth, left TMJ: slight increase in condylar head excursion and shape.

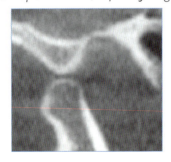 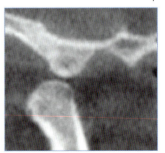

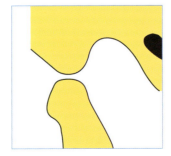 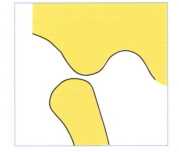

COMPARISON

BEFORE

AFTER ARS

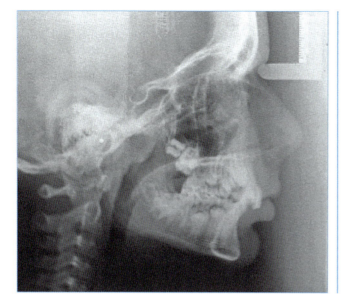

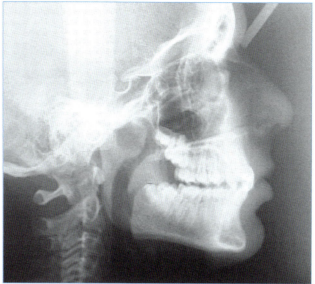

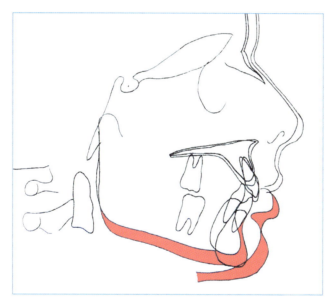

Superimposed before and after head film outlines.

NOTE: In this case, the ARS played a dual role:
- It resolved the musculoarticular problems, especially by remodeling the condylar heads (PHASE I).
- It corrected the Class II malocclusion by integrating the action of the fixed appliances (PHASE II).

CHECKUP (2 years posttreatment; 2007)

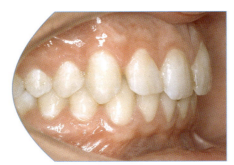
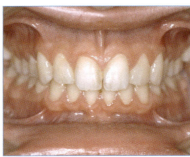
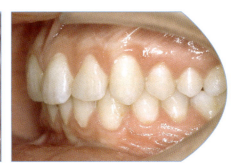

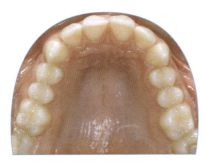
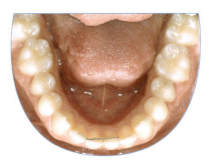

COMPARISON

PRETREATMENT | CHECKUP (2007)

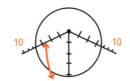
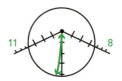

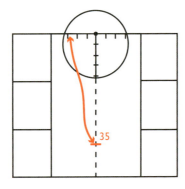
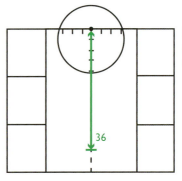

Slight grating on opening and closure

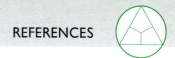

REFERENCES

1. Pancherz H, Michailidou C. Temporomandibular joint growth changes in hyperdivergent and hypodivergent Herbst subjects. A long-term roentgenographic cephalometric study. Am J Orthod Dentofacial Orthop. 2004;126:153-61

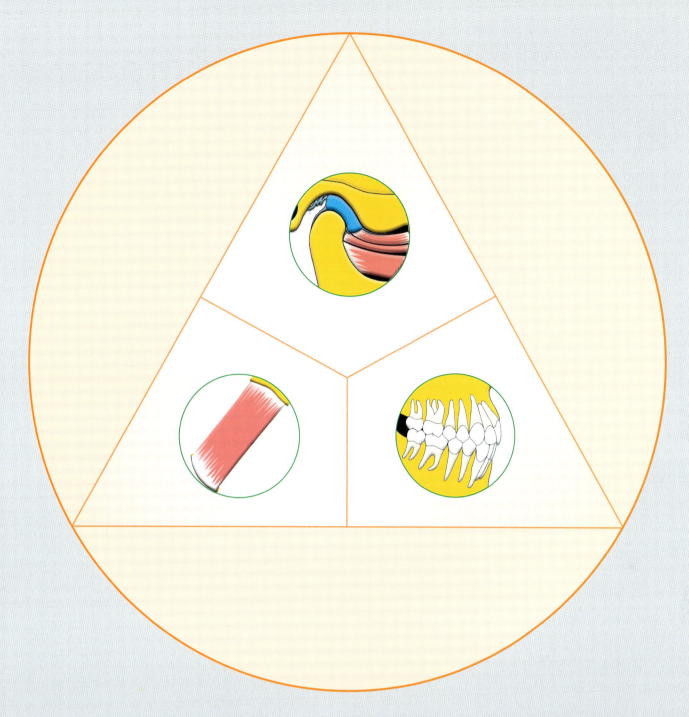

INNOVATIVE ORTHODONTIC TREATMENT OF TEETH, MUSCLES, AND TEMPOROMANDIBULAR DISORDERS

PRESENTATION OF PROSPECTS

ANCHORAGE WITH MINISCREW IMPLANTS (SPIDER SCREWS)

It is important to maintain stable anchorage without having to depend on the patient's cooperation.

Patient: M. M.

Case records kindly provided by Dr B. Giuliano Maino

The patient presented with dental asymmetry: Class II on the right side, and Class I on the left side.

PRETREATMENT RECORDS

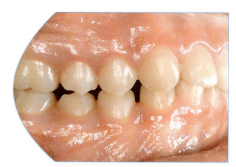
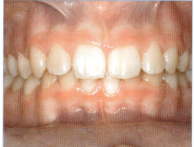
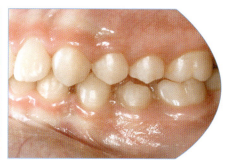

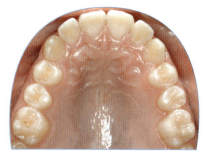
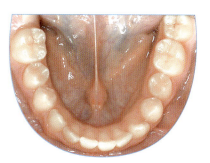

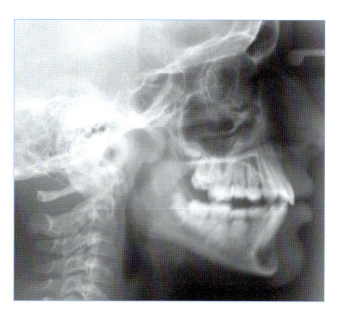
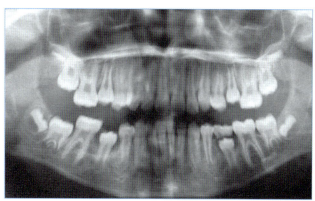

Pretreatment cephalogram and OPT.

INITIAL STEP

Distalization with Sentalloy coil springs

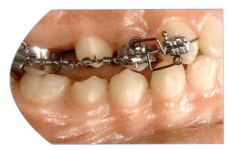 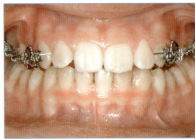 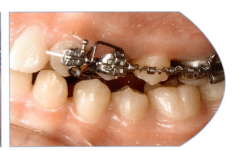

After a first tooth alignment stage, Spider Screws are inserted between the second premolar and first molar, both left and right.[1-5] With the aid of the anchorage thus obtained, distalization of all the teeth in the maxillary arch can proceed. (Documentation is kept to a minimum.)

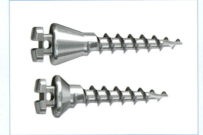 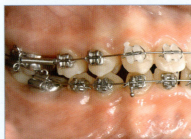 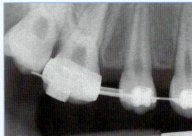

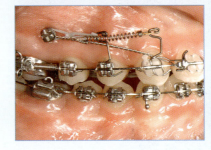 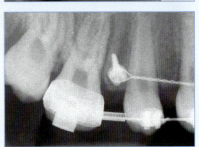

POSTTREATMENT

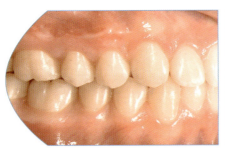 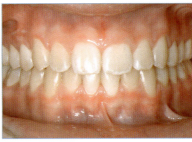 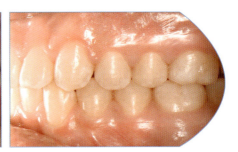

COMPARISONS

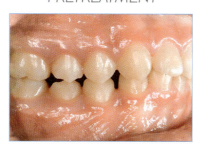 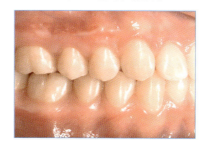

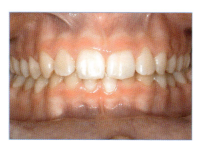 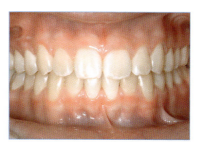

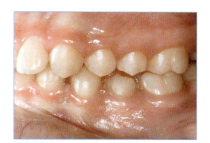 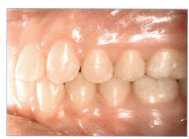

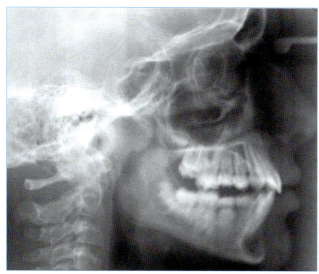 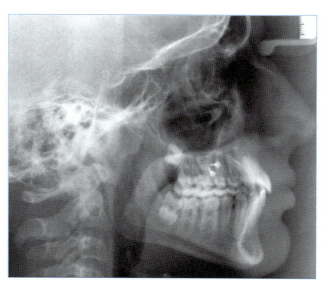

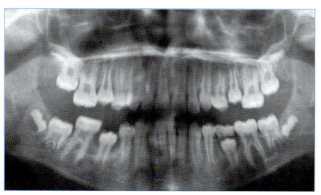 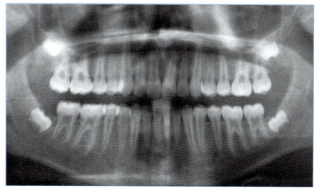

ORTHODONTIC TREATMENT OF CLASS II MALOCCLUSION WITH AN ARS

The case of N. warrants attention because this was the first time (1997) that the authors used an ARS with the intention of applying Class II orthodontic treatment. When treating TMDs, it was realized that positive results were gained not only in disorder therapy but also in terms of dental and skeletal improvements in adult patients with Class II malocclusion. In this case, the patient achieved a successful outcome after 11 months of ARS therapy; in contrast, several years of fixed braces had yielded only disappointing results, despite the patient's active cooperation.

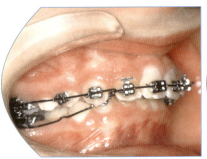

February 1997: The patient's condition on suspension of fixed appliance treatment.

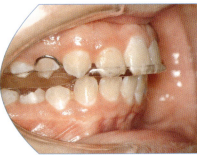

June 1997: ARS fitted.

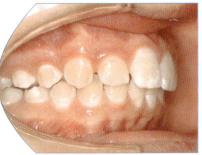

May 1998: End of ARS therapy (11 months later).

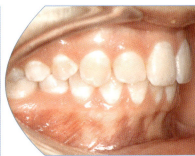

2003: Check-up 5 years after completion of treatment.

COMPARISON OF PROFILE

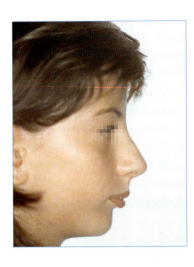

June 1997: Start of ARS therapy.

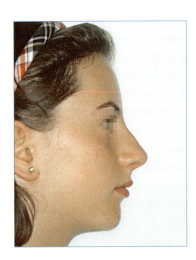

May 1998: Posttreatment.

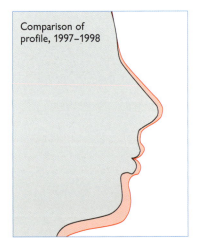

Comparison of before and after profile.

Comparison of profile, 1997–1998

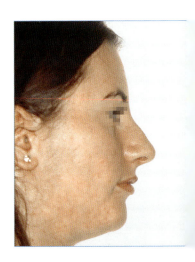

2003: Check-up.

GI. CO. INTRA-ARCH SYSTEM: RESEARCH PROJECT

ORTHODONTICS IN TMD TURNS OUT TO BE INNOVATIVE ORTHODONTICS

Orthodontic occlusal finishing with normal appliances requires that the patient always wear an ARS, which limits the use of traditional treatment devices to the buccal side. This new proposal makes use of the same appliances, but treatment is planned and applied on a new basis. The basic principles and technical procedures may also be applied in traditional orthodontics, when a splint is not necessary.

The principal reference point is to establish areas of anchorage and areas of movement that will later be reciprocally inverted. While acting within the individual arches, this makes it possible to achieve correct intercuspation.

INTERESTING PROSPECTS IN TRADITIONAL ORTHODONTICS

This method simplifies traditional orthodontic procedures and opens up an endless range of solutions to more efficiently personalize treatment for each patient. Another significant advantage of this method is that it reduces the need for patient cooperation.

GI. CO. INTRA-ARCH SYSTEM: FUNDAMENTAL ELEMENTS OF THE RESEARCH PROJECT

1. The possibility of using simple procedures to create the space necessary to move teeth. The main archwire is almost always suitably longer than the arch being treated, with stops mesial to the back teeth. A key factor specific to each patient is the progression in which the teeth are ligated to the archwire.

2. Application of continuous forces within the same arch to move the teeth three-dimensionally, with particular care to ensure that the roots do not go beyond their biologic barriers.

3. Anchorage stabilization:
   - Skeletal, affecting part of the jaw being treated.
   - Dental, involving all the teeth in the arch (or hemi-arch) except the tooth requiring movement at that particular stage of progression.

4. Simultaneous application of more than one therapeutic procedure, beginning with the most challenging, while attempting to drastically reduce length of treatment (see page 294).

5. Requires minimal cooperation from the patient.

6. Limitations:
   - Traditional fixed and removable orthodontic appliances can only be fitted to the buccal face.
   - The two arches, though treated separately, must be harmonized by the end of treatment.

This particular section is part of the more general and complete RESEARCH PROJECT referred to elsewhere in this book.

INVISALIGN

THE INVISALIGN METHOD IN PATIENTS WITH DYSFUNCTION
Prof. Giuseppe Siciliani and Dr Maria Paola Guarneri

University of Ferrara, Italy
Department of Specialization in Orthognathodontics
Director: *Prof. Giuseppe Siciliani*

The quest to improve the "smile area," especially in adults, has generated an ever-increasing demand over the past few years for esthetic appliances with state-of-the-art materials and methodology. Today's orthodontist is able to satisfy patients' requirements with less visible means ranging from ceramic brackets to lingual braces to the even more recent Invisalign method with its clear removable aligners.

A patient's request to improve his or her facial esthetics often goes hand in hand with the need for a functional improvement, the latter objective being of primary importance for the orthodontist not only on completion of the therapy but also during diagnosis and throughout the treatment.

For a clinician sensitive to the problems of TMDs, the most significant difference between Invisalign and other invisible fixed orthodontic devices is that the latter do not put any interocclusal device in place. Therefore they do not interfere with nor change in any way the patient's physiologic masticatory dynamics during treatment. In contrast, the Invisalign method relies upon the occlusal placement of a thin aligner (approximately 0.75 mm), a molded plastic shell that exactly reproduces a person's dental morphology. This aligner concerns orthodontists who speculate that it may interfere with articular function in dysgnathic patients. However, bites and other oral planes are also used by clinicians to reposition the condyle in a therapeutic position.

Setting aside clinical beliefs, it is worth noting that any thickness interfering with occlusion causes trigeminal motor neuron excitability and triggers the masseter inhibitory reflex (MIR) and its related recovery curve. Researchers at the University of Ferrara investigated whether Invisalign aligners caused interference with neuronal circuits by using diagnostic tests on healthy patients versus bruxers. The neurophysical tests used in the first study attempted to ascertain whether patients fitted with clear aligners showed altered neurological control of mastication, thereby evaluating the aligners' potential to interfere with interocclusal function during treatment. This evaluation was based on analysis of trigeminal excitability and the MIR recovery curve. The data enabled the investigators to detect any potential interference of this type of orthodontic device on the encephalic trunk neuronal circuits commanding masticatory activity.

The MIR is an inhibitory reflex. Its afferent pathway consists of one of the three branches of the trigeminal nerve, with the V3 being of main interest since its efferent branch is formed by the trigeminal fibers that carry signals to the masticatory muscles.

The physiologic function of the MIR is voluntary suppression of masticatory muscle action as soon as an unexpected change in food consistency is noted (such as biting on a cherry stone) or in response to harmful stimuli to the mouth and/or face. This mechanism prevents damage caused by an involuntary contraction of the masticatory muscles, and consequently, mechanical stimulation within the oral cavity provoked by the aligner would evoke precisely this reflex during voluntary bite contraction.6

Thirteen volunteers (average age, 28.33 years; Vertical Dimension of 5.68) were fitted with an Invisalign series according to a protocol previously approved by the ethics committee.

Patients were always assessed late in the afternoon while sitting with their head in median position to avoid excessive contraction of cervical extensor and/or neck flexor muscles. This was to ensure that they did not assume any lateroversion positions of the neck that would interfere with masticatory motor efference modulation.[7] The patients were then asked to contract their mandibular elevator muscles bilaterally in an intercuspid occlusal position and maintain a constant submaximal force of approx 80%, partly aided by audiovisual electromyography (EMG) feedback. Between recordings, patients were asked to unclench their bite for at least 20 seconds. If they felt fatigue or muscle or joint pain, as frequently occurs with bruxers, the test was interrupted for a longer time (30 minutes).

The patients were subjected to two types of neurophysiologic assessment:
- MIR in response to a single electrical stimulus to the right and left mentalis nerves, duration 0.1 milliseconds and intensity over 120% of the excitability threshold for a completely silent period. The stimulator cathode was placed over the mental foramina and the anode laterally.
- MIR in response to a single magnetic stimulus using a figure-of-eight (butterfly) coil placed at chin height with stimulation intensity 120% of the excitability threshold for a completely silent period.

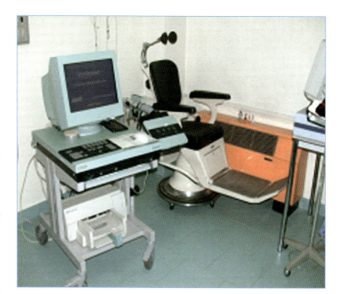

EMG and stimulator.

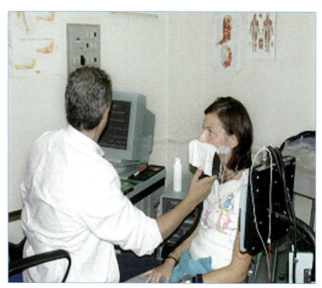

Magnetic stimulation.

Of the two methods, the following parameters were taken into consideration:

- Latency during silent periods, late silent period (SP2) latency compared to the early silent period (SP1) latency taken as 100%.
- MIR recovery curve from dual-pulse electric stimulus obtained by delivering two identical-intensity stimuli with a 300-millisecond interstimulation interval on one side only, with stimulation parameters described for the single stimulus.
- MIR recovery curve from dual-pulse magnetic stimulus obtained by delivering two identical-intensity stimuli with a 300-millisecond interstimulation interval, with the stimulation parameters described

For the latter two tests, the following parameters were taken into consideration:

- Duration and latency of the early silent period from test stimulus (IIsp1) compared with duration and latency of the early silent period from conditioning stimulus (Isp1) taken as 100%
- Duration and latency of the late silent period from test stimulus (IIsp2) compared with duration and latency of the late silent period from conditioning stimulus (IIsp2) taken as 100%

Previous studies have shown that EMG measurements are similar between the two sides,[8,9] so the research team evaluated data from the side with fewer stimulus artifacts. Surface EMG activity was recorded for the right and left masseter muscles using Ag-AgCl disk electrodes, with the active electrode placed over the motor point and the reference electrode placed over the angle of the mandible. The EMG readings were processed according to suggestions found in the literature[10]: The signal was rectified, and at least eight recordings were added up for each type of assessment.

The reference value was determined by a line representing 80% of maximum EMG activity during voluntary contraction. The points of intersection between this line and the patient's rectified EMG total

were taken as the beginning and end of the silent period, and used to calculate duration. The height of this perpendicular at the minimum electrical activity achieved for each silent period was taken as its latency.

Magnetic stimulation was done with a Dantec stimulator (MagLite-r25-Twin Top, Dantec Medical) able to deliver single- and dual-pulse stimuli. A butterfly coil was used (magnetic field outer diameter 9 cm; magnetic field peak intensity 2.3 T). Stimulus intensity was expressed as a percentage of the stimulator's maximum output. The magnetic stimulator coil was maintained in situ to reduce as far as possible any involuntary movements from the point of magnetic stimulation.

The parameters applied were assessed according to the following protocol:

- Baseline assessment, without Invisalign, prior to treatment
- Assessment a few minutes after initial aligner fitting
- Assessment after approximately 3 months of treatment without Invisalign
- Assessment after approximately 3 months of treatment with Invisalign
- Further assessment with and without Invisalign after approximately 6 to 10 months for some patients

The results of this study show that aligner wear does not alter the encephalic trunk neuronal circuits involved in commanding masticatory activity. More explicitly, there appears to be no importance and even less relevance in the patient's neurophysiologic behavior before commencing treatment with Invisalign. The data indicate that no neurophysiologic alterations occur as a result of Invisalign treatment. A comparison of similar conditions treated "with" and "without" Invisalign, between readings 1 and 2, indicate a lack of statistical significance (Wilcoxon matched-pairs test, alpha-error: $P < .05$).

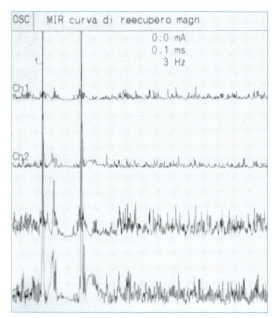

Magnetic stimulus without Invisalign.

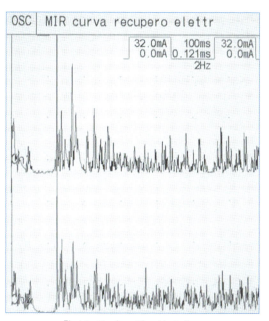

Electric stimulus without Invisalign.

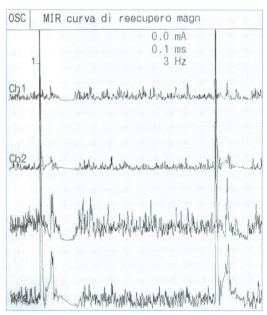

Magnetic stimulus with Invisalign.

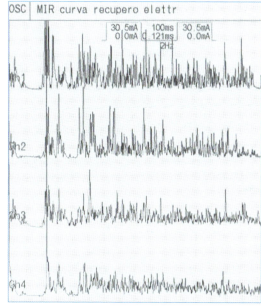

Electric stimulus with Invisalign.

Despite a minimal effect on patients' interocclusal bite, the Invisalign method does not introduce any significant alteration to masticatory dynamics or to the function of the encephalic trunk circuits responsible for commanding occlusal muscle activity. The authors attribute this lack of interference to the perfect way in which Invisalign reproduces occlusal morphology, which compensates for the minimum 0.75 mm thickness that the aligner adds to the bite.

SLIGHT SKELETAL MOVEMENTS IN BOTH PHASE I AND PHASE II

Clinical investigation at the Training Center in La Spezia, coordinated by Dr Pietro Petroni

Patients with TMJ dysfunction who are treated with an ARS often show considerable improvement in their pain symptomatology, which corresponds to changes in their TMJ anatomic structures. During posttreatment physical examination, it is not uncommon for clinicians perceive that the mandible has advanced from its original position, even in adult patients. This observation led to the decision to establish a method of assessing whether cephalometric variations actually occurred. Therefore, cephalometric outlines were collected from a group of 23 patients with intracapsular pathology who met the following requirements:

• The onset of TMJ dysfunction and ARS therapy happened after the patients stopped growing (pretreatment age > 18 years).
• The ARS was worn consistently for about 22 hours per day for more than than 9 months.
• The full treatment plan included simultaneous orthodontic occlusal finishing in conjunction with use of the ARS.

Documentation for each case examined in the study included a triple set of cephalograms. These were taken pretreatment (group 1); on completion of the ARS articular rehabilitation, which coincided with commencement of orthodontic treatment (group 2); and on completion of orthodontic occlusal finishing treatment (group 3). At each of these three distinct stages of treatment, each patient's cephalometric values were assessed using the following skeletal and dental parameters:

Skeletal:	ANB angle
	Wits appraisal
	SN-Go/Gn
	Sn-Po
	Po-Go/Gn
Dental:	Go/Gn-mandibular incisor

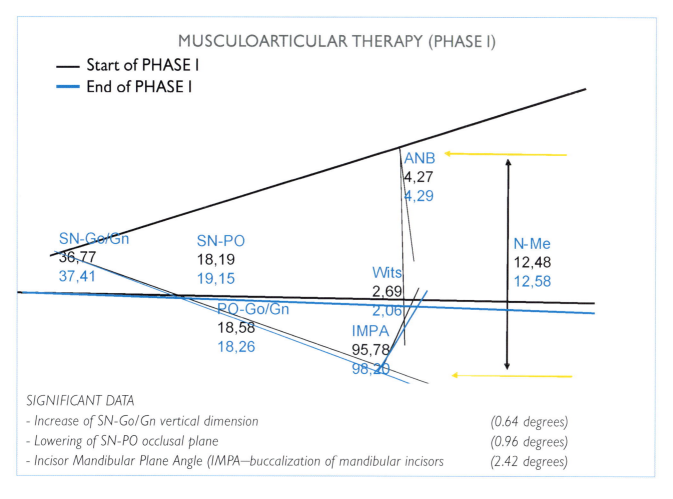

MUSCULOARTICULAR THERAPY (PHASE I)

— Start of PHASE I
— End of PHASE I

ANB
4,27
4,29

SN-Go/Gn
36,77
37,41

SN-PO
18,19
19,15

N-Me
12,48
12,58

Wits
2,69
2,06

PO-Go/Gn
18,58
18,26

IMPA
95,78
98,20

SIGNIFICANT DATA

- *Increase of SN-Go/Gn vertical dimension*	*(0.64 degrees)*
- *Lowering of SN-PO occlusal plane*	*(0.96 degrees)*
- *Incisor Mandibular Plane Angle (IMPA—buccalization of mandibular incisors*	*(2.42 degrees)*

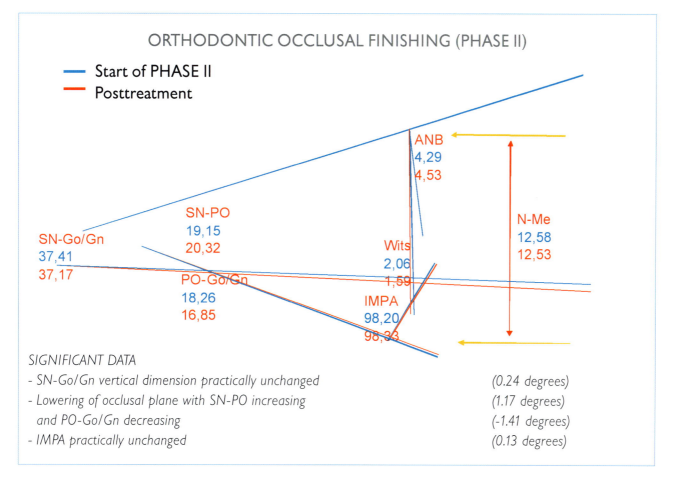

ORTHODONTIC OCCLUSAL FINISHING (PHASE II)

— Start of PHASE II
— Posttreatment

ANB
4,29
4,53

SN-PO
19,15
20,32

SN-Go/Gn
37,41
37,17

N-Me
12,58
12,53

Wits
2,06
1,59

PO-Go/Gn
18,26
16,85

IMPA
98,20
98,33

SIGNIFICANT DATA

- *SN-Go/Gn vertical dimension practically unchanged*	*(0.24 degrees)*
- *Lowering of occlusal plane with SN-PO increasing*	*(1.17 degrees)*
and PO-Go/Gn decreasing	*(-1.41 degrees)*
- *IMPA practically unchanged*	*(0.13 degrees)*

401

TABLES AND BOXES

	ANB	SN-Go/Gn	SN-PO	PO-Go/Gn	Wits	IMPA	N-Me
——— Pretreatment, PHASE I	4.27	36.77	18.19	18.58	2.69	95.78	12.48
——— Pretreatment, PHASE II	4.29	37.41	19.15	18.26	2.06	98.20	12.58
——— Posttreatment	4.53	37.17	20.32	16.85	1.59	98.33	12.53
Difference ———	+0.02	+0.64	+0.96	-0.32	-0.63	+2.42	+0.1
Difference ———	+0.24	-0.24	+1.17	-1.41	-0.47	+0.13	-0.05
Difference ———	+0.26	+0.40	+2.13	-1.73	-1.1	+2.55	+0.05

COMPARISON OF PRETREATMENT AND POSTTREATMENT RESULTS

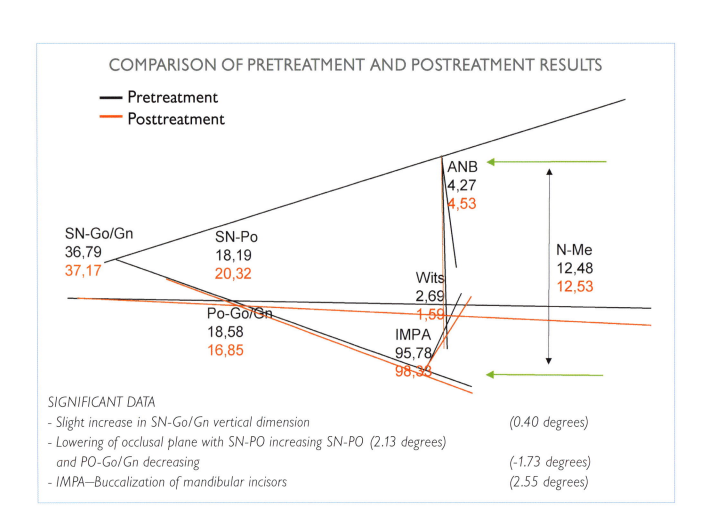

— Pretreatment
— Posttreatment

SIGNIFICANT DATA
- *Slight increase in SN-Go/Gn vertical dimension*   *(0.40 degrees)*
- *Lowering of occlusal plane with SN-PO increasing SN-PO (2.13 degrees) and PO-Go/Gn decreasing*   *(-1.73 degrees)*
- *IMPA—Buccalization of mandibular incisors*   *(2.55 degrees)*

DISCUSSION

To assess whether any statistically significant differences existed between the three treatment stages, a Student's t-test was used to compare groups 1 and 2, groups 2 and 3, and groups 1 and 3. There was no conclusive evidence of statistically significant skeletal changes ($P >$ .05) between any of the groups nor of significant intramandibular relationships. Thus it may be hypothesized that the effects of "dysfunctional" therapy take place primarily within the joint, with some remodeling and/or regrowth of anatomic structures in addition to other benefits.

Nevertheless, some interesting data were obtained from the investigation:

• Mean buccalization of mandibular incisors, from pretreatment to overall postreatment (after both PHASE I and PHASE II), was measured at approximately 2.55 degrees. This is explained by pressure on the lower incisors from the mandibular repositioning flange. Go/Gn-1 changes from 95.78 to 98.20 after phase I, becoming 98.33 after phase II.
• The mean Po-Go/Gn change of 2.13 degrees from pretreatment to after overall therapy and the 1.10-degree reduction in Wits appraisal may be explained by the flattening of the curve of Spee, which was accentuated before treatment commenced in the majority of the cases studied.

Extrusive effects leading to an increase in vertical height act on the maxillary posterior teeth, which are vertically freed from the ARS acrylic. Simultaneously, the mandibular posterior teeth contact the splint wedge freely where it passes from an inclined plane to a vertical position.

To conclude, musculoarticular therapy and orthodontic finishing cause the mandible to shift, only slightly, downward and sometimes backward. What the clinician perceives to be an advance of the lower third of the face can mainly be attributed to buccal inclination of the mandibular incisors, which explains an apparent contrast between advance as a result of mandibular incisor inclination and retrusion of the chin as a result of clockwise rotation of the mandible. These small changes do not affect the underlying treatment principle—the importance of maintaining a consistent fixed therapeutic splint position from initial pretreatment planning through to its completion.

Note: Different results may be achieved by taking wax bite registration in a position aimed at mandibular stimulation (see pages 380 and 394).

FINAL CONSIDERATIONS

Disorders affecting the teeth, muscles, and TMJs as a unit have been the main focus of this book. Likewise, the importance of formulating an individual diagnosis and treatment plan for each patient has been shown to be an essential part of effective therapy.

To summarize, the procedure to follow when diagnosing and treating a patient with TMJ dysfunction is to:

- Obtain a thorough patient history.
- Complete a new patient examination.
- Conduct specific tests as required, especially MRI.
- Perform diagnostic-therapeutic manipulation.
- Assess the patient's psychologic attitude and behavior.
- Look for signs of dual bite:
–A muscle-led bite with normal tone is considered valid even if there is minimal intercuspation.
–A dental bite, even with maximum intercuspation, is not valid since it is accompanied by muscle tension.

At every appointment, the clinician must work to progressively eliminate the dental bite, replacing it with the muscle-led position such that the jaws achieve a single, stress-free, consistent intercuspation pattern. This alone will ensure correct anatomical and functional relationships between the three components of the stomatognathic apparatus.

THERAPY

Some solutions to stomatognathic problems include the following:

- Chemical, physical, neurologic, and pharmacologic approaches.
- Treatment with splints, especially transitioning from an SS to the more complete ARS.
–If worn for the entire duration of treatment, an ARS provides the best long-term support for maintaining the therapeutic position for the musculoarticular structures as established at the outset of treatment.
- A two-stage therapeutic plan that applies the correct strategies in separate procedures:
–PHASE I: musculoarticular
–PHASE II: orthodontic occlusal finishing with careful

ongoing reference to anchorage, which in turn is divided into:
–Skeletal, when a whole jaw or part of it is involved
–Dental, when involving all the teeth excepting that requiring movement in turn along the main archwire (Gi.Co. System as part of the broader orthodontic research project)
- Temporary anchorage devices (Spider Screws).

The combination of the balanced management of one or more types of anchorage and consequent tooth movement wherever necessary in either jaw, the use of continuous forces, and the tridimensional control of each tooth moved within the biologic limits of the main jaw body basal bone allow the clinician to conclude treatment satisfactorily, within a reasonable timeframe, and with minimum cooperation from the patient.

In addition to orthodontics, other procedures that help the clinician to achieve these goals include:

- Limited selective grinding of as few teeth as possible, done in one sitting after preparation on articulator-mounted casts
- Complete occlusal harmonization, both "plus and minus," practiced on an articulator and then repeated on the patient's teeth in one sitting
- Complete rehabilitation with prosthodontics to provide a statically and functionally valid new occlusion
- Maxillary surgery, provided that it maintains correct TMJ relationships following damage repair

These therapies have other applications as well:

- Therapy of whiplash injuries, to rearrange condyle-disc-fossa relations according to the type of trauma suffered by the condyles.
- Use of an ARS to improve sports performance.
- Therapeutic recommendations or specific retention therapy for patients with ligamentous laxity.
- Prevention of musculoarticular damage in children, especially if they have had a head injury. Systematic investigation of children's conditions reveals a surprising percentage of TMJ damage, which indicates the need to propose fundamental rules for prevention.
- Orthodontics helps to prevent TMD, correct oral habits, treat malocclusion, and rearrange altered dental and skeletal relations. It interrelates systematically with

other branches of dentistry, including pre-prosthodontic work, preparation for maxillary surgery, and periodontology.

The results of treatment may not always appear perfect, and clinicians regularly have to accept that, for various reasons, sometimes they must accept a compromise outcome. For this reason, the book includes a number of cases describing how to achieve the best outcome possible when an ideal solution cannot be reached. These difficulties also help to drive the field forward. Challenges such as moving the teeth of a patient who is

always wearing a splint spur clinicians to create innovative solutions, which develop into new prospects for traditional orthodontics, too.

THE PURPOSE. To achieve a posttreatment outcome in which the inseparable unit of teeth, muscles, and TMJs is in a state of anatomic, functional, and esthetic harmony that also enhances facial and smile esthetics.

NEW SPLINTS

ARS: ADAPTATION "A" (SIMPLIFIED SPLINT)

DESCRIPTION

Adaptation A is an ARS that is less inconvenient for patients yet still cures the same type of pathology with three-dimensional control of articular structures.

Key features

- Immobilization of the maxilla is limited to the posterolateral districts while the anterior area remains free.
- A smooth plane in the maxilla contacts the mandibular teeth in only the posterolateral districts.
- Two acrylic bridges extend from the lingual faces of the maxillary premolars and support an anterior flange for the mandibular anteriors.

The principal benefit of this adaptation is greater freedom for the tongue. It makes social interaction considerably easier, especially for those who need to make a good impression when speaking.

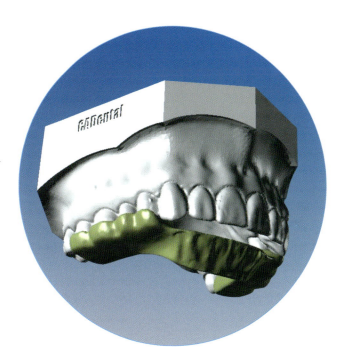

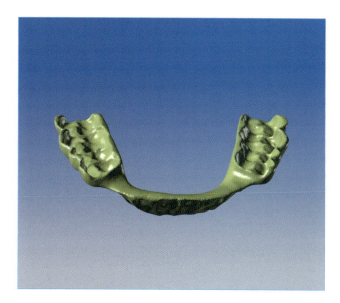

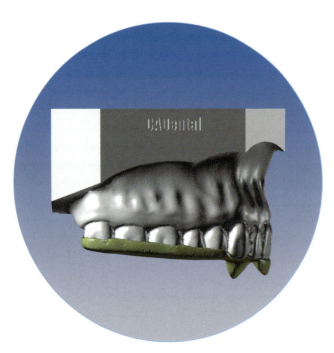

ARS: ADAPTATION "B" (MANDIBULAR STABILITY SPLINT)

DESCRIPTION

This is a variation of a traditional ARS, with a lingual and buccal stopper to prevent the mandibular incisors from anterior or posterior sliding.

PURPOSE

As previously highlighted, ligamentous laxity contributes to the risk of musculoarticular pathology, and in cases of whiplash, it is even more detrimental. Frequently, a first recommendation is that patients avoid opening their mouth by more than 20 to 22 mm. This precaution is sufficient prevention in a high percentage of relatively uncomplicated cases.

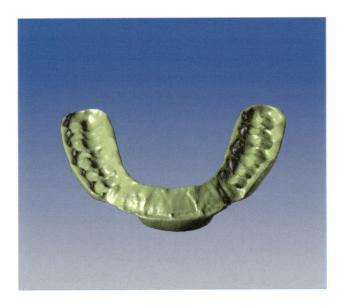

The ARS illustrated here is designed to safely limit mandibular excursions by the addition of a buccal extension to the normal lingual flange. A downward-facing groove creates a "nest" for the mandibular anteriors when the jaws are closed, thus ensuring greater mandibular incisal stability. Patient appreciate the greater comfort and security that this provides. (See patient C. T., pages 346 through 350.)

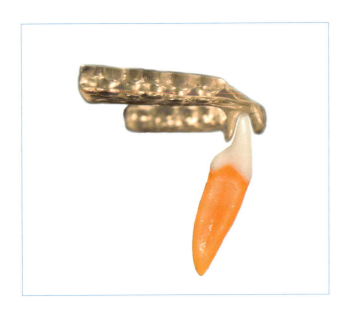

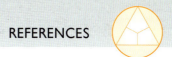

REFERENCES

References

1. Maino B G, Mura P, Gianelly A.A. A Retrievable palatal implant for absolute anchorage on orthodontics. World J Orthod 2002; 3,2: 125-134

2. Maino BG, Bednar J, Pagin P, Mura P. The Spider Screw for skeletal anchorage. J Clin Orthod 2003;37; 90–97.

3. Maino BG, Maino G, Mura P. Transitional anchorage devices in orthodontics: Miniscrews. Semin Orthod 2005;11:32–39.

4. Maino BG, Gianelly AA, Bednar J, Mura P, Maino G. MGBM system: New protocol for Class II non extraction treatment without cooperation. Prog Orthod 2007;8:130–143.

5. Maino BG, Bednar J, Mura P. The spider screw. In: Cope JB (ed). Orthotads: The Clinical Guide and Atlas. Dallas: Under Dog Media Dallas, 2007:201–212.

6. Godaux E, Desmedt JE. Exteroceptive suppression and motor control of the masseter and temporalis muscles in normal man. Brain Res 1975;85:447–548.

7. Miralles R, Palazzi C, Ormeño G. Body position effects on EMG activity of sternocleidomastoid and masseter muscles in healthy subjects. Cranio 1998;16:90–99.

8. Gastaldo E, Graziani A, Paiardi M, et al. Recovery cycle of the masseter inhibitory reflex after magnetic stimulation in normal subjects. Clin Neurophysiol 2003;114:1253–1258.9. Gastaldo E, Quatrale R, Graziani A, Eleopra R, Tugnoli V, Tola MR, Granieri E. The excitability of the trigeminal motor system in sleep bruxism: a transcranial magnetic stimulation and brainstem reflex study. J Orofac Pain. 2006 Spring;20(2):145-55.

10. Cruccu G, Inghilieri M, Fraioli B, Guidetti B, Manfredi M. Neurophysiology assessment of trigeminal function after surgery for trigeminal neuralgia. Neurology 1987;37:631–638.